Vitreous Microsurgery

Third Edition

Vitreous Microsurgery

Third Edition

Steve Charles, M.D.
Clinical Professor, Department of Ophthalmology
University of Tennessee
Vitreoretinal Surgeon-Private Practice
Charles Retina Institute
Chairman, Micro Dexterity Systems
Memphis, Tennessee

Adam Katz, M.D.
Board Certified Ophthalmologist
Mid-Hudson Retina Consultants, PLLC
Middletown and Newburgh, New York
Attending, Horton Medical Center
Middletown, New York
Attending, Arden Hill Hospital
Goshen, New York

Byron Wood
Owner, Delta Angiography
Chief Photographer and Director of Graphics
Charles Retina Institute
Memphis, Tennessee

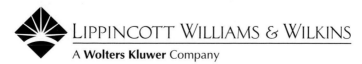

LIPPINCOTT WILLIAMS & WILKINS
A **Wolters Kluwer** Company
Philadelphia · Baltimore · New York · London
Buenos Aires · Hong Kong · Sydney · Tokyo

Acquisitions Editor: Jonathan Pine
Developmental Editor: Stacey L. Baze
Production Editor: Thomas J. Foley
Manufacturing Manager: Colin J. Warnock
Cover Designer: Joan Greenfield
Compositor: Lippincott Williams & Wilkins Desktop Division
Printer: Quebecor World Color-Taunton

© **2002 by LIPPINCOTT WILLIAMS & WILKINS**
530 Walnut Street
Philadelphia, PA 19106 USA
LWW.com

All rights reserved. This book is protected by copyright. No part of this book may be reproduced in any form or by any means, including photocopying, or utilized by any information storage and retrieval system without written permission from the copyright owner, except for brief quotations embodied in critical articles and reviews. Materials appearing in this book prepared by individuals as part of their official duties as U.S. government employees are not covered by the above-mentioned copyright.

Printed in the USA

Library of Congress Cataloging-in-Publication Data

Charles, Steve.
  Vitreous microsurgery / Steve Charles, Adam Katz, Byron Wood. — 3rd ed.
    p. ; cm.
  Includes bibliographical references and index.
  ISBN 0-7817-3306-5
  1. Vitreous body—Surgery. 2. Microsurgery. I. Katz, Adam, 1967- II. Wood, Byron.
III. Title.
  [DNLM: 1. Microsurgery. 2. Vitreous Body—surgery. WW 250 C477v 2002]
  RE501 .C48 2002
  617.7′46059—dc21

                                                            2002016155

Care has been taken to confirm the accuracy of the information presented and to describe generally accepted practices. However, the authors and publisher are not responsible for errors or omissions or for any consequences from application of the information in this book and make no warranty, expressed or implied, with respect to the currency, completeness, or accuracy of the contents of the publication. Application of this information in a particular situation remains the professional responsibility of the practitioner.

The authors and publisher have exerted every effort to ensure that drug selection and dosage set forth in this text are in accordance with current recommendations and practice at the time of publication. However, in view of ongoing research, changes in government regulations, and the constant flow of information relating to drug therapy and drug reactions, the reader is urged to check the package insert for each drug for any change in indications and dosage and for added warnings and precautions. This is particularly important when the recommended agent is a new or infrequently employed drug.

Some drugs and medical devices presented in this publication have Food and Drug Administration (FDA) clearance for limited use in restricted research settings. It is the responsibility of the health care provider to ascertain the FDA status of each drug or device planned for use in their clinical practice.

10 9 8 7 6 5 4 3 2 1

To the memory of Edward W.D. Norton, M.D., my mentor
and the founder of the Bascom Palmer Eye Institute; to my grandfather,
Clayton Charles, M.D., a hard working surgeon; to my father,
Clayton Henry Charles, who was a creative genius; to my father's
oldest brother, John D. Charles, M.D., a wonderful surgeon;
and to Harry G. Johnson, my grandfather and a brilliant
mechanical engineer.

Contents

Preface

During the thirty year history of vitreoretinal surgery, many new techniques and technologies have been introduced. Many of these techniques and technologies have proven successful; some, quite frankly, have failed, while others are still under evaluation. Since the second edition of this volume was published fifteen years ago, we have seen the incredible success of macular hole surgery, the rise and fall of macular translocation, and we have found that submacular surgery is moderately successful in certain non-AMD cases. Yet, the efficacy of laser tissue cutting, enzyme assisted vitrectomy, ICG staining of ILM, branch vein decompression, central vein cannulation, and visco-dissection has not yet been determined in spite of significant promotion. After a large study of longterm visual outcomes of surgery for Stage 5 ROP, I no longer perform nor recommend this procedure. Fortunately, early intervention with the laser has proven to be a great success story in ROP, and a few Stage 4B cases can be successfully operated on.

Patients who are blind often ask what techniques or procedures the future will bring to give them hope. There are three broad strategies that are currently being studied: transplantation, implantable electrical stimulation of the retina, and tissue regrowth. It is my belief that rejection, as well as neural and vascular connection issues, make transplantation a very complex problem, which is not close to a solution at this point. Stability of electrical connections, the marked complexity of the retinal architecture, and many other issues make a retinal "implant" also very unlikely despite the enormous publicity concerning the early, primitive research efforts in the field. Regrowth of retinal and/or RPE tissue using advanced tissue engineering techniques is very complex as well, but seems to offer some real hope.

Since the last edition was published, vitreous cutters, fluidics, scissors, forceps, fragmentation, laser photocoagulation, and exchange techniques have continued to evolve. It is likely, in my opinion, that any revolutionary advances will ultimately come from molecular biology, biotherapeutics, tissue engineering, and related technologies.

Steve Charles, M.D.

Acknowledgments

The original idea for this edition was that it would be published only on the internet, but the encouragement of my friend, former fellow and co-author, Adam Katz, M.D., led to the decision to publish a third edition in book format. Adam diligently edited all of the chapters to this edition and also provided all of the references. Byron Wood, my long time friend, photographer, and graphic artist, did an incredible job with the 3-dimensional color illustrations and provided further editorial input. My wonderful colleague, Sandy Brucker, M.D., founder and editor of *Retina*, read the initial manuscript and provided excellent advice concerning the style of this edition. He also encouraged the publisher to move forward with this project. Special acknowledgment is also extended to Lisa Fogel, M.D., for her editing assistance and to Gary Fanning, M.D., for his assistance with the anesthesia section.

Fellow vitreo-retinal surgeons, fellows, residents, visiting doctors, and engineers at Alcon Surgical provided valuable input; and The Macula Society, Retina Society, Vitreous Society, and Club Jules Gonin provided an environment that encouraged an ongoing interchange of ideas between colleagues.

1

Presurgical Decision Making

Vitreous surgery has been applied successfully to a wide spectrum of ocular diseases. The complex set of biologic and systemic risks, techniques, and technology considerations confronting the surgeon creates a difficult decision-making environment. Rather than emphasizing a search for good prognosis or easy cases, the goal must be to avoid bilateral or irreversible blindness. Many potential vitreous surgery patients have profound socioeconomic problems as a result of blindness and/or systemic disease. An intensive attempt to understand the patient's medical and socioeconomic situation is essential to effective and compassionate health care delivery. The surgeon must examine the patient completely and, preferably, perform most assessments personally to reach the best clinical decision. The surgeon must develop an open, direct, and warm relationship with the patient before surgery can be considered. It is probably better to discuss specific statistical results of surgery on similar patients than to discuss the details of a specific methodology. Rather than using qualitative words such as *excellent* or *poor,* using a percentage success rate is more meaningful. The frequency of the most important complications should be mentioned, as well as the range and mean of postoperative vision in functional and numeric terms. All available family members and the surgeon's secretary, technician, or nurse should witness this conversation. A complex, legalistic permission document is far less important than meaningful, compassionate personal communication with the patient. The patient should be informed about inpatient/outpatient status, postoperative positioning, pain, medications, operating time, type of anesthesia to be used, the requirement for postoperative examinations, and limitations on activity. The surgeon must take personal responsibility for obtaining financial support for the economically disadvantaged patient and act as a consumer advocate concerning facility fees. It is unconscionable to turn away a patient or permit the facility to do so because of the patient's financial status.

It is the surgeon's responsibility to organize the scheduling process so that the preoperative assessment or logistical/bureaucratic delay does not affect the prognosis. Waiting lists are highly inappropriate for patients with significant visual problems. If surgery is performed within a few days of the original examination, the surgeon will be more acutely aware of significant aspects of the patient's history and findings during surgery.

SYSTEMIC FACTORS

Age

Age is a consideration at both extremes of the timeline. Although age cannot be used as an arbitrary criterion, it is clear that both the neonate with pulmonary problems and the elderly patient with multisystem systemic disease are poor surgical risks. In both circumstances, anesthesia risk factors determine the decision. Surgery on the premature infant can be delayed until pulmonary function and body weight increase, allowing safer anesthesia. Most vitreoretinal surgery today is performed under local anesthesia, but children and certain adults must have general anesthesia.

Sensory deprivation from poor vision may contribute to disorientation and agitation in certain elderly patients. Unilateral visual loss is well tolerated in many elderly patients because of less demanding occupational and recreational needs. While it is the surgeon's obligation to determine ocular status and needs, medical consultants and anesthesiologists can help determine and manage systemic risk.

Diabetes

As diabetes is common in vitrectomy patients, the vitreous surgeon must be quite familiar with the ramifications of this multisystem disease. An individualized approach is superior to arbitrary surgical criteria. The presence of systemic infection is a contraindication to vitrectomy. All ocular conditions except endophthalmitis and severe glaucoma can wait until a systemic infection has been treated. End-stage renal disease decreases life span and creates difficult socioeconomic as well as medical problems. The stable transplant patient can undergo successful vitrectomy, although immunosuppressant drugs create increased infection risk, especially with general anesthesia. The dialysis patient is a poor general anesthesia risk and may have increased bleeding with vitrectomy. Although surgical conservatism is indicated for patients with end-stage renal disease, many carefully selected patients can benefit from vitrectomy.

Cardiopulmonary Disease

Specific guidelines in the area of cardiopulmonary disease again must be replaced by an individualized approach with reliance upon medical and anesthesia consultation. Although local anesthesia is safer than general, a significant risk is associated with local anesthesia, which points to the need for careful medical assessment and the monitored approach with an anesthesiologist or Certified Registered Nurse Anesthetists (CRNAs) present. Pulse oximetry, electrocardiogram, continuous blood pressure monitoring, and frequent blood glucose assessments are mandatory.

OCULAR FACTORS

Examination of the vitrectomy patient embodies the same steps, but with different emphasis than that required for other ophthalmic specialties. A problem-oriented approach studying specific factors that have a high impact on decision making is more effective than "routine" examination.

Visual Function Testing

Visual function testing can be the most difficult component of previtrectomy evaluation unless approached properly. Careful, precise measurement of visual acuity is more relevant than an array of laboratory tests.

VISUAL ACUITY

The inherent subjectivity of visual acuity testing demands random presentation of stimuli, multiple repetitions, and sophisticated examiners. Specifically, the examiner cannot ask, "Can you see the light?" but should say instead, "Tell me when the light goes on and off." The patient must describe the direction of randomly presented motion when testing for "hand motion." Multiple repetitions increase reliability because of problems stemming from patient guessing. The patient's neurologic/psychologic status and educational level may interfere with accurate testing. The light perception determination is of particular significance because patients without light perception should *never* have eye surgery unless it is clearly understood that the procedure is to prevent the spread of cancer, to prevent infection, or possibly to provide cosmetic preservation of the globe. Dense opaque media require a bright testing light such as that from an indirect ophthalmoscope at 7.5 volts. The finger-counting method is fraught with error because of the great variance in finger size, position, color, and illumination. It is preferable to use a printed, 20/200-sized "E" on a white card. This can be presented in random orientation with multiple repetitions, and the distance can be measured to determine acuity as a fraction (e.g., 1/200). A patient with 1/200 vision typically cannot see well enough to walk, whereas a 5/200 patient typically is ambulatory, and an individual with 9/200 vision can read large print with magnification. Placing all these patients into the finger-counting category is misleading. Vision testing devices based on the cathode ray tube (CRT), liquid–crystal display, or the Titmus system are accurate and rapid ways of testing visions of 20/300 or better and can replace more traditional projector charts (1). The printed charts with special illumination used by the Early Treatment of Diabetic Retinopathy Study (2) are very accurate but somewhat cumbersome. A current refraction must be in place for visual acuity testing at the 20/400 or better level. Pinholes are difficult for retinal patients to use and may reduce contrast sensitivity in the presence of organic retinal disease, resulting in testing errors. Near vision testing is essential because of hereditary myopia and induced myopia from nuclear sclerosis and encircling buckles.

Projection and Field Testing

Marked opaque media create light scatter and false projection, whereas recent retinal detachments can have normal projection. Occasionally, an advanced glaucoma patient with opaque media will respond only in the temporal field, but frequently, the patient indicates a larger field due to light scattering.

Entoptic Phenomenon

The shadows of the retinal vessels can be seen by the patient if a focal light source (transilluminator) is rubbed against the closed lids. Care must be taken because these lights generate heat. If the light source is turned on after skin contact is made and the skin contact is never broken, heat dissipation is usually adequate. Cooperative patients report the shadows as appearing like leaves or cracks, and there appears to be excellent correlation with attachment of the posterior 30° of retina. However, many patients with normal retinas cannot respond in a positive manner to this test, greatly reducing its value.

Color Discrimination

Patients with recent total retinal detachments and many long-term, low detachments have excellent color discrimination with large targets. Because 90% of the cones are extramacular, large macular scar patients have normal color function with large targets. Standardized color-testing methods are highly dependent on 20/200 or better visual acuity, negating their value in opaque media cases. Hemorrhagic vitreous acts as a red filter, altering color discrimination.

Maddox Rod

Detection of the orientation of a Maddox rod is said to correlate with good postoperative function in opaque media cases. Patients with recent total detachments and advanced glaucoma can provide accurate answers to this test, thereby reducing its value. Certain inoperable patients respond positively to this test, further decreasing its value.

Two-Point Discrimination

Two-point sources of light (transilluminators) can be moved laterally, initially touching and then progressing to a distance of 1 m. Reporting of "two lights" at close distance (<2.5 cm) corresponds with better retinal function. Patients with recent or partial retinal detachments can respond normally to this test, and light scatter can cause false negatives, dramatically reducing the value of this test.

Laser Interferometry

Dense cataracts and vitreous hemorrhage prevent visualization of laser interference fringes. Although laser interferometry can be used with minimally opaque media, it measures vernier-type acuity, with only moderate correlation with Snellen acuity.

VALUE OF PSYCHOPHYSIC TESTING

In general, patients with a positive response to all the preceding psychophysic tests show better postoperative results; conversely, those with a negative response typically achieve poor visual function (3). The subjective nature of these tests and the many instances of false positives and false negatives greatly decrease their value. Examiners may use these methods to seek out good-prognosis cases, some of which do not really require surgery, but a negative response to these tests frequently indicates an operable retinal detachment demanding immediate vitrectomy. At present, the authors use only visual acuity testing to assess function.

PUPIL TESTING

An afferent pupillary defect discovered with the swinging flashlight test can be of value in preoperative evaluation. The relative frequency of bilateral iris disease decreases the utility of this test. Glaucoma, retinal detachment, ischemic optic neuropathy, and optic nerve trauma are the most frequent factors in an abnormal response. If one afferent and one efferent loop are intact, the test can have value. As in psychophysical methods, a negative response may indicate an operable retinal detachment rather than an inoperable eye. Large macular disciform scars can cause a moderate afferent pupillary defect.

SLIT-LAMP EXAMINATION

A problem-oriented examination is far more effective than a "routine" examination. Specific, subtle details can have a major impact on presurgical decision making.

Cornea

Epithelial erosions are common in diabetics and patients that have had recent surgery. Stromal edema may preclude the excellent visualization required for vitrectomy. Unless vitreous touch, lens touch, or glaucoma to be treated by vitrectomy is present, the net effect of vitrectomy will be to further decrease endothelial function. Guttata and low endothelial cell counts indicate the possibility of postoperative corneal edema and suggest more rigid vitrectomy indications. Blood staining, scarring, or edema, if very extensive, is an indication for penetrating keratoplasty or endoscopic surgery. Vitrectomies can frequently be performed by working around central corneal or lenticular opacities.

Iris/Anterior Chamber

The extent of pupillary dilation is important if the lens is to be retained. On occasion, a clear lens lensectomy will be necessary in an emergency vitrectomy only to allow the removal of anterior chamber or perilenticular blood or fibrin.

Iris neovascularization is subtle in its early stages but of extreme importance. The iris surface overlying the sphincter should be examined using magnification of 24× to 40× *prior* to dilation. Large vessels, ectropion uveae, and peripheral anterior synechia (PAS) are late changes and are not required for a diagnosis of iris neovascularization. Capillaries on the iris surface indicate activity, while larger vessels will persist after involution of the capillary activity. Examiners with red-green color discrimination problems find it difficult to recognize iris neovascularization, and make this condition a negative factor in the decision to become a vitreous surgeon. Dilated stromal vessels or exposed iris vessels with lens implants are usually quite easy to differentiate from iris neovascularization. Topical phenylepherine decreases the visibility of iris neovascularization due to vasoconstriction.

While significant trabecular meshwork neovascularization can be present with minimal iris neovascularization, this is unusual. Because gonioscopy is time-consuming and may damage the corneal epithelium, the iris is usually used as an indicator of anterior segment neovascularization. Cells and flare are present in the anterior chamber of many patients requiring vitrectomy and are not a contraindication. Fibrin syndrome usually contraindicates all but emergency vitrectomies for endophthalmitis.

Lens Opacities

Blood or pigment on the anterior or posterior surface of the lens or lens implant may necessitate lens or implant removal for adequate visualization. Many vitreous hemorrhage cases have posterior subcapsular cataracts. The lens should be removed if significant posterior subcapsular changes are present to provide excellent surgical visualization and because these changes virtually always rapidly progress postoperatively. Cortical changes, if moderate, can be tolerated. Moderate nuclear sclerosis will permit adequate visualization and progresses more slowly than posterior subcapsular opacities following vitrectomy.

Intraocular Pressure

Indentation (Schiotz) tonometry is generally inadequate and outdated for the measurement of intraocular pressure (IOP). Applanation tonometry is adequate but is inaccurate with irregular corneas. The Tonopen is more accurate with irregular corneas and ocular rigidity problems, causes less corneal trauma, and does not result in fluoroscein in the tear film and anterior chamber. Tonopen tonometry is easier than applanation tonometry for patients with marked blepharospasm.

Low pressure (hypotony) has an undeserved bad reputation. Most low pressures are due to reparable wound leaks or reparable retinal detachments with increased uveoscleral outflow. Low pressure does not cause phthisis; rather, phthisis may cause hypotony. Phthisis might best be defined as ocular collapse from a cyclitic membrane. In no instance should hypotony delay an otherwise indicated vitrectomy. Ciliary body shutdown is an overrated, theoretical cause of hypotony, which occurs only after massive destruction of the ciliary epithelium by cryopexy, ultrasound, laser, or infection.

Elevated IOP has many causes, and a complete discussion is beyond the scope of this book. Pupillary block, hemolytic (erythroclastic), and phakolytic glaucoma are treated by vitrectomy. Neovascular glaucoma (NVG), unless moderate, is usually made worse by vitrectomy unless panretinal photocoagulation or retinal reattachment can be accomplished during the procedure, thereby decreasing vascular endothelial growth factor (VEGF).

SLIT-LAMP BIOMICROSCOPY OF THE RETINA

An understanding of the vitreous anatomy and the forces acting on the retina is far more important than vitreous drawing in evaluation of potential vitrectomy cases. In large part, vitreous drawing is a useless exercise; the traction forces are evident from retinal contours, and visibility of the vitreous is far better at the time of surgery. Small retinal breaks, macular edema, macular holes, epimacular membranes (EMM), subretinal neovascular membranes, and subtle neovascularization are best observed with slit lamp biomicroscopy. Cloudy media decreases the value of slit lamp biomicroscopy. Contact lenses are optically superior to the 18 to 90 diopter lenses and provide better depth of field and therefore stereopsis, although the latter are very effective, easy to use, and comfortable for the patient.

INDIRECT OPHTHALMOSCOPY

An understanding of vitreoretinal anatomy and the forces acting on the retina is a necessity in clinical decision making. The examiner cannot be a passive observer of vitreous "bands" but must grasp the concepts of the continuum of the anterior and posterior vitreous cortex and the forces causing retinal contour changes.

The indirect ophthalmoscope is essential to vitreoretinal examination because of the stereopsis, wide field, and contrast obtained even with nonoptimal media. It should be used on its brightest setting (7.5 V) in most instances. The +20-D larger lenses are preferable because greater light-gathering ability increases contrast. If possible, the pupil should be widely dilated, the room dark, and the examiner well dark-adapted. Continued dark adaptation, by keeping the entire examining unit dimly illuminated, is far more efficient than waiting for dark adaptation to occur during each examination.

VITREOUS CONFIGURATION

The examiner must make a specific effort to look *at* rather than *through* the vitreous with the indirect ophthalmoscope. Much can be learned from the geometric configuration of an opaque or semiopaque vitreous. A common tendency is for the clinician to give up and describe the opaque media case as "no view, "no retinal detail," or "red reflex."

The normal shape of the vitreous is roughly spherical with a small anterior concavity for the lens. The continuity of the outer surface (cortex) is the most essential concept in developing an understanding of surgical anatomy. The vitreous base is not a space-occupying structure but a zone of adherence between retina and vitreous. The vitreous base is a flat, ring-shaped surface. The vitreous base represents a zone connecting the anterior vitreous cortex (AVC) and posterior vitreous cortex (PVC).

Degenerative changes (syneresis), hemorrhage, inflammation, thermal effects, and cellular migration and proliferation can cause shortening of vitreous surfaces, which is best termed *hypocellular vitreous contraction.* Dense hemorrhagic vitreous has been described as "organized" by many but should be termed, more correctly, "opacified." *Organization* is a specific term applied to the proliferation of fibroblasts. It is usually observed only with severe ocular trauma or retinal necrosis. Clear vitreous is fully capable of creating sufficient force to cause a total traction retinal detachment. Many examiners refer to "vitreous bands" in their analysis of vitreoretinal pathology. Discrete vitreous bands are markedly overemphasized and typically represent only a more opaque section of the continuous PVC. The clear contiguous portions of PVC create a tremendous force on the retina, demonstrating that "band"-oriented vitreous description or surgical approach is useless.

As the vitreous contracts, it pulls away from the posterior retinal surface but remains adherent to the vitreous base. The vitreous is normally more adherent to the optic nerve, foveola, and vessels. Abnormal adherence will occur in areas of chorioretinal scarring, neovascularization, trauma sites, and photocoagulation. Further vitreous contraction will create a conical configuration of the PVC because of the posterior adherence areas. Epiretinal membranes (ERM) may occur along the attachment sites but also occurs independent of the vitreous in the form of star folds, epimacular membranes, or the ridge or sheetlike ERM seen in diabetes and retinopathy of prematurity. Frequently, the vitreous will separate from the retinal surface in some areas, leaving scattered zones of adherence.

Saccadic motion of the eye and a change in head position can help differentiate between flaccid PVC with retinal adherence and taut PVC causing traction on the retina. Saccadically induced motion can create a form of dynamic traction capable of creating a retinal break but incapable of causing traction retinal detachment (TRD). The traction referred to in this book might more correctly be termed *static traction.*

The conical configuration (the cone) may have one or more apices created by zones of adherence. The most typical apex of the single point cone is the optic nerve. Two-point cones are usually attached to the optic nerve and a vascular arcade (most frequently superotemporal). It is essential to understand that the PVC must bridge these vitreoretinal attachment points. Nasal location of the cone apex usually precludes traction detachment of the macula. The apices can be acute angles or broad truncations of the conical PVC, indicating small or larger zones of adherence. If the vitreous is taut, the shape of the PVC apex is the mirror image of the shape of the traction detachment. Single acute-angle apices result in simple conical traction detachments. Ringlike apices along the arcades and disk create ringlike traction detachments. Truncated, taut PVC cones result in "table-top" traction detachments with a truncated conical configuration of the retina. Again, the continuity of the PVC across and between each apex must always be kept in mind. If the retina can be seen in some areas but not others, the shape of the retina in the visible areas can be used to extrapolate the position of nonvisible retina.

VITREOUS CLARITY

Some assessment of the age of a vitreous hemorrhage should be made. Discrete blood clots must go through thrombolysis and dispersion phases before clearing occurs. Subposterior vitreous detachment (sub-PVD) and preretinal hemorrhage clear much more rapidly than does vitreous hemorrhage and should be designated accordingly. The retina can frequently be seen through semi-opaque vitreous. It is useful to grade vitreous hemorrhage from 1+ to 4+ (clear, semiopaque, opaque; or slight, moderate, dense and opaque) to permit subsequent examiners to assess the rate of clearing.

RETINAL CONFIGURATION

The transition from retinal to vitreoretinal surgery necessitates a change in examination goals. A methodic quest for retinal breaks must be replaced in large part by an approach, which emphasizes understanding of the forces acting on the retina. Retinal breaks eliminate the pressure gradient normally existing across the retina resulting in rhegmatogenous retinal detachment. Damage to the retinal pigment epithelium (RPE) pump mechanism results in loss of the transretinal pressure gradient and a convex configuration of the retina. In contrast, the transretinal pressure gradient remains in traction retinal detachment cases, which explains the concave shape of the retinal surface. The presence of a retinal break with concave retina is, hydraulically, a traction, not rhegmatogenous, retinal detachment. In contrast, convex retinal detachment with no visible retinal break has a rhegmatogenous component or RPE pump failure.

Perpendicular or oblique traction on the retina is best recognized by alterations in retinal contour. Conical areas of retinal elevation result only from PVC adherence and traction to the apex of the cone. Broader zones of PVC adherence create truncated cones of retinal elevation. Ridgelike changes in the retinal surface result from perpendicular (vitreous sheet) or tangential traction. Star folds or incarceration result from traction directed inward toward a central point, whereas macular holes result from radial, surface traction, directed outward.

RETINAL BREAKS

The detection of retinal breaks assists in surgical planning but can be more difficult in the patient with decreased vitreous clarity. In contrast to conventional retinal surgery, the view is always far better in the operating room than in the office. The reward for prolonged examination of the patient can be examiner fatigue and patient discomfort.

Retinal breaks are frequently located adjacent to abrupt changes in retinal contour associated with vitreous traction. If the retina is concave, it is certain that these breaks have played a minor role in the retinal detachment. As any break may contribute to postvitrectomy detachments, all breaks must be recognized at the time of vitrectomy and treated accordingly. Retinal breaks are frequently located adjacent to retinal/RPE adherence areas or previous retinopexy sites acted on by vitreous traction. A record of the position of all retinal breaks should be made preoperatively and reviewed moments before or during surgery to avoid overlooking areas needing retinopexy.

RETINAL NEOVASCULARIZATION

Active neovascularization of the disk (NVD) or "elsewhere" (NVE) can be thought of as a marker for the presence of vascular endothelial growth factor (VEGF) in the vitreous cavity. Assessment of neovascularization is important not because of intraoperative bleeding, which is usually easy to control, but because it correlates with postoperative neovascular glaucoma and fibrovascular proliferation on the anterior vitreous cortex and is an indication for PRP. Large vessels in an epiretinal membrane without active capillary budding remain present even after PRP decreases VEGF. These larger vessels are more impressive but are not as significant as capillary activity.

EPIRETINAL MEMBRANE

Since "fibrosis" in the vitreous cavity is only present in the context of severe trauma or inflammation, this term should rarely be used. It should be recognized that an epiretinal membrane is usually contiguous with the posterior vitreous cortex in areas not having a posterior vitreous separation. ERM should be examined for color: a brownish pigment may indicate RPE etiology, whereas white coloration points more toward a glial mechanism. It is essential to assess the relationship of the ERM to any retinal elevation. Broad areas of ERM, when contracted, cause more significant retinal elevation than do very small epicenters of ERM.

The epiretinal membranes in PVR are typically less opaque than the membranes associated with diabetic traction retinal detachment or retinopathy of prematurity. For this reason, they are frequently overlooked, and such misnomers as "retinal stiffening" are applied. Retinal stiffening in most disease processes is from periretinal membrane proliferation, even if the ERM or subretinal membranes are transparent. Every fixed fold or star fold must have an ERM, subretinal membrane (SRM), or incarceration as its cause unless the problem is developmental. The surgical approach can only be planned by determination of the location of these membranes. The exact indications for removal are discussed in the chapters on appropriate disease states.

FOREIGN-BODY LOCALIZATION

Localization of an intraocular foreign body (IOFB) has become somewhat of an end unto itself in the work-up of trauma cases. Vitreous surgery has radically changed the approach to IOFB patients. For this reason there is little need for extensive localization studies in most instances. If the fundus cannot be seen, in most cases, vitrectomy will be performed and accurate visualization of the foreign body will become possible intraoperatively. The relative inaccuracy of preoperative localization of foreign bodies near the ocular wall can contribute to mismanagement. The nature of the injury causing the foreign body assists in localization. Most steel foreign bodies are created by hammering and seldom have the velocity to double-penetrate the globe. For this reason they may be assumed in most cases to be intraocular and managed with vitrectomy and forceps removal. In contrast, most shotgun injuries are double perforating because of the high velocity, and even if a lead pellet is intraocular, it need not be removed for 10 to 14 days. Computerized axial tomography is expensive and only moderately accurate, and MRI is contraindicated because a magnetic foreign body may be moved by the magnetic field. Foreign-body localization techniques not utilizing a contact lens are extremely inaccurate and can give false information. Foreign-body localization methods using a contact lens carry the risks of infection and prolapse of ocular contents from the pressure of application of the contact lens. Ultrasonic methods, although better, are difficult to interpret when the foreign body is near the ocular wall. This will be discussed further in the section on diagnostic ultrasound. Anteroposterior and lateral x-rays of the orbit are important, however, to determine the presence and number of IOFBs but are not as useful in localization.

DIAGNOSTIC ULTRASOUND

Diagnostic ultrasound has greatly improved the management of the opaque media patient. This method, however, is best utilized in the hands of the potential surgeon rather than in a distant laboratory setting. The surgeon has the entire clinical picture in mind at the time of ultrasonic examination, making possible better integration of the ultrasonic diagnosis into the thought process. If the ultrasound equipment is located in the surgeon's primary examining room, it will be utilized much more frequently and can be done without charge. Technicians should not be used for what should be thought of as acoustic ophthalmoscopy.

Clinical Acoustic Physics

An understanding of the physical principles involved in the interaction between ultrasonic energy and biologic materials is essential for accurate ultrasonic diagnoses. Ophthalmic ultrasonography utilizes pulse-echo reflection ultrasound. Brief pulses of ultrasonic energy having a 10 MHz, or greater, center frequency are repeated at a rate of 1 to 5 KHz, allowing time for the same transducer to receive the reflected echoes. Knowledge of the average speed of ultrasonic energy propagation through tissue (1,540 m/s) permits the display of the distance between the transducer and echo-producing structure as a dimension on the cathode ray tube (CRT). Acoustic energy is reflected and refracted at interfaces between materials of different acoustic densities (Fig. 1.1).

If the face of the piezoelectric transducer crystal has a small radius of curvature, the result is a point focus with poor depth of field. The depth of the eye (25 mm) requires a

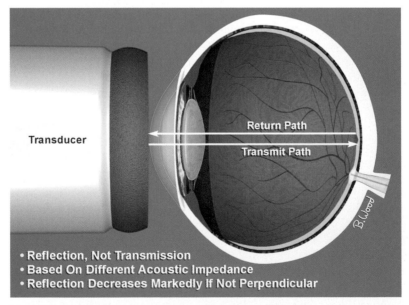

FIG. 1.1. Materials of different acoustic densities reflect and refract acoustic energy at their interfaces.

weaker focusing to obtain an appropriate depth of field. This wide beam width (3 mm at the 6-dB point) creates poor lateral resolution (Fig. 1.2): Targets in the near field are displayed as double, while far-field targets are displayed as spread out laterally. This is inescapable without using computed sonography, which is currently not available in ophthalmic ultrasound systems.

Axial resolution is a function of frequency, with higher frequencies resulting in better axial resolution. Higher frequencies are absorbed more by biologic structures, mandating higher powers to obtain the same small echo sensitivity. The risk of cataract formation determines the maximum power limit than can safely be utilized. In practice, this compromise results in the use of 10-MHz ultrasound with about 0.15-mm axial resolution, which is more than an order of magnitude better than lateral resolution (Fig. 1.3). Axial resolution can also be degraded when the wide beam is reflected from curved surfaces.

The greatest reflection of ultrasound is obtained when the beam strikes the interface perpendicularly. Beams reflecting tangentially from the equatorial ocular wall result in little reflection back to the transducer. With accurate representation of echo amplitudes, an entire circular eye cross section cannot be displayed.

Because the speed of sound is greater in denser tissues such as the lens, structures behind the lens are displayed as being closer, and refraction occurs at the edge of the lens (Fig. 1.4). Dense structures such as lens, intraocular lens (IOL), IOFB, and scleral buckles have multiple internal reflections, and display evenly spaced false echoes of decreasing amplitude behind the structure (Fig. 1.5). The echoes have paradoxical movement with transducer repositioning that aids in their recognition. Dense structures such as calcified cyclitic membranes, intraocular lenses, and foreign bodies create significant shadowing behind them because of absorption of acoustic energy.

The absorption of ultrasonic energy as it passes twice through the tissue results in distant echoes being displayed with relatively less amplitude. Increasing the gain for distant targets can compensate for this absorption. This method is called time-varied gain.

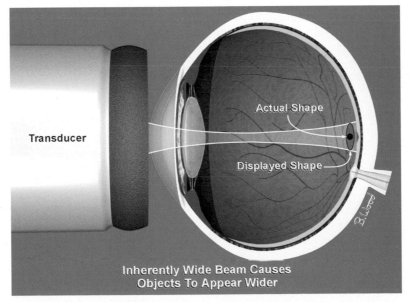

FIG. 1.2. Poor lateral resolution results from the inherently wide ultrasound beam.

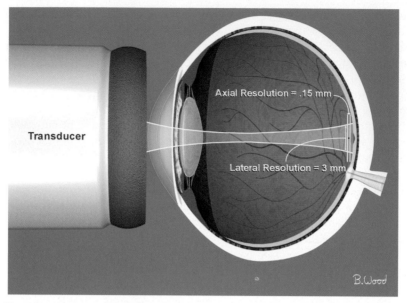

FIG. 1.3. Ten-megaherz ultrasound frequency produces axial resolution an order of magnitude greater than the lateral resolution.

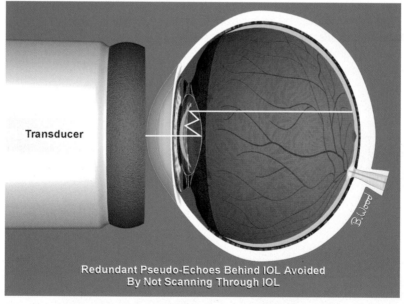

FIG. 1.4. Evenly spaced false echoes of decreasing amplitude result from the multiple internal echoes of dense structures such as IOLs.

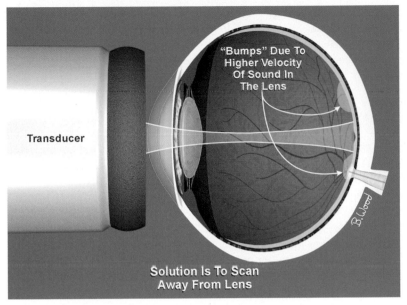

FIG. 1.5. Structures behind denser tissues appear closer than they really are, because of the increased speed of sound through these denser materials.

An emphasis on only displaying interfaces, such as cornea, lens capsule, retina, and sclera, has resulted in inaccuracies in the display system. Increasing the amplitude and clipping the peaks means that all echoes are displayed as equal amplitude. With this approach the vitreous and retina can easily be confused. Similarly, electronic differentiation to detect interfaces eliminates the more subtle echoes within lens, vitreous, and tumor.

A-Scan Versus B-Scan

Time amplitude ultrasonography (A-scan) was the original method of ultrasonography but has little utility in the opaque media work-up. A-scan information is one-dimensional and is analogous to a "needle-in-the-haystack" approach. Extremely experienced A-scan ultrasonographers can spatially integrate the one-dimensional information and obtain some limited value. The typical clinician, however, has far more difficulty with this approach. Quantitative A-scan echography has been overemphasized as being capable of a tissue diagnosis. A-scan echo amplitude is highly dependent on the angle at which the ultrasonic beam strikes the reflecting structure. Oblique angles cause marked attenuation of the reflected echo. Highly convoluted retinal detachments will have areas of high and low reflection. For this reason there is a large sampling error in this one-dimensional approach.

B-Scan

Sector-type B-scan ultrasonography is a two-dimensional approach in which a knife-like slice or plane of acoustic section is made through the tissue, as opposed to the one-dimensional needle approach of A-scan. Echoes are displayed as intensity-modulated dots on the screen. As with A-scan ultrasonography, the best reflections are from those structures roughly perpendicular to the beam. For this reason the cornea, anterior and posterior lens, retinal and scleral surfaces are the best-displayed structures. The equatorial sclera and lens are seen less well, except when the eye is rotated or approached from different angles, emphasizing the need to move the eye and probe during the examination.

Real Time

Real time is defined as appearing virtually continuous and instantaneous to the human observer. It is accomplished by a scanning rate of 5 to 30 scans per second. Real-time ultrasound has many advantages in presurgery decision making. As opposed to a static scan captured with photography, continuous tomography is possible by moving the transducer. As the transducer is moved with respect to the eye, the examiner can observe the screen and integrate multiple two-dimensional scans into a three-dimensional cerebral picture of the intraocular contents. Any attempt to reconstruct this picture from individual photographs taken at discrete intervals is much more difficult and inaccurate.

Real-time ultrasound is of great value in detecting rigidity or, conversely, mobility of ocular structures. The PVC, when detached from the retinal surface in a PVD configuration, is highly mobile. Loose vitreous cones attached at a single point to the retina are nearly as mobile but become immobile if they are taut with resultant TRD. Rhegmatogenous retinal detachments are somewhat less mobile than the detached vitreous but have a definite undulation motion during saccadic motion of the eye. Retinal detachments with PVR have much less mobility than a typical rhegmatogenous retinal detachment (4). Giant breaks have marked retinal mobility (5).

With real-time capability, moving patients and those with nystagmus can easily be examined. In fact, it is advantageous to elicit repeated saccadic motion in all directions to decrease sampling error and to test the rigidity and mobility of ocular structures.

Preretinal hemorrhage can be seen to flow from one position to the other, and dislocated lenses, implants, and foreign bodies can be seen to move with saccadic motion. Real time adds the fourth dimension (time) to the three-dimensional image reconstructed in the examiner's cerebral cortex. When the posterior vitreous has detached from the retina, it will lie in contact with the retina when the patient is in the supine position. Saccadic motion can then demonstrate with real-time ultrasound that the apparent adherence is only gravity-induced contact of the vitreous with the retina. Disciform scars and preretinal hemorrhage can be differentiated by the saccadic-induced motion of the latter.

Gray Scale

Gray-scale B-scan relates echo amplitude to the brightness of specific areas on the display. The vector positional data from the sector scan are displayed as a sector on the screen. Very reflective echoes have white dots on the screen; less reflective echoes have a dimmer shade of white; and absence of echo is displayed as black. Simply stated, the more sound reflected from the ocular structure, the more light emitted from the corresponding area of the screen. Earlier ultrasound units had static scanning with bistable storage CRTs, and the echo amplitude information was therefore not displayed two-dimensionally. Combined A-scan was utilized to obtain a limited, one-dimensional impression of echo amplitude. If a combined A-scan approach was used and the A-scan intersected the retina obliquely, it might be called vitreous. The pattern recognition capabilities of the examiner, however, can, in effect, join the dotted lines between the highly reflective areas using a gray-scale B-scan. With low noise and high dynamic range signal processing, even diffuse red blood cells and normal vitreous can be seen. Long-term retinal detachment causes atrophy, decreasing acoustic density just as cellular proliferation in the vitreous can increase reflection, making amplitude alone an insufficient criterion to distinguish retina from vitreous.

When gray scale is coupled with real time (Charles S, Griffith J, Lindgren W, unpublished paper, 1974), it permits a further appreciation of retinal structures, such that diagnosis is made in a Gestalt manner rather than by itemization of individual diagnostic criteria. The authors consider a real-time, gray-scale B-scan to be an absolute necessity for the work-up of the opaque media patient (6,7).

Technical Limitations

Diagnostic ultrasound has certain limitations:

1. The typical semifocused B-scan transducer creates a beam that is 2 to 3 mm in width; as a result, the target is displayed widened in the lateral orientation. A target is imaged before and after the beam center is lined up with the target during the sector scan. Highly focused beams improve lateral resolution but markedly decrease depth of focus.
2. Axial resolution is a function of the frequency of the ultrasound. Higher-frequency ultrasound, however, is absorbed more by tissue, thus requiring dangerous power levels to achieve the same sensitivity or imaging limited to the anterior segment. Practical 20-MHz retinal B-scan technology is now available (Alcon Ultrascan II).
3. Beam inclination to a reflecting "surface" markedly decreases the amplitude of the reflected echo. The complex topography of vitreoretinal disease prevents quantitative echography because of this beam inclination–induced decrease in echo amplitude.
4. Denser structures such as a nuclear sclerotic cataract, IOL, or calcified tissue absorb sound but increase the speed of sound within the tissue. Because distances are measured in ultrasound by use of an assured speed of sound, increased tissue density causes more distant echoes to be displayed as being closer to the transducer.
5. The human eye observing a CRT has only a 20-dB dynamic range, whereas ultrasound interpretation of ocular tissue produces a 60- to 100-dB dynamic range. For this reason, high gain must be used for minimal vitreous hemorrhage or normal vitreous surfaces, while the gain must be turned down to avoid clipping large echoes such as IOLs.

Vector Scanning

The process of electronically removing a line from a real-time B-scan and displaying it in the typical time amplitude, A-scan manner is called vector scanning or simply simultaneous A-scan and B-scan. It makes possible the combined A-scan approach with its wide dynamic range combined with the real-time, gray-scale, two-dimensional topographic information. It is of more value in looking at internal tumor architecture than it is in the typical opaque media previtrectomy work-up.

Image Archiving and Viewing

Hard-copy images can be used to establish to the reimbursement or legal community that an ultrasound examination was performed. On occasion, old digital or hard-copy images can be compared with the current on-screen image to determine if a change has occurred. The authors again emphasize that ultrasound is a key component of the clinician's examination, not a test, archival, or photo opportunity.

Examination Methods

Contact scanning on the eyelid is used in most opaque media examinations before vitrectomy. A monolithic blob of highly viscous acoustic coupling material is applied to the probe before application to the upper lid for the contact scan. The patient is asked to look multiple times in every direction, and the scan is made both in the anteroposterior direction through the lens for the classic picture and then outside the lens for better resolution and to aid in three-dimensional thinking. It is best that this examination be performed in the standard examining room and that an ultrasound unit be readily available. Putting the unit on a wheeled cart will increase utilization. Ultrasound should be used at every visit in which the patient has opaque media, since the retinal situation can change very rapidly from one visit to the next (8,9).

BRIGHT FLASH ELECTRORETINOGRAPHY

Bright flash electroretinography was originally developed in the context of recording the human early receptor potential (ERP) (10). It was discovered that bright strobes could overcome the light-absorbing property of dense vitreous hemorrhage and allow the elicitation of an electroretinogram (ERG) in these densely opaque media patients. There are many problems with this method, however (11,12). Many examiners incorrectly think that a retinal detachment will still have a recordable ERG that can be used to determine retinal viability. However, because of conduction problems, a total retinal detachment of any age does not produce a recordable ERG. Similarly, some examiners believe that a nonrecordable bright flash ERG means that a vitrectomy should not be done. In most cases, the remaining part of the clinical and ultrasound examinations will reveal a total detachment, which requires immediate vitrectomy. In contrast, many surgeons wish to do cases that have a recordable BF ERG. While this is certainly easier for the surgeon, if they are unilateral moderate vitreous hemorrhages, they are just the cases that do *not* require vitrectomies. Use of this test therefore as a prognostic means must be thought of in terms of the complete clinical picture.

Although it is true that a decreased B-wave correlates with ischemic inner retinal layers, this is also not a valuable criterion because the small portion of the retina around the macula can be well perfused and capable of good vision after vitrectomy. Further, false negatives occur in extremely dense vitreous hemorrhage cases because even the bright strobes used cannot penetrate the ocular media sufficiently. Extensive panretinal photocoagulation (PRP) may cause a nonrecordable ERG similar to that in retinitis pigmentosa. Therefore a patient that had a vitreous hemorrhage after a successful PRP would have a nonrecordable bright flash ERG, causing some examiners to think that surgery was not indicated. If protocol mentality allows the bright flash ERG to be utilized in a patient with clear media just because his or her initial ERG testing was not recordable, permanent damage to the retina can result from the bright strobe.

Because of the many false positives and false negatives described earlier and the possibility of technical laboratory error, bright flash ERG has very little value in the preoperative evaluation. Certainly, if it is recordable and if other clinical factors suggest surgery, the patient has a better prognosis. Having a better prognosis, however, in many clinical situations is not the reason to have a vitrectomy.

VISUAL EVOKED POTENTIAL

The visual evoked potential (VEP) also has limited value because of difficult interpretation, equipment complexity, false negatives, and false positives. As with ERG testing, a patient with severely decreased preoperative VEP might not be considered for vitrectomy, when in reality, he or she could have ambulatory vision after vitrectomy.

REFERENCES

1. Timberlake GT, Mainster MA, Schepens CL. Automated visual acuity testing. *Am J Ophthalmol* 1980;90:369.
2. NAS-NRC Committee on Vision and Recommended Standard Procedures for the Clinical Measurement and Specification of Visual Acuity. Report of Working Group 39. *Adv Ophthalmol.*
3. Michels RG, Ryan SJ. Preoperative evaluation of patients for vitreous surgery. In: Gitter KA, ed. *Current concepts of the vitreous, including vitrectomy.* St Louis: CV Mosby, 1976:121–128.
4. Han DP, Lewandowski M, Mieler WF, et al. Echographic diagnosis of anterior hyaloidal fibrovascular proliferation. *Arch Ophthalmol* 1991;109:842–846.
5. Genovesi-Ebert F, Rizzo S, Chiellini S, et al. Echographic study of the vitreoretinal interface in giant retinal tears. *Ophthalmologica* 1998;212[Suppl 1]:89–90.
6. Capeans C, Santos L, Tourino R, et al. Ocular echography in the prognosis of vitreous hemorrhage in type II diabetes mellitus. *Int Ophthalmol* 1997–98;21: 269–275.
7. Kumar A, Verma L, Jha SN, et al. Ultrasonic errors in analysis of vitreous hemorrhage. *Indian J Ophthalmol* 1990;38:162–163.
8. Jack RL. Ultrasonographic ocular evaluation prior to vitrectomy. In: Irvine AR, O'Malley C, eds. *Advances in vitreous surgery.* Springfield, IL: Charles C Thomas, 1976:100–112.
9. Jack RL, Hutton WL, Machemer R. Ultrasonography and vitrectomy. *Am J Ophthalmol* 1978;78:265.
10. Galloway NR. Early receptor potential in the human eye. *Br J Ophthalmol* 1967;51:21.
11. Fuller DG, Knighton RW, Machemer R. Bright flash electroretinography for the evaluation of eye with opaque vitreous. *Am J Ophthalmol* 1975;80:214.
12. Fuller D, Knighton R, Machemer R. Bright flash ERG. In: Irvine AR, O'Malley C, eds. *Advances in vitreous surgery.* Springfield, IL: Charles C Thomas, 1976;97–99.

2

Instrument Considerations

High-technology vitreous surgery requires intensive and continuous attention to the equipment and operating environment. Equipment, supplies, training, staffing, and storage of the equipment are ultimately the surgeon's responsibility. The requirements for effective difficult surgery should outweigh logistical considerations. Blaming problems on equipment, companies, nurses, technicians, administrators, or managed care is irresponsible and ineffective.

OPERATING ROOM ENVIRONMENT

Scheduling

Every attempt should be made to schedule vitrectomies when the surgeon and team are not rushed or heavily burdened mentally. If this means early, late, day-off, or weekend surgery, it must be done. Many surgeons become tense if they are heavily committed for time following a surgery. As vitrectomies can be lengthy, especially during the learning phase, time must be available to facilitate concentration on the surgery rather than on a subsequent event. A designated operating room is preferable to ad hoc room utilization as it facilitates equipment accessibility, maintenance, stocking, and storage of disposables.

Preoperative Evaluation

Regardless of the type of anesthesia contemplated for vitreoretinal (VR) surgery, the patient should undergo a thorough preoperative evaluation before the procedure. Under most circumstances this evaluation should occur well before the day of surgery so that required adjustments can be performed in advance to help ensure that the patient is in optimal condition before surgery. Specific investigations, such as chest x-ray, electrocardiogram (ECG), and blood chemistries, should be performed only when dictated by the findings of thorough history and physical examinations. So-called screening labs are not indicated when the appropriate history and physical examinations are negative.

General Versus Local Anesthesia

Both general and local anesthetic techniques are acceptable for VR surgery; however, I prefer to do the vast majority of my cases using local anesthesia for a variety of reasons: (a) local anesthesia offers increased safety for patients, especially those in high-risk categories; (b) local anesthesia saves time and reduces cost; and (c) local anesthesia provides rapid recovery and prolonged analgesia, both of which are especially important in the outpatient population.

Not all patients are appropriate candidates for VR surgery under local anesthesia. Immature, mentally deficient, claustrophobic, and uncooperative patients are best managed with general anesthesia. Patients with language barriers, however, can frequently be managed extremely well with local anesthesia if a competent translator can be found. Estimated surgical time is an additional consideration when choosing general versus local anesthesia. Surgeons requiring more than 90 minutes for a given VR procedure ought to consider general anesthesia over local anesthesia, as patients frequently become restless and uncomfortable when asked to lie completely still for such long periods. An additional indication for general anesthesia is the patient who absolutely insists upon it, although these patients will be rare if properly informed and reassured by a sympathetic surgical team.

Monitoring During Surgery

Regardless of the type of anesthesia used, the patient must be carefully monitored during surgery. Appropriate monitoring begins with the continuous presence of an anesthesiologist or certified registered nurse anesthetist during the entire procedure. If sedation is given, it is not in the patient's best interest to have the surgeon or circulating nurse monitor the patient, as may be the case in a brief procedure performed under strictly local anesthesia without sedation. Basic monitoring includes continuous ECG, noninvasive blood pressure (NIBP), and pulse oximetry. End-tidal CO_2 monitoring is additionally essential during general anesthesia and can be helpful during local anesthesia. Core temperature monitoring is indicated during longer procedures under general anesthesia to help ensure that thermal preservation procedures are successful and to help monitor for the rare occurrence of malignant hyperthermia. In diabetic patients, the ability to monitor blood glucose in the perioperative period is also essential to recognize and treat extremes of both hyper- and hypoglycemia.

Blood Pressure Considerations During General Anesthesia

It is common for VR surgeons to become angry if the patient moves at all during surgery. An unintended consequence of this tendency is for the anesthesia provider to maintain deeper levels of anesthesia to prevent movements, which may result in low enough systemic blood pressures to compromise retinal profusion. During VR surgery intraocular pressure (IOP) is carefully controlled in the ranges of 35 to 45 mm Hg. Ocular ischemia and central retinal artery occlusion can occur if low systemic blood pressures are allowed to persist during the procedure. To ensure adequate levels of general anesthesia and immobility of the patient, adequate, monitored muscular relaxation combined with processed electroencephalogram (i.e., bispectral analysis) monitoring should be considered, so that excessively deep levels of general anesthesia can be avoided.

Sedation During Local Anesthesia

In general, patients having VR surgery under local anesthesia should have minimal sedation, most of which should be given at the time of the block. Patients should not be sedated too deeply during VR surgery for a number of reasons. In the first place, airway obstruction may occur, requiring manual support and interruption of the procedure. This has been described as anesthesia without airway control. Second, respiratory movements during sleep or near sleep often result in magnified movements of the head, which greatly hinder the progress of the surgeon who is seeing these movements magnified 20 to 40 times through the operating microscope. Third, some patients become quite talkative and social when overly sedated. It may be impossible for them to quit talking and moving despite the most vigorous admonitions to do so. The only way to manage these patients is to stop all sedation completely or to convert to general anesthesia. Finally, patients who are asleep or nearly asleep are prone to awakening suddenly and being totally disoriented, resulting in movements that can be devastating, even in the hands of the finest surgeon.

Judicious amounts of sedatives and/or opioid agents can be helpful during local anesthesia for VR surgery, especially in the patient who is very apprehensive or slightly claustrophobic. Brevital, thiopental, midazolam, propofol, alfentanil, remifentanil, ketamine, and others have been promoted to provide good operating conditions and acceptable patient satisfaction for a variety of procedures performed under local anesthesia. For VR surgery, the emphasis must be placed on balancing patient comfort and satisfaction while providing the most stable conditions for surgery. In general, this means using small doses of rapid- and short-acting drugs given continuously with very careful monitoring of effect. The goals are to assist the patient in lying perfectly still for 60 to 90 minutes without falling asleep, to enhance analgesia, and to provide a measure of amnesia. These are not easily achieved, but they can be accomplished in most patients by an experienced and knowledgeable anesthesia provider.

Psychologic Preparation for Local Anesthesia

In preparing patients for VR surgery under some form of local anesthesia, it is important to give them specific details about the experience so that they will suffer no surprises. They need to know about the drape and about not being able to see during the procedure. They also need to know that plenty of fresh air will be provided for them under the drape and that breathing under the drape will not be a problem. This is the perfect opportunity to discuss the patient's fears, such as claustrophobia, positional dyspnea, positional pain, and so on. One may discern during these discussions that a particular patient might be better managed with general anesthesia.

The patient should also be given a realistic estimate of the length of the procedure and the need for lying extremely still. Almost anyone can lie still for 30 to 45 minutes, but for longer procedures the patient must be reassured that short "time outs" can be arranged to allow some movement.

Patients must also be aware that an anesthesia provider will be constantly present and dedicated to monitoring their condition and to act as liaison with the rest of the team. It is extremely important for the anesthesia provider and surgeon to communicate freely during the procedure, both with each other and with the patient. Simple means for communication with minimal movement, such as hand-holding or hand-held signaling devices, give the patient a feeling of comfort in knowing that it is possible to alert the team to a problem while not jeopardizing the surgical field. If the patient cannot speak English, it is imperative to have a translator in the room who is fluent in the patient's native language.

Choice of Local Anesthesia

Essentially four types of local anesthesia are commonly used in ophthalmic surgery: topical, retrobulbar, peribulbar, and sub-Tenon's. Topical anesthesia is useful in a variety of operations, but it has limitations in VR surgery because of the need for complete akinesia during many VR procedures, such as macular surgery and membrane peeling. The terms *retrobulbar* and *peribulbar* are confusing and imprecise, and should be replaced by the terms *intraconal* and *extraconal,* which more accurately describe the intended location of the needle in the orbit. These techniques carry a risk, albeit small, of major complications, such as ocular perforation, bleeding, and brain stem anesthesia, but both are very useful for VR surgery, providing excellent akinesia, anesthesia, and prolonged postoperative analgesia. Sub-Tenon's anesthesia offers an increased level of safety over intraconal and extraconal techniques, and can provide suitable conditions for VR surgery. We especially prefer it in the patient with a long eye, who represents an increased risk of ocular perforation with the intraconal and periconal techniques. Sub-Tenon's may not be appropriate for patients who have had previous scleral buckling, as scleral perforation with a sub-Tenon's cannula has been reported in such a patient.

The following scheme presents our current thoughts for choosing a local anesthesia technique for VR surgery:

1. *Reblocking during the procedure.* Sometimes during surgery local anesthesia must be supplemented. This can occasionally be accomplished with topical anesthesia, but we most commonly supplement intraoperatively by placing a flexible cannula into Tenon's space and injecting additional local anesthetic. An additional intraconal injection can also be performed by placing the needle between Tenon's capsule and the sclera to enter the intraconal space. Most often reblock is necessary when the block has been inadequate, when the patient is a re-op, and when the procedure is prolonged.
2. *Facial nerve blocks.* Separate facial nerve blocks are rarely indicated, especially if a well-performed extraconal block is used. Avoiding a facial nerve block spares the patient a very painful injection and prevents the bleeding, swelling, and other complications that occasionally accompany these blocks. If the patient is a marked "squeezer," the orbicularis oculi can be easily and effectively blocked by inserting a 0.5-inch 30-gauge needle transconjunctivally into the lower lid just beneath the orbicularis and injecting about 1.5 mL of local anesthetic.

Sources of Pain During VR Surgery

Local anesthesia needs to be quite solid during VR surgery if the experience is to be pain-free. Manipulation of the iris, ciliary body, and sclera can all be painful, especially if blunt instruments are being used. Thermal stimulation is also an important source of discomfort. Cryosurgery is very painful, more so than laser or even radio-frequency cautery. Lasers in the near-infrared range are more painful than the argon laser at 514 nm or the diode-pumped, frequency-doubled continuous wave (CW) YAG laser at 532 nm. As one or more of these modalities may be employed during VR surgery, it is important that the patient receive adequate anesthesia.

Carbon Dioxide Issues

Patients lying awake under the drape frequently complain that they cannot get enough air. As pulse oximetry routinely records a normal oxygen saturation in these patients, their complaints are frequently attributed to anxiety. In fact, CO_2 often builds up under the drape, resulting in hypercarbia and a feeling of air hunger. This may be noted by a rise in the baseline if capnography is being used, even though the peak expired CO_2 may be normal or only slightly elevated. An easy solution to this problem is to ensure adequate air/oxygen supplementation near the patient's nose and mouth as well as active evacuation of the exhaled gases by way of a vacuum line placed under the drapes.

Air/Gas and General Anesthesia

If gas and/or air are introduced into the eye during VR surgery, nitrous oxide should be turned off at least 10 minutes beforehand, and fresh gas flow into the anesthesia machine should be increased to ensure adequate washing out before introduction of the gas. Failure to do so results in a smaller than desired gas bubble within the eye and lower than desired IOP postoperatively when nitrous oxide diffuses out of the bubble. Conversely, if a patient has a bubble in the eye from a previous procedure, nitrous oxide should be avoided from the beginning to prevent expansion of the bubble by diffusion of nitrous oxide into it, thus raising IOP. In fact, patients must be warned to alert physicians to the presence of the bubble should they require emergency surgery.

Anesthetic Considerations for Specific Procedures

Endophthalmitis

Endophthalmitis is an acute situation in which cultures must be taken and therapy instituted as quickly as possible. In many situations cultures and even core vitrectomy can be performed under topical anesthesia. If general anesthesia is required, surgery cannot be delayed to allow the stomach to empty.

The Open Globe

Each patient must be thoroughly evaluated, as choice of anesthesia will depend on the extent of the injury and the ability of the patient to cooperate. Often initial wound closure can be accomplished under topical and intracameral anesthesia. In cooperative patients with limited damage, orbital regional anesthesia can be safely used, provided that the person performing the block has had sufficient experience, uses limited volumes of anesthetic, and injects very slowly (i.e., 1 mL every 30 to 60 seconds) while closely watching the eye. When general anesthesia is required, the issue of whether to use a depolarizing muscle relaxant arises. The choice must be left to the anesthesia provider, who will decide based on the total clinical picture.

Scleral Buckles

Many patients presenting for scleral buckling procedures will be high myopes. These patients have long axial lengths, often accompanied by posterior staphylomata and scleral thinning. Sub-Tenon's cannula techniques might be considered in these patients to lessen the risk of perforation.

Regional anesthesia for scleral buckling procedures may be complicated by the fact that the retractor can cause significant orbital rim pain even in the presence of complete ocular anesthesia. Additionally, with traction of the extraocular muscles the oculocardiac reflex may occur. Most commonly, the resulting bradycardia will return to normal when traction is released, and the reflex will diminish over time. Intravenous atropine is more effective than glycopyrrolate in blocking the reflex, but its use is associated with a higher incidence of subsequent tachyarrhythmias. Local anesthetic injection may block the bradycardia, but the reflex is also seen in the presence of a complete block.

Patients who have had previous scleral buckles and present for another procedure may be difficult to block. As the buckling may slightly elongate the eye, one must be aware of an increased danger for perforation. As scarring occurs, normally "safe" procedures may become less safe, and ocular perforation has been reported with sub-Tenon's anesthesia in a patient with a previous scleral buckle.

Anticoagulation Issues

In our practice we virtually never stop anticoagulation before VR surgery, although it is wise to ensure that the patient taking warfarin compounds has an international normalized ratio (INR) in the therapeutic range (generally 2 to 3). Stopping anticoagulants risks causing morbidity or mortality from a variety of causes, including stroke, myocardial infarction, pulmonary embolism, and deep venous thrombosis. The dangers of intraoperative hemorrhage are grossly overemphasized when compared with the dangers of stopping therapeutic anticoagulation. Use of cannula techniques for local anesthesia greatly reduces the risk of hemorrhage in these patients, as does the use of short needles (1.25 inch or less) placed in the less vascular areas of the orbit (i.e., avoiding the superior half of the orbit in general and especially the superonasal quadrant) for orbital blocks.

Postoperative Pain

One source of postoperative pain is the injection of antibiotics and steroids into the periocular tissues at the end of the procedure. This can be totally eliminated by injecting these substances into the sub-Tenon's space with a cannula. In addition, injection of a long-acting local anesthetic, such as bupivacaine, at the end of the procedure can greatly reduce postoperative pain. This is especially important in the occasional patient who requires general anesthesia for VR surgery.

Summary

The vast majority of VR procedures can be safely, comfortably, and efficiently performed under local anesthesia with minimal sedation. Compared with general anesthesia, properly performed local anesthesia offers the patient an increased level of safety, reduced recovery times, and prolonged postoperative pain relief. Nonetheless, the choice of anesthesia technique must be based on the needs of the patient, the requirements of the surgeon, and the skills of the anesthesia provider, ever keeping in mind that our ultimate goal is a satisfied patient with a good visual outcome.

Instrument Storage

The approach in which instruments are assembled from various sources just before the case is inadequate for high-technology vitreous surgery. It is not optimal to share these specialized instruments with other surgeons and procedures. A tray that is equipped for all basic vitreous, retinal, and microsurgical methods should be prepared and stored. The removal of dense lenses, intraocular lenses, and large intraocular foreign bodies through the limbus requires that the appropriate instruments be present on the basic vitrectomy tray. Similarly, scleral buckling techniques are required frequently and probably should not dictate the use of a second tray. An identical sterile backup tray should be available at all times in the operating room or adjacent storeroom.

All fragile instruments, such as intraocular scissors, forceps, contact lenses, and the like, must be kept sterile at all times in transparent peel-packs stored in well-labeled trays, cabinets, or boxes. These instruments are then stored in a lockable cabinet in the operating room or a movable cabinet that is taken to the operating room before use. They should be stored in specific places in the cabinet to permit daily inventory control and maintenance. If not stored in a single cabinet, the instruments tend to become lost and unavailable at a critical time in vitrectomy.

All disposable materials such as patient drapes, microscope drapes, sutures, needles, and tubing sets should be stored in sufficient numbers in a specific place. In this way, faulty or inadvertently contaminated materials and instruments can be instantly replaced without having to be ordered from a central supply area. The many steps in a complex procedure should not be delayed while waiting for instruments or materials to be delivered.

A fast para-acetic acid (Steris) and/or gas plasma (Sterad) as well as a fast cycle steam autoclave should be immediately available to the operating room personnel to speed case turnover and resterilization of inadvertently contaminated equipment if sufficient backups are not available.

Presurgical Equipment Testing

All equipment should be set up and tested before the administration of any form of anesthesia. If needed vitrectomy, lensectomy, endophotocoagulation, operating microscope, or scissors equipment are not functional, the case must be postponed. Infusion fluid should be run copiously through all tubing to remove any bubbles or particulate material. Only after all equipment is tested and the surgeon is present can the team begin local or general anesthesia.

Operating Room Personnel

Preferably, a single surgical technician or nurse should be responsible along with the surgeon for all instruments as well as for the ordering, maintenance, and inventory of disposable materials. Preferably, this individual should also function in the office environment to enhance information transfer and patient confidence. This same individual can assist in the recording and compilation of pre-, intra-, and postoperative data for outcome testing, medical records, and billing. Participation in the follow-up care provides personal evidence of the impact of surgical success and failure. This individual should then be in command of the remainder of the team and should be responsible for backup personnel in their absence. A friendly, cooperative atmosphere with a sense of humor is conducive to the team-play attitude, which is as necessary in the operating room as it is for a successful sports team. This is preferable to a tense, angry, chauvinistic, find-someone-to-blame attitude unfortunately so prevalent in operating rooms.

Video Recording

Although certain cases may have teaching value, video recording should not become a time- and concentration-consuming concern in the operating room. Centering the microscope and producing the best photo opportunity should not consume costly labor dollars or a surgeon's mental focus. At best, it is a moderately efficient way to teach and is often used for promotional purposes.

VITRECTOMY INSTRUMENT SYSTEMS

Characteristics of the ideal vitrectomy system include excellent cutting capability, reliability, lightweight, small size, cool operation, and accurate control of suction and infusion. These goals are compatible but place high demands on design, manufacture, and maintenance. Each of these factors will be discussed separately.

Infusion Site Options

Infusion instruments, as well as other vitreous surgery instruments, can enter the eye through the limbus, ciliary body, or pars plana.

Full-Function Probes

The generic term *vitreous infusion suction cutter* implies the full-function probe concept. While having all functions on one probe was an original goal in the design of vitrectomy instruments (2–6), in almost all situations, separation of functions is more flexible and permits smaller incisions (7,8). Restated, three-port vitrectomy is preferred to one-port vitrectomy for the vast majority of situations.

Infusion Cannulas

Although an infusion sleeve can be slipped over a 20-gauge cutter to restore the full-function probe concept (Fig. 2.1), this is useful only in some anterior vitrectomy scenarios. Sew-on infusion cannulas through the pars plana create far less turbulence and decrease fluid throughput (Fig. 2.2). Separation of the infusion function from the vitreous cutter decreases its size and enhances flexibility. Proportional (linear) suction connected to various extrusion cannulas (see Chapter 4) is far more efficient with separate infusion and does not require that the vitrectomy instrument be in the eye to provide infusion. The wide separation of the infusion and egress ports decreases turbulence and operating time when removing blood products from the eye. Internal fluid/gas exchange and internal drainage of subretinal fluid (SRF) (see Chapter 4) are similarly more efficient with a separate infusion system. If a retinal break is present or occurs during vitrectomy, the

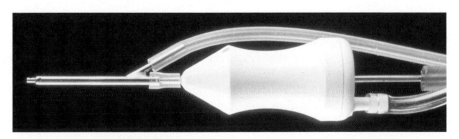

FIG. 2.1. Infusion sleeve over vitrectomy probe.

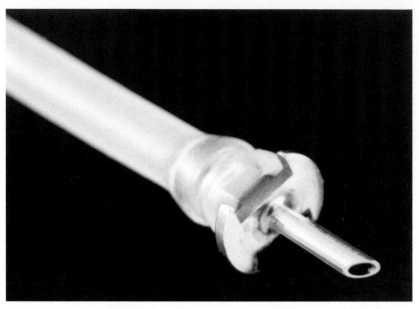

FIG. 2.2. Sew-on infusion cannula.

SRF will increase when exposed to the infusion of the full-function probe, whereas the separate infusion system approach results in decreased SRF if the cutter is brought near the break. The sew-on infusion system is placed without the vitrectomy probe, following the "first in, last out" rule to provide infusion and pressure control throughout the case.

Infusion into the suprachoroidal or subretinal space is the only complication unique to the infusion cannula system. These complications are manageable but, more important, preventable by careful technique (see Chapter 4). Longer (4-mm) cannulas than the 2-mm cannulas originally recommended reduce the chance of inadvertent suprachoroidal or subretinal infusion and do not interfere with the lens, unless the cannula is rotated into the lids or there is traction on the tubing. The maintenance of the standard 20-gauge (0.89-mm) size throughout all components is the best compromise between wound size and flow rates. Interchanging 1.0-mm, 19-gauge, and 20-gauge instruments creates wound leaks; the larger sizes are technically unnecessary and disadvantageous.

Infusion Devices

A 30° bend in a blunt, end-opening, 20-gauge cannula (May) permits access to the anterior chamber via a pars plana entry site over the bridge of the patient's nose (Fig. 2.3) (9). These cannulas are used for infusion when the pars plana cannot be visualized, in most retinopathy of prematurity (ROP) cases, and in some cases of anterior vitrectomy. Infusion sources smaller than 20-gauge provide inadequate infusion rates for 20-gauge removal systems and create hypotony and ocular collapse.

Sharp infusion needles risk inadvertent puncture of ocular structures and damage to the cutter. The bevel can leak fluid when the tip is near the wound and can infuse into the

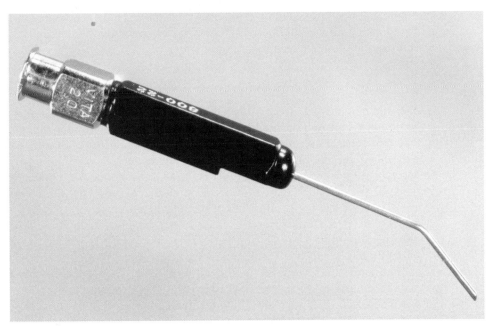

FIG. 2.3. May infusion cannula.

choroid or cornea. Scalp veins and silicone tubing can inadvertently contact the corneal endothelium and should be avoided.

Infusion Fluid

Infusion fluids that include a bicarbonate buffer, dextrose, and glutathione in addition to the usual components of Ringer's solution should be considered mandatory in all cases (Alcon Laboratories BSS Plus) (10). The tubing and connectors must be handled with meticulous, sterile technique. Flushing should be used to prevent bubbles, and care should be taken to avoid negative pressure in infusion bottles. Certain surgeons use lactated Ringers or BSS rather than BSS Plus in a misguided attempt to save money. High labor cost due to slow surgery, not infusion fluid, is the most significant cost driver, yet it receives less emphasis because it points back to the surgeon. Glucose was initially added to the infusion fluid before the advent of frequent blood glucose testing during surgery. The procedure 20 years ago was to utilize intravenous dextrose 5% in water to prevent hypoglycemia during local or general anesthesia. The principal author has not added anything to the infusion fluid for more than 25 years and has not observed significant posterior subcapsular changes. The safety of the cumulative dose of antibiotics or epinephrine in the infusion bottle has not been established. The principal author has performed more than 16,000 vitrectomies with only three cases of postoperative endophthalmitis. The author (SC) had two cases of endophthalmitis in 1975; one case had severe oral sepsis and multilayer drapes were used, permitting the patient to exhale on the operative site. The second case had an infected suprapubic cystotomy and, in retrospect, should have been postponed until the systemic infection had been successfully treated. The third case occurred when no subconjunctival antibiotics were used at the end of the case, an experiment that was immediately terminated. The authors never add epinephrine or any other agent to the infusion fluid because of the risk of contamination, toxicity, and iatrogenic administration of the incorrect dose or agent.

Infusion Pressure

Gravity-fed (bottle height) and air-pressure-driven (Alcon GFI, VGFI) infusion systems imply but do not result in a defined IOP. The actual IOP is highly dependent on flow. An analogy to electrical current (flow) created by a voltage difference (pressure) acting on a resistance (cannula/tubing size and length) enhances understanding (Fig. 2.4). The 84-inch infusion lines currently in use coupled with stopcocks, connectors, and the resistance of the cannula create significant pressure losses. The pressure decreases by 1 mm Hg for each 1 mL/min flow. With typical vitrectomy variables, this equates to a pressure drop of 10 mm Hg or greater. Many surgeons have the false impression that the IOP should be 15 to 25 mm Hg during vitrectomy. These are the surgeons who frequently have "soft eye" problems when vacuum is applied. It should be common sense that using a 20-gauge system at 20 mm Hg to supply fluid while removing fluid using vacuum levels that far exceed that infusion pressure is going to result in a soft eye. There is no scientific or clinical evidence that an IOP of 35 to 45 mm Hg causes any damage during cases lasting several hours. The authors set the Accurus VGFI system at 45 mm Hg, except for neonates (30 mm Hg) and patients with very low diastolic blood pressures.

High IOP can overcome perfusion pressure and create vascular occlusion. For this reason the pressure is only elevated above 45 for a few minutes to control bleeding. Low IOP creates miosis, astigmatism, and striate keratopathy, which greatly limit surgical visibil-

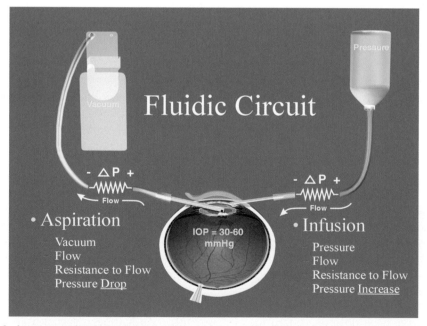

FIG. 2.4. Intraoperative intraocular pressure is determined by the interaction of pressure, suction, flow rate, and tubing resistance.

ity. If the IOP exceeds the pump capacity of the corneal endothelium even for a few minutes, the result is corneal edema.

Pressure and perfusion must be monitored continuously during vitrectomy. The apparent resistance of the eye to deformation by the instruments (bimanual feel), the appearance of striate keratopathy, and fourth-digit tactile methods enhance awareness of IOP. When the retinal vessels become visible, they should be carefully observed for evidence of the perfusion pressure being exceeded by the IOP, especially in situations of low perfusion pressure, such as in infants, low diastolic blood pressure, and general anesthesia.

The so-called gas-forced infusion (GFI, Alcon Laboratories, Morris & Witherspoon) system has the same dynamics as the gravity-fed infusion but is advantageous because it provides a direct, digital readout of the infusion pressure in the familiar mm Hg notation. Alcon has developed the vented "gas-forced" infusion (VGFI) system to enable rapid increase *and* decrease of infusion pressure via console or foot pedal without moving the bottle. The VGFI system enables the Accurus foot-controlled "tamponade" system to prevent or control bleeding or manage low pressure due to wound leaks or poor fragmenter port occlusion on hard nuclear fragments.

Suction Systems

A pressure difference across the suction port of a vitrectomy instrument is necessary to cause substances to enter the port. The term *passive egress* is incorrect because there is no physical difference between transorifice pressure (also called *delta P*) achieved by high infusion pressure and that achieved by negative pressures (vacuum) on the inside of the port. Semirigid materials such as membranes and lenses must be deformed to pass through a suction port in response to a transorifice pressure gradient. Markedly low transorifice pressure will prolong the process of vitreous removal; large gradients create traction on the vitreoretinal interfaces. In general, a maximum suction setting of 150 mm Hg should be used for lensectomy and a setting of 100 mm Hg or less should be used for core vitrectomy. The lowest suction force possible to accomplish vitrectomy should be used to reduce vitreoretinal traction. Air lock should be cleared by flushing the system outside the eye, and not by increasing the suction force. After the vitreous has been removed, higher suction force can be used to carefully remove adherent or previously delaminated epiretinal membranes. Suction-induced vitreoretinal traction is a key factor in the production of post- and intraoperative retinal breaks. A baseline incidence of aphakic-like retinal detachments will exist as long as vitreous is removed using suction force. Factors other than suction force such as lattice degeneration, preexisting retinal breaks, and vitreous incarceration in the sclerotomies also cause postvitrectomy retinal detachments.

There has been an evolution of systems utilized to control suction force for vitreous surgery. Manually operated syringes controlled by the assistant provided excessive, pulsatile control of suction force because of syringe friction and a volumetric primary controller. Large swings in transorifice pressure ultimately related to vitreoretinal traction with all manual syringe methods. Use of the mechanical syringe drive offered better control because of its mechanical advantage. Peristaltic pump systems primarily control flow rather than pressure and typically undergo transient peaks of high transorifice pressure as materials are impacted in the port. As the material deforms and moves rapidly through the port, this excessive pulse of "residual" suction force is transmitted to the surrounding vitreous, creating undue vitreoretinal traction. Venturi pumps are safer than most peristaltic- or scroll-pump-based vitrectomy systems.

Vacuum systems controlled by the surgeon's foot offer a major advantage over surgeon's hand or assistant control. Suction force is analogous to the pressure one places on a knife or scissors to cut and should be directly controlled by the surgeon. The maximum vitreoretinal traction is under constant control with a controlled vacuum system. Controlling the vacuum with a button on the cutter causes inadvertent hand movements and operator fatigue. Foot-controlled solenoid valves interrupt the connection of the suction port to a collection bottle at a preset vacuum level, but create an abrupt onset of suction and inability to decrease suction without stopping the process. Better control is made possible by having the foot pedal proportional to the suction force. Simply stated, pedal position correlates with suction force. Proportional suction control, frequently called *linear suction* (11,12), permits continuous optimization of the suction force. Rather than using the circulating nurse for resetting the level of suction, a preset maximum is utilized, with a constant use of just enough suction to remove vitreous as judged visually. Readout of this force on the console is available but is seldom observed because the correct force is judged by viewing vitreous and retinal movement into the port. A distinct advantage of this method is the control over the rate of increase of the suction force. The suction force is gradually increased until vitreous movement into the port is just achieved. Fast response time, also known as tracking, is essential for proportional (linear) suction systems. The Alcon Accurus system has been optimized to decrease the vacuum rapidly (25 ms) in response to a foot-pedal command to reduce suction, without the need to stop cutting (Fig. 2.5). This precise control requires matching dynamic port resistance, cut rates, tubing resistance, and console fluidics. A real-time operating system implemented on a dedicated fluidics processor provides guaranteed latencies. The Accurus system coupled with the Alcon Innovit cutter (Charles) enables safe dissection with the probe virtually touching the retinal surface. Other systems using a single processor and non–real-time operating systems such as

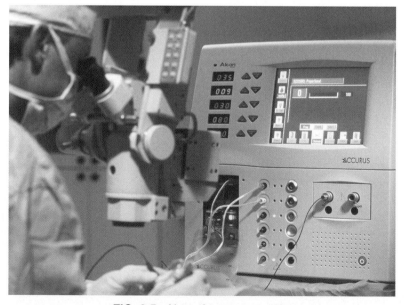

FIG. 2.5. Alcon Accurus console.

Windows have poor tracking, resulting in delays between the foot-pedal command and vacuum change. At times, the vacuum will rise for 250 ms after the command to decrease vacuum with Windows-based operating systems.

Cutter Type

Vitreous cutters can be grouped into axial (guillotine) and rotational (continuous or oscillatory) types of cutters. All cutters can cut well when at peak efficiency. If an axial cutter becomes worn, it simply chops ineffectively on the fibers but creates no vitreoretinal traction unless the probe is moved with the suction activated. In contrast, rotating and multiturn oscillating cutters, when worn, wind the vitreous around the rotating needle, creating excessive vitreoretinal traction. The Innovit cutter utilizes a double-acting piston-cylinder and rack-and-pinion drive (Fig. 2.6). This actuation system produces a very high cutting rate (cuts/minute), gives a high cutter velocity, and rotates just enough to open and close the port, eliminating winding. Self-sharpening instruments (MVS, Accurus, and Innovit) have larger frictional forces requiring more powerful motors-actuators than nondisposable cutters. Reusable, non–self-sharpening systems require more precision in manufacture and maintenance and frequent resharpening. Reusable cutters often are used when they are in need of resharpening, creating excessive vitreoretinal traction. Pneumatically driven cutters are much smaller, lighter, and cooler in operation, and have no electrical hazards compared with electrically driven cutters. Disposable, self-sharpening cutters remain sharp for the entire procedure and are then discarded.

Cutting Speed and Frequency

Vitreous cutters are best operated at the fastest cutting rate available during core vitreous removal to minimize suction-induced vitreous fiber movement before cutting takes place (Fig. 2.7). This effect is thought to be more significant than the inertial cutting effect associated with high cutter velocities. Slowing the cutting rate increases flow and is used by many surgeons for cutting membranes and lens material. Low cut-

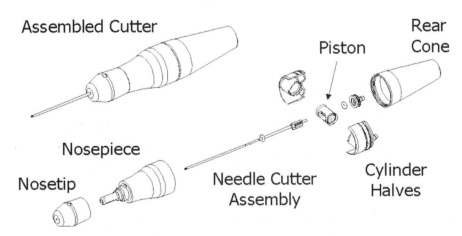

FIG. 2.6. Exploded view of the Alcon Innovit vitreous cutter.

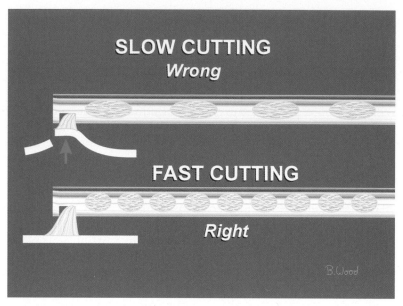

FIG. 2.7. Maximum cutting rates minimize suction-induced vitreous fiber movement.

ting rates increase the likelihood of dangerous, sudden elastic deformation through the port analogous to occlusion break in phaco surgery. There is a misconception that slower is safer, when actually slowness results in more traction on the retina during core vitrectomy because uncut vitreous moves through the port. Low moving mass allows higher cutting speed with less vibration, just as it is an advantage in audio transducers and car suspension systems. High cutter speed increases the resistance to flow and reduces the chance of retinal damage when cutting dense membrane near mobile retina. The cutting rate modulates resistance and therefore flow rates, with a given vacuum. Higher cutting rates result in decreased flow per port opening cycle, less fluctuation in pressures, and greater fluidic stability. Fluidic stability is particularly important when working near mobile and peripheral retina.

Endoillumination

Full-function probes utilize a coaxial fiberoptic illumination system. Although this is vastly superior to microscope illumination, it is inflexible and illuminates only the cutter tip and surrounding vitreous. A separate endoilluminator can be used bimanually with intraocular instruments other than the cutter and allows illumination of any area of interest. Retroillumination with the endoilluminator allows better visualization of clear vitreous with less glare. Safety is increased by the ability to illuminate remote areas of vitreous during membrane or vitreous removal. Infusion, manipulation, and diathermy can be added to the endoilluminator, which is ideal for diabetic cases. Various divergence angles can be used for a spot- or floodlight effect. Wide-angle illumination probes (bullet) produce more uniform contrast on video images but make visualization of clear vitreous more difficult. They are often used with wide-angle visualization systems.

Handpiece Configurations

All hand instruments should be held in three fingertips and rest on the web of tissue extending from the base of the thumb to the second digit. Fingertips are softer and have better tactile sensation than the bony portions of the fingers. Triangulation of instruments between three fingertips and this web is the most stable grip and occupies approximately 35 mm of handle length. Any handle or cable extending beyond this grip moves the center of gravity behind the grip point and creates torque on the fingers. Extension beyond 35 mm gives dangerous leverage to an assistant inadvertently striking the handle or pulling on the cable/tubing.

The lightest probe is the best probe. While a heavier, metal, electrically driven cutter may appear to be well made, the weight creates excess loading of the proprioceptive sense (Weber-Fechner law) and decreases sensitivity. Excess weight coupled with excessive length is extremely muscle fatiguing and tremor inducing. Mental fatigue, tension, and caffeine accentuate tremor. An hourglass-shaped probe (Charles, Wang) wedges between the fingers, reducing the force required to prevent slippage in either direction. Pneumatically driven, disposable, self-sharpening, hourglass-shaped, lightweight, 35-mm-handle probes are the best compromise at this time (Fig. 2.8).

Cutter Movement

Some surgeons have recommended pulling the cutter away from vitreous while cutting, but this technique is dangerous because the force created by probe movement is added to the force created by transorifice pressure (Fig. 2.9). This is particularly dangerous when slow cutter speeds, relatively high suction levels, or malfunctioning cutters are used. In cataract or penetrating keratoplasty, vitrectomy cutting while pulling the probe out of the

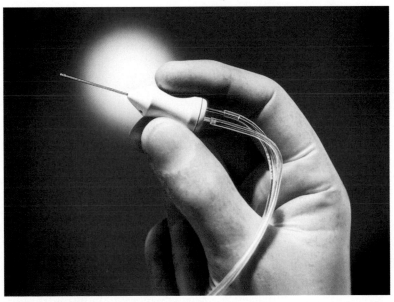

FIG. 2.8. Lightweight, ergonomically designed probes enhance proprioceptive response while reducing tremor and fatigue.

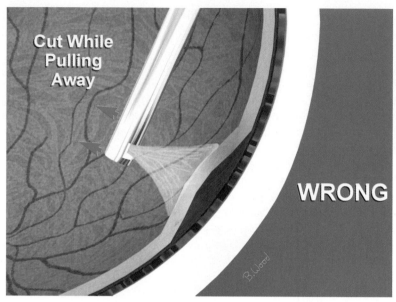

FIG. 2.9. Cutting while pulling away increases vitreous traction forces by adding physical displacement to transorifice pressure.

vitreous has the added disadvantage of creating airlock as air is introduced into the system. If material becomes caught in the port, the surgeon should *not* jerk the probe back ("burned-hand" reflex) but should wait and have an assistant squeeze the suction tubing or better yet, use the Accurus foot-pedal reflux mode or equivalent.

With the Accurus or equivalent suction systems, accurately controlled low suction force allows the port to be turned toward the retina or at 90 degrees rather than 180 degrees away. The probe should be moved toward the tissue to cut, just as one would use any other power tool. Excessive suction must be applied if the port is turned anteriorly, away from the vitreous to be cut. The combination of the high-performance cutters and advanced fluidics achieves the ultimate goal of cutting tissue in its original position. Surgeons accustomed to the vitreous being drawn to the port at first may think these systems are not cutting but later learn to move the cutter to the tissue to be removed (Fig. 2.10).

Port Configuration

Large ports decrease the force per unit area but allow the entry of larger tissue pieces without cutting or deformation of the tissue. Ports closer to the tip are advantageous only when high cutting rates and high-performance cutter/fluidic systems permit safe operation near the retina. Although most epiretinal membranes are removed by delamination or forceps peeling, cutter operation near the retina is especially advantageous in diabetic traction detachments.

Self-Sharpening

Higher force-to-weight-ratio pneumatic actuators are preferred to drive self-sharpening cutters. Self-sharpening cutters remain sharp throughout the procedure. Any self-sharpening cutter must be disposable because self-sharpening results in loss of metal and, ultimately, failure of the probe.

2 INSTRUMENT CONSIDERATIONS

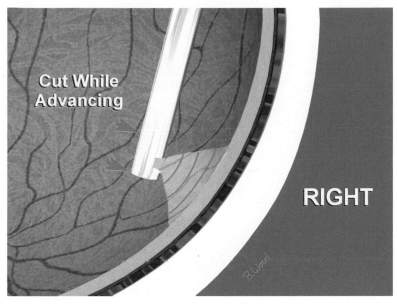

FIG. 2.10. Cutting while advancing severs the tissue in its original position, minimizing traction forces.

OPERATING MICROSCOPE

An operating microscope with power zoom, focus, and two-axis power translational (XY) or rotational (pitch, yaw) movement is necessary for vitrectomy (13). A beam splitter (50/50) that allows the assistant to share the surgeon's view is a necessity. Assistant's microscopes are inappropriate for vitrectomy because of noncoaxial viewing. Although 30/70 beam splitters allow better television images, they decrease the surgeon's contrast and should be avoided. The power XY system can be controlled by a three-axis, six-direction chin switch (14) (Charles and McCarthy), but this can cause temporal-mandibular joint discomfort. Zoom and light on/off must be on the foot pedal. Speech recognition systems have been used to control microscope position but are ill suited to control any of these real-time tasks. The observer tube is essential for the assistant if hand-held contact lenses are used and can be utilized for teaching other clinicians, technicians, or nurses. Many current observer tubes have limited stereopsis, reducing their value. High-quality television in the operating room is very advantageous for team coordination and in-room teaching, but recording is over utilized.

DIATHERMY

Bipolar diathermy systems for cautery should be present in the operating room and incorporated into most vitrectomy systems (see Chapter 4). Forceps-type diathermy tips are excellent for control of bleeding on the sclera, conjunctiva, and Tenon's capsule. The so-called eraser leads to excessive areas being treated compared with the forceps. Diathermy sources can also be used for intraocular bipolar bimanual diathermy (BBD), diathermy combined with illumination (Fig. 2.11), or the much more commonly utilized unimanual, bipolar diathermy (UBD) (see Chapter 4).

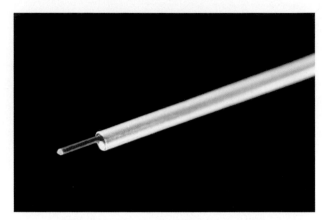

FIG. 2.11. Illuminated diathermy probe.

RETINOPEXY

Laser endophotocoagulation is preferred to any transscleral retinopexy in most instances because of the elimination of scleral damage. Cryopexy causes more cellular migration and proliferation, and increased vascular permeability than laser or diathermy (Fig. 2.12), and is used only in those rare situations in which endophotocoagulation is impossible. The authors usually do not use laser indirect treatment in conjunction with vitrectomy procedures because light scattering from the cornea and lens can cause retinal damage, iris damage, and absorption in the nucleus, increasing cataract. LIO also increases cervical spine problems for the surgeon because of weight on the head and unusual head positions.

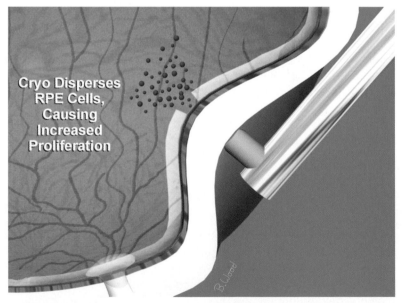

FIG. 2.12. Cryopexy causes excessive cellular migration and proliferation, and is used only when laser endophotocoagulation is impossible.

Transscleral diathermy with a fiberoptic unit can be utilized for retinopexy when the sclera is exposed and endophotocoagulation is unavailable. Minimal scleral damage occurs if air/gas is present because of the thermal and electrical insulation effects of air.

Visualization Systems

The Machemer plano-concave contact lens with a handle was the original method of visualization during vitrectomy. This method remains the most cost-effective and practical method if a steady-handed assistant is available. The authors have learned that technicians can do a superior job of contact lens holding if they are comfortably seated, view through an observer tube, and are treated with respect. Assistant surgeons frequently mentally focus on the case instead of the contact and require reminders to center the lens. Neither wide-angle viewing systems nor the indirect ophthalmoscope is suitable for macula cases. Prism lenses can be used for viewing the periphery but slow down the surgery because of paradoxical movement. Indirect ophthalmoscope viewing for vitrectomy is grossly inferior to operating microscope-endoilluminator viewing.

Sewed-on contact lenses were developed to eliminate the need for an assistant but can create problems as well. Bleeding and bubbles under the lens, use of expensive viscoelastics, cost of sutures, suboptimal centering, and damage to the conjunctiva are all potential problems with sewed-on lenses.

Wide-angle viewing systems are primarily useful for peripheral dissection; internal drainage of subretinal fluid through peripheral breaks in phakic or pseudo-phakic eyes, and cyclophotocoagulation. They are available in contact and noncontact varieties. The contact lens–based systems provide a field of view that is approximately 10° wider and eliminate corneal astigmatism but require a very steady hand because of prism shift. Only recently have autoclavable, contact lens–based systems become available. Scleral depression can accomplish peripheral viewing with no cost and with the added advantages of viewing the retina in contour and relaxing traction to enable better dissection. Wide-angle viewing systems have become popular in part because of overemphasis on video production. Wide-angle viewing systems are inadequate for macular surgery, decrease contrast, and increase inadvertent lens contact. Head repositioning during surgery facilitates peripheral viewing.

Endoscope Systems

Endoscope systems are rarely needed in vitreous surgery. Theoretically, they can be of value to dissect, drain SRF, and laser peripheral retinal detachments in phakic eyes with small pupils. If capsular fibrosis limits the view, it can be dissected with the scissors to enlarge the opening, eliminating the need for an endoscope. The authors never use iris clips or sutures because of iris damage, postoperative inflammation, and cost. If the pupil is small, the periphery can be seen by careful positioning of the head and eye, scleral depression, and sphincterotomies (in aphakic eyes). Endophotocoagulation of the ciliary body can be performed using scleral depression or with endoscopic viewing. Gradient index (GRIN) rod endoscopes have 15 times more pixels than fused coherent fiber-bundle-based systems but have limited optical resolution. Combining white light illumination, laser endocoagulation, and a fluid channel can increase the utility of an endoscope. The fluid channel plugs easily if used for aspiration and is seldom, if ever, needed for infusion. The authors find little practical value for endoscopic vitreous surgery.

OPERATING ROOM SETUP

The operating table and head support must be very rigid and stable and have minimal thickness between the patient's head and the surgeon's knees. The surgeon must sit up very straight, stretching to reach the microscope in order to decrease all-too-common cervical and lumbar spine problems caused by leaning and bending forward. No perfect chair seems to have been designed for the operating room. The ideal chair would have a back and no armrests, exert no pressure on the sciatic nerves or perineum, and not allow the surgeon to slip off.

The surgeon's hands rest on the patient's face during vitrectomy and not directly on the "wrist rest." The wrist rest should be padded to prevent pain and be adjustable in height. One of the authors (SC) has built a wrist rest that attaches to the side rails of the operating table rather than being held down by the patient's body. Paired vertical rods support the wrist rather than the single central post, which can put pressure on the patient's head. The wrist rest is used primarily to create a trough in conjunction with the drape, permitting continuous aspiration of fluid runoff from the eye. The trough is a necessity to protect the foot pedals from water damage, to contain contaminated fluids, and to catch dropped instruments.

The microscope should usually be placed on the patient's right side to create a tent with the drape under which the anesthesia personnel can visualize the airway. An assistant can be located opposite either of the patient's ears. Hand instruments are best kept on a Mayo stand between the surgeon and the assistant on the left, with a back table placed behind for other surgical tools and disposables. The vitrectomy system and 532-nm diode pumped laser are stacked on a cart at the patient's left hand, with a sterile Mayo stand in front for the associated handpieces and tubing. This stand should be placed over the patient's chest with the bipolar handpiece, contact lens, contact lens suction, and infusion tubing, after the patient is prepped and draped. The Mayo stand over the patient's chest creates a tent that allows the anesthesiologist to visualize the chest wall movement, abdomen, airway, and EKG leads. This setup is used regardless of which eye is to be operated upon, thus permitting more rapid and consistent setting up. A right-handed assistant holds the contact lens from the right, regardless of the eye to be operated on, to keep the hand out of the surgeon's way. The assistant should always use the dominant hand to hold the contact lens; thus a left-handed assistant sits on the left. This approach is not practical with smaller operating rooms or certain microscope arrangements.

Placing the equipment on a rack over the patient prevents the surgeon from viewing the console display. In addition, access to the patient is limited in the case of a medical emergency or restless patient. This approach is to be avoided.

Microscope drapes are essential to prevent fibers, wires, tubing, and instruments from being contaminated. The microscope is handled by many people, is directly over the patient, and is therefore a potential source of contaminated particles on the eye.

Powder-free gloves should be used on all cases. Specific care must be taken for patients with latex allergy. Care should be taken to prevent cotton fibers, plastic particles, and cellulose material from touching the instruments. The authors almost never touch the eye with cellulose sponges or cotton-tipped applicators to avoid particulate matter being left in the eye. Masks with an integral plastic flap to prevent fogging are easier on the skin than foam rubber or adhesives. It has been reported that the incidence of facial basal cell carcinoma is elevated in surgeons who taped their mask for many years.

A single-piece drape with an integral suction connection at the lowest point of a preformed trough is the most efficient method of draping. The drape should be transparent over the airway and face for safety. The drape should be thicker than typical drapes to avoid inadvertent perforation. Head drapes and other drapes are not needed, saving time and money. No opening should be made in the drape for the eye. A cut should be made in the drape after the drape is applied with the lids open. The flaps created by this method are then folded over the lid margins and held in place by the speculum to keep cilia and lid bacteria away from the operative site. The skin must be degreased and dry or the drape will not adhere. The drape must first be applied to the superior orbital ridge, then the nasal canthus, and finally the zygoma and outer portion of the orbital ridge in order to have a complete seal. A complete seal prevents water from running into the patient's hair and ears, and more important, prevents exhaled air from reaching the eye. Exhaled air is a sterility risk and causes fogging of the contact lens. Benzoin can be used to increase drape adherence.

Prep Technique

Povidone iodine (Betadine 5%) prep should be used unless the patient has an iodine allergy. Betadine drops should be used for the cul-de-sac before and immediately after surgery. Lash trimming is no longer performed because it has been reported that it increases bacteria in the cul-de-sac, emphasizing the need to cover the lashes with the drape. The corneal epithelium should be covered with the lids or irrigated frequently with BSS to markedly reduce the need for scraping. The authors almost never need to remove the corneal epithelium.

REFERENCES

1. Abbott PJ, Sullivan G, Cardiovascular toxicity following preincisional intra-articular injection of bupivicaine (letter). *Arthroscopy* 1997;13:282.
2. Banko A. Apparatus for removing blood clots, cataracts, and other objects from the eye. United States Patent 3,732,858. Filed February 14, 1969.
3. Machemer R, Buettner H, Norton EW, et al. Vitrectomy: a pars plana approach. *Trans Am Acad Ophthalmol Otolaryngol* 1971;75:813.
4. Peyman GA, Dodick NA. Experimental vitrectomy. *Arch Ophthalmol* 1971;86:548.
5. Douvas NG. The cataract roto-extractor (a preliminary report). *Trans Am Acad Ophthalmol Otolaryngol* 1973;77:792.
6. Federman JL, Cook K, Bross R, et al. Intraocular microsurgery 1: new instrumentation (SITE). *Ophthalmic Surg* 1976;7:82.
7. O'Malley C, Heintz RM. Vitrectomy via the pars plana. *Trans Pac Coast Otoophthalmol Soc* 1972;53:121.
8. O'Malley C, Heintz RM. Vitrectomy with an alternative instrument system. *Am Ophthalmol* 1975;7:585.
9. May DR. Anterior chamber infusion with the 30-degree bent needle. *Ocutome Fragmatome Newsletter* 1979;4:4.
10. Edelhauser HF, VanHorn DL, Schultz RO, et al. Comparative toxicity of intraocular irrigating solutions on the corneal endothelium. *Am J Ophthalmol* 1976;81:473.
11. Charles S, Wang C. Linear suction control system for the vitreous cutter. *Arch Ophthalmol* 1981;99:1613.
12. Charles S, Wang C. Motorized gas injector for vitreous surgery. *Arch Ophthalmol* 1981;99:1398.
13. Parel J-M, Machemer R, Aumayr WA. New concept for vitreous surgery for automated operating microscope. *Am J Ophthalmol* 1974;77:161.
14. Charles S, McCarthy C, Eichenbaum DA. Chin operated switch for motorized three-axis microscope movement. *Am J Ophthalmol* 1975;80:150.

3

Vitrectomy Techniques and Technology
for Anterior Segment Problems

Although developed for posterior vitreoretinal surgery, the vitrectomy instrument has widespread application to anterior segment surgery (1–8). Every anterior segment microsurgeon must have vitrectomy techniques and equipment at his or her fingertips to manage vitreous loss at cataract surgery and other common problems. The anterior segment microsurgeon with extensive knowledge of corneal physiology, aqueous dynamics, intraocular lenses, cataract complications, and microsurgical techniques need not rely on a posterior segment surgeon to manage all anterior segment vitreous problems. Similarly, an anterior segment surgeon should not delve into complex vitreoretinal problems just because the technology is available. The demands are so complex that it is a very unique individual who is an expert in both arenas.

VITRECTOMY INSTRUMENT CHOICE

The large size and fluid flow characteristics of full-function probes make them as inappropriate for anterior segment surgery as they are for posterior segment surgery. Microsurgical size (20-gauge) advanced cutters, and high-performance proportional (linear) suction control are a necessity for anterior segment surgery, just as they are for vitreoretinal procedures (see Chapter 2).

INFUSION SYSTEMS FOR ANTERIOR VITRECTOMY

Infusion can be provided by the infusion sleeve (S. Charles, unpublished data; 9), which slips over the vitrectomy instrument for a one-incision technique (see Chapter 2). This method is easy to use but results in a return to the turbulent fluid flow observed with full-function probes (Fig. 3.1). Use of the infusion sleeve should be limited to vitrectomy in soft eyes with no sideport, a rare situation.

A bimanual approach (10) with a blunt 30° bent 20-gauge infusion needle as the infusion device is used if the pars plana cannot be seen, as well as for retinopathy of prematurity (ROP) (5). This technique allows the independently movable infusion to hydrate and mobilize the lens material for aspiration. By using 20-gauge infusion, ocular collapse is reduced and the infusion needle can be interchanged with a cutter to provide better access to the posterior chamber and periphery.

Unsupported butterfly needles or silicone tubing should not be used for anterior chamber infusion because they may damage the endothelium and offer no help in accessing the posterior chamber for manipulation of cortex. Sew-on corneal infusion cannulas do not permit changing the active instrument from one hand to the other, and can cause corneal damage.

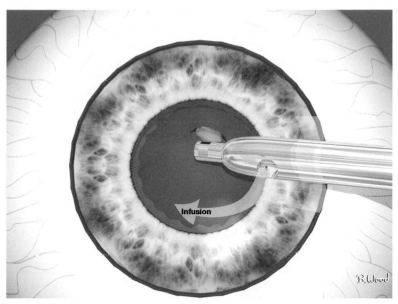

FIG. 3.1. Infusion sleeves increase infusion fluid turbulence, resulting in endothelial cell damage.

ULTRASONIC FRAGMENTATION

Aspirating ultrasonic fragmenters permit 20-gauge incisions to be used for relatively dense cataracts (11,12). Twenty-gauge aspirating fragmenters require a separate infusion cannula identical to modern vitrectomy systems. The phakoemulsifier is analogous to the full-function vitrectomy approach and similarly requires a larger incision and creates more turbulence.

Infusion Sources

Infusion can be accomplished with the same options used with the vitrectomy instrument: bimanual, with 20-gauge, 30° bent, blunt cannula, infusion sleeve, or sew-on infusion cannula.

The metal infusion sleeve, which has the potential of dampening the sonic energy, is not intended for use with the fragmenter. Bimanual infusion with the angulated, blunt cannula can be kept away from the suction port, decreasing turbulence, and may be used for selective mobilization and hydration of lens material in certain cases. Pars plana, sew-on infusion cannulas cannot be used until they can be visualized with the microscope.

The pars plana infusion cannula, with a 20-gauge ultrasonic fragmenter, is the optimal approach for pars plana lensectomy. It decreases turbulence, utilizes 20-gauge incisions, and adds to surgical flexibility.

Vacuum Sources

Syringes, peristaltic pumps, or venturi-based systems can provide suction for the vitrectomy probe or aspirating fragmenter. For the reasons discussed in Chapter 2, venturi-based vacuum systems are far superior to the other approaches because they reduce vitreoretinal traction and ocular collapse. A vitrectomy system with proportional (linear) suction control of a venturi source offers the most precise control over suction level currently available. Leaving the fragmenter lumen open to the atmosphere (incorrectly called "passive egress") is inappropriate because precision, foot control, and reflux capability are lost. The tubing can be squeezed to create reflux, if the iris or retina becomes impacted in the port. Certain vitrectomy systems (Accurus made by Alcon Surgical, Inc.) offer foot-pedal-controlled reflux.

Modern phako technique(s) utilizing high suction and limited flow rates can be used with the fragmenter, especially for harder nuclei.

Intermittent Versus Continuous Sonification and Aspiration

Bursts of intermittent sonification alternated with aspiration have been recommended for fragmenter use, but they prolong the procedure and cause unnecessary heating of the sclera (13). Aspiration without sonification is ineffective and time-consuming. Luminal fluid flow is the most effective means of dissipating frictional heat generated by the fragmenter in the wound. Squirting fluid on the needle shank externally does not cool the internal scleral wound. By combining continuous sonification with continuous aspiration, a safe and rapid lensectomy can be performed using the continual luminal fluid flow for scleral cooling.

Limbal Versus Pars Plana Approach for Anterior Vitrectomy

Elective anterior vitrectomy during routine cataract removal should be reserved only for those cases in which the anterior vitreous cortex and an opaque posterior capsule resistant to polishing are firmly adherent. Complete posterior capsulectomy from the limbal approach almost always results in anterior vitrectomy because of the approach angle and posterior displacement of the posterior capsule from the infusion system.

Although the limbal approach to anterior vitrectomy is more comfortable for the anterior segment surgeon, it creates more endothelial and iris trauma than pars plana surgery. Peripheral anterior synechiae frequently form at the limbal wounds postoperatively. The pars plana approach allows more complete removal of peripheral membranes and vitreous without iris trauma. (See the section entitled "Pupillary Membranes" later in this chapter.) If conversion to posterior vitrectomy becomes necessary, the limbal approach is inappropriate because the angulated instruments cause striate keratopathy. Most pupillary or retro–intraocular lens (IOL) membranectomies should be done through the pars plana. Translimbal bimanual lensectomy can be used for radiation cataracts in retinoblastoma patients and in some cases of severe iris–retinal adherence when pars plana entry is unsafe.

PARS PLANA LENSECTOMY

Indications

Pars plana lensectomy is not indicated for elective cataract removal. The obligatory interruption of the anterior vitreous cortex increases retinal complications (cystoid macular edema [CME] and retinal detachment) and is not in keeping with modern phako surgery techniques. The role of pars plana lensectomy is in combination with indicated pars plana vitrectomy.

Many phakic, proliferative vitreoretinopathy (PVR) and giant break cases require pars plana lensectomy even if the lens is clear (see Chapters 7 and 10). Many trauma cases require removal of the lens because of associated lens damage or ciliary body damage.

Aphakic eyes allow better visualization, better approach to the anterior vitreous cortex and peripheral vitreous, and easier fluid/gas exchange; eliminate the substrate for cyclitic membrane formation; and permit faster egress of cells, protein, fibrin, fibrinectin, hemorrhage, and cytokines. Clear lenses should not be removed in a vitrectomy performed for proliferative diabetic retinopathy (PDR) because of the increased risk of neovascular glaucoma unless there is fibrin syndrome, postoperative bleeding is highly probable, or silicone is used for large retinectomies. It is thought that the anterior vitreous cortex and the lens act as a barrier to diffusion of vascular endothelial growth factor (VEGF) to the anterior segment, causing neovascularization of the iris and trabecular meshwork. For this reason the anterior vitreous cortex should be avoided in diabetic vitrectomies in which the lens is left in place, unless it is opaque. The indications for elective clear lens and anterior vitreous cortex removal without IOL implantation in the diabetic patient will be explained in a subsequent chapter

Endocapsular Lensectomy

The development of vitrectomy and phakoemulsification has an intertwined and interesting history. Anton Banko patented the first vitrectomy cutter in 1969 in response to vitreous complications of early phakoemulsification. Banko had apparently learned of the need for a vitreous cutter because he developed the fluidics for Kelman's early phakoemulsifier. Machemer developed the trans pars plana vitrectomy procedure in 1970 and shortly thereafter performed lensectomy with the Vitreous Infusion suction cutter (VISC). It was soon discovered that the vitreous cutter would not handle significant nuclear sclerosis. Girard developed the fragmenter with Sparta in 1972 as a phakoemulsifier alternative without the coaxial infusion sleeve. The principal author (SC) was the first advocate of trans pars plana lensectomy using the Girard fragmenter with aspiration. Girard advocated vitrectomy with his unit and later recommended using the fragmenter for routine cataract surgery. The author believes that ultrasonic vitrectomy and pars plana lensectomy for routine cataract surgery are unsafe. Shock adapted a dental unit to cataract surgery just as Kelman had at an earlier date, but like Girard could not use a coaxial infusion sleeve, which had been patented by Kelman. The Shock technique required a large, intentionally leaky wound and was used with infusion through the fragmenter needle rather than suction. Machemer used the Shock system with a large, leaky pars plana incision when nuclear sclerosis was too great for the VISC.

Conventional Fragmenter Techniques

Current practice for trans pars plana lensectomy with the fragmenter begins with placement of the infusion cannula. The cannula is then inspected with the microscope to ascertain that it has penetrated the choroid and nonpigmented ciliary epithelium. It is very dangerous to inspect the cannula with the unaided eye, even using the endoilluminator.

The next step in conventional lensectomy is to incise the equatorial lens capsule with the microvitreoretinal (MVR) blade. The principal author (SC) used the fragmenter to incise the lens capsule before endocapsular lensectomy was developed. The fragmenter method was initiated to avoid the stress that capsular incision with the MVR blade creates on the zonules. Many surgeons advocate penetration of the nucleus with the MVR blade. This step is unnecessary if the nucleus is soft, and it creates excessive stress on the zonules if the nucleus is hard.

After incising the lens capsule, the fragmenter is used in what phako surgeons would call a sculpting mode to remove lens material. The author has advocated sculpting in a plane parallel to the iris, starting on the temporal side adjacent to the entry site. An initial thick sheet of cortex and nucleus is removed while being careful to avoid the cortex near the anterior and posterior lens capsules. The posterior capsule is much weaker than the anterior capsule and is usually not intact by the time the posterior cortex has been removed.

Many surgeons recommend alternating aspiration and sonification. Unlike the phakoemulsifier, the fragmenter has no infusion sleeve and must rely on fluid flow through the lumen for cooling. The needle has approximately 0.003 in. of longitudinal movement and generates significant frictional heat. In contrast, the author has always recommended continuous and simultaneous sonification and aspiration. The constant fluid flow cools the needle and therefore the sclera. If white, particulate matter ("lens milk") appears at the needle, the surgeon must release the foot pedal immediately to avoid scleral burns. If the needle becomes clogged, it should be back-flushed with a syringe filled with Balance salt solution (BSS), with the ultrasound activated after double-checking to determine that the needle is outside the eye. Aspiration of saline from a cup is never effective, nor is it necessary to clean the needle with a stylet or replace the needle if it becomes plugged.

Infusion Options

Many surgeons recommend placing a separate infusion into the lens rather than using the pars plana infusion cannula. If the lens is soft, infusion directly into the lens is not necessary. If the lens is hard, infusion into the lens will not reach the temporal side where the sculpting must begin. Infusion into the lens tends to force lens material through ever-present defects in the posterior capsule. For this reason, the authors use only the pars plana infusion cannula for lensectomy cases except during hydrodissection.

Lens Capsule Removal

Most surgeons use the vitreous cutter to remove the capsule. The principal author has recommended end-opening forceps to remove the capsule since the late 1970s. The author has used the diamond-coated forceps developed with Grieshaber since they became available in the late 1980s. Zonulorhexis is performed in a circular motion identical to capsulorhexis (Fig. 3.2). Care must be taken to avoid engaging the vitreous so as to prevent undue force on the retina. Using the vitreous cutter to remove the lens capsule frequently damages the iris, causes miosis, prolongs operating time, is a possible cause of bleeding, and leaves residual lens material.

Fragmenter Performance

Fibrasonics made all the original fragmenter handpieces sold by Berkley Bioengineering, Coopervision, Sparta, Fibrasonics, MidLabs, Storz, and Alcon. These fragmenters were useful but had less power than the phakoemulsifier and hence more difficulty with dense nuclear sclerosis. Alcon introduced a Four Crystal Fragmenter (Fig. 3.3) in the early 1990s that uses the same ultrasonics as the Legacy phakoemulsifier. The Alcon Accurus fragmenter will handle dense nuclear sclerosis just as well as the phakoemulsifier.

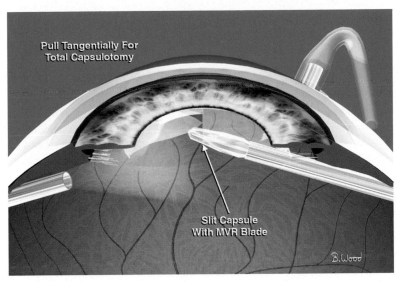

FIG. 3.2. Zonulorhexis is performed in a circular fashion with the diamond-coated end-opening forceps.

Phakoemulsification with Pars Plana Vitrectomy

Many surgeons now recommend using a phakoemulsifier to remove visually significant cataracts through a conventional cataract incision before initiating vitreous surgery. If this is done as a separate operation, it adds risk and cost. If a cataract surgeon is brought in to operate with the vitreous surgeon, it adds cost and operating time. Phako at the time of vitrectomy frequently causes miosis, retained viscoelastics in the anterior chamber, and usually slight corneal haze, some striate keratopathy, and pigment in the anterior chamber. Viscoelastics are contraindicated if silicone is to be used because they decrease the interfacial tension, which increases emulsification of the oil. If iris clips or sutures are used because of miosis created by transpupillary phako, there

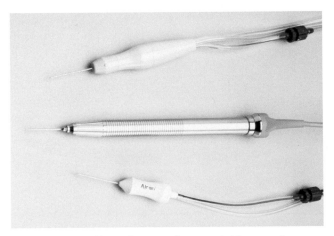

FIG. 3.3. Alcon Accurus four-crystal fragmenter.

will be more postoperative inflammation, increased operating time, and greater cost. The authors never use iris clips or sutures.

Anterior Lens Capsule Retention and Lens Implantation in the Sulcus

The late Ron Michels was long an advocate of preserving the anterior lens capsule until the end of the vitrectomy to reduce damage to the endothelium and trabecular meshwork induced by erythrocytes, infusion fluid, and turbulence. Kokame and Blankenship reported retention of the anterior lens capsule to permit implantation of posterior chamber lens in the ciliary sulcus at the end of the vitrectomy. They recommended performing an anterior capsulotomy after lens implantation. Some phako surgeons have been critical of this procedure because endocapsular implantation has better results than ciliary sulcus placement in elective cataract surgery. The authors have had very good results with this method with no cases of decentration. Capsular fibrosis occurs rapidly if the capsule is in contact with silicone oil. The authors have found that polishing the capsule increases the chance of preserving a clear capsule. The authors have recently started using the Acrysoft foldable acrylic lens from Alcon through a 3.2-mm keratome, clear corneal incision with implantation in the sulcus, anterior to the retained anterior capsule after the vitrectomy. One should avoid the use of silicone lenses, as they absorb silicone oil and have marked condensation problems (Fig. 3.4) during fluid/air (gas) exchange.

Endocapsular Lensectomy Method

Conventional lensectomy, as described earlier, has many of the attributes of endocapsular phako except that it starts with a risky, equatorial capsular incision. This equatorial defect frequently leads to capsular tears that extend into the anterior capsule. Extension of

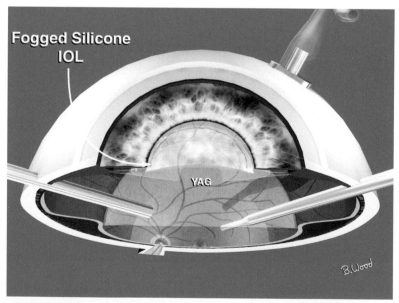

FIG. 3.4. Silicone IOLs may exhibit marked condensation problems during fluid/air exchange, resulting in reduced visibility.

capsular tears was a frequent problem in phako surgery until the continuous capsulorhexis was developed. Cataract surgery has seen a progression from intracapsular to extracapsular surgery, and ultimately, phakoemulsification. Phako has evolved from anterior chamber phako, to iris plane phako, to endocapsular surgery. Continuous capsulorhexis has dramatically reduced problems with capsular tears for the cataract surgeon.

Endocapsular Lensectomy Surgical Sequence

The principal author (SC) has been using posterior capsulorhexis, cortical cleaving hydrodissection, and sculpting since 1994, and has found these techniques of great value in lensectomy. He calls this approach *endocapsular lensectomy.*

Endocapsular lensectomy begins with conventional placement and inspection of the infusion cannula. All sclerotomies are made with the MVR blade, 3.0-mm posterior to the limbus, unless pars plana pathology demands a more anterior location. The second sclerotomy is made superonasally for the endoilluminator. The endoilluminator is essential to stabilize the eye and provide a controllable red reflex. The endoilluminator can be touched to the lens capsule in various locations to aid in visualization without the light toxicity associated with retina-reflective red reflex methods. The third sclerotomy is made superotemporally for the capsulorhexis, hydrodissection, sculpting, and cortex-aspiration tools. A capsulorhexis is made with vitreous cutter (Fig. 3.5) after a limited anterior vitrectomy. The vitrectomy is performed to prevent vitreoretinal traction from the fragmenter. Cortical cleaving hydrodissection is the next step. A blunt, 27-gauge cannula attached with a short length of tubing to a 5-mL syringe operated by the assistant is used for this step (Fig. 3.6). Sculpting is then initiated at the temporal margin of the nucleus to avoid damaging the capsule with the fragmenter. The Alcon, 20-gauge, four-crystal fragmenter is used to sculpt the nucleus, epinucleus, and finally the cortex (Fig. 3.7). This fragmenter has the same ultrasonics as the Legacy. The anterior cortex is avoided to prevent damaging the anterior cap-

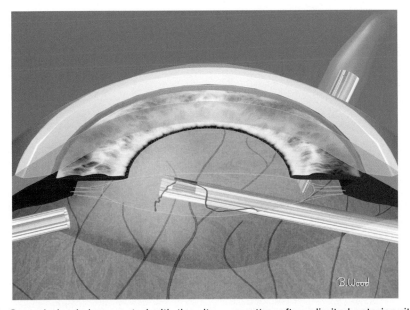

FIG. 3.5. Capsulorhexis is executed with the vitreous cutter, after a limited anterior vitrectomy.

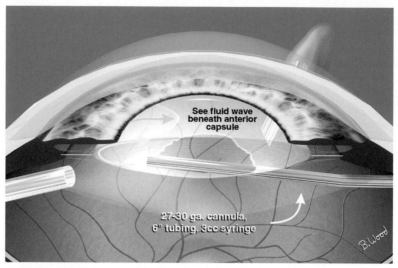

FIG. 3.6. Cortical cleaving hydrodissection is performed with a blunt, 27-gauge cannula attached to a 3- to 5-mL syringe via a short length of tubing.

sule. The vitreous cutter is used for aspirating the remaining cortex. The vitreous cutter is better than classic Irrigation/Aspiration (I/A) tools because of the cutting capability, which acts like chopping. The anterior capsule is polished after aspirating the cortex (Fig. 3.8). Almost any posterior chamber lens could theoretically be utilized, but foldable IOLs offer the advantage of a smaller incision. The acrylic (Alcon Acrysoft) lens is currently being utilized. Scleral tunnel or clear cornea incisions can be used (Fig. 3.9). Silicone lenses, as previously stated, should not be used because they have severe condensation problems during fluid/air exchange and they adsorb silicone oil.

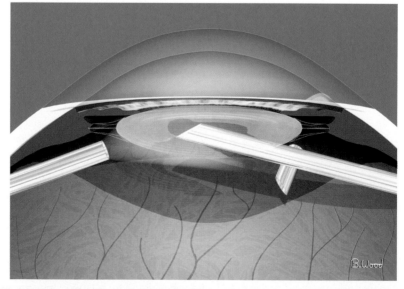

FIG. 3.7. The nucleus, epinucleus, and cortex are sculpted with the fragmenter.

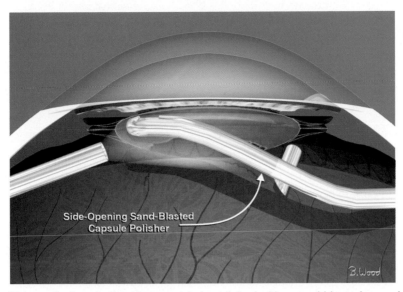

FIG. 3.8. After cortical aspiration, the capsule is polished with a sand-blasted capsule polisher or the vitreous cutter.

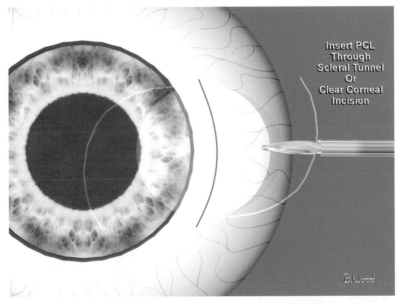

FIG. 3.9. A foldable acrylic IOL is inserted through either a scleral tunnel or a clear corneal incision.

Pars Plana Capsulotomy After Lensectomy

Capsulotomy is used if the intent is complete capsule removal. An MVR blade is placed through the sclerotomy and used to incise the anterior and posterior capsules centrally to create an "edge." The fragmenter almost always ruptures the posterior capsule, eliminating the need for posterior capsulotomy. The forceps used for total capsule removal requires an "edge."

Pars Plana Capsulectomy After Lensectomy

Diamond-coated, end-opening forceps should be used to remove the anterior and posterior capsules after capsulotomy. Iris contact should be avoided. A circular, zonulorhexis approach is better than pulling across the eye because it reduces traction on the peripheral retina.

Avoidance of Vitreous in the Fragmenter

The fragmenter emulsifies formed vitreous gel but does not emulsify collagen fibers, giving a false impression of vitrectomy. The vitreous fibers remain intact, and suction applied with the fragmenter creates dangerous vitreoretinal traction. When vitreous enters the fragmenter, the vitrectomy probe, not the fragmenter, should be used to remove the vitreous. The fragmenter should never be used for emergency or elective vitrectomy.

Subluxated Lenses During Vitrectomy

Subluxated lenses are best managed by completing the vitrectomy through the pars plana before approaching the lens. Posterior dislocation is frequently seen and presents no problem with the pars plana approach. After the vitreous surrounding the lens is removed, the 20-gauge aspirating ultrasonic fragmenter can safely be used to complete the lensectomy, as described earlier (Fig. 3.10). Rhexis and hydrodissection are very difficult if the lens is subluxated or dislocated and may be omitted.

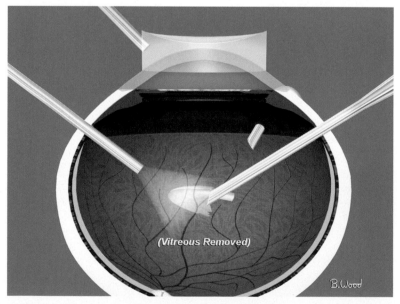

FIG. 3.10. Subluxated lens material can be safely removed with the 20-gauge fragmenter after the vitreous has been removed.

Posterior Dislocation of Lens Material During Cataract Surgery

Surgical Psychodynamics

Cataract surgery has been one of the most frequently performed surgical procedures worldwide for more than a century. While inexperience is known to cause a higher complication rate, high surgical volumes and phenomenal success rates can also cause surgeons to become complacent and make judgment errors when complications do occur. Busy schedules, observers, and video may contribute to faulty decision making when the capsule ruptures and lens material and the vitreous exchange locations. High success rates, outpatient surgery, no stitch, no patch, emmetropia, and topical anesthesia elevate patient expectations unrealistically, which can place more pressure on the surgeon.

Early Recognition and Management of Defects in the Lens Capsule

Modern optical systems enhance the red-reflex, allowing early recognition of capsular defects. The surgeon must admit that the defect has occurred rather than rationalize because of the psychologic factors described earlier. When a capsular defect is recognized, the first action should be to construct a barrier between the posterior capsule and the anterior vitreous cortex. Colvard has proposed a plastic barrier that can be deployed in this space, but none are available at this time. High-viscosity, cohesive viscoelastics injected into the defect can serve as a temporary barrier, enabling removal of remaining lens material (Fig. 3.11). If the lens implant can be placed over the defect and posterior to the lens material, it can function as a barrier. Many surgeons focus exclusively on prevention or management of posterior dislocation of lens material rather than on the more serious matter of reducing vitreoretinal traction and subsequent retinal detachment. Any maneuver designed to prevent posterior dislocation that increases vitreoretinal traction should not be employed. Kelman has described the use of a needle inserted through the pars plana to prevent lens material from falling posteriorly. This method ignores the pressure that must be placed on the eye to place the needle and the anterior movement of the vitreous that occurs without a barrier. The next section discusses management of vitreous that prolapses through the capsular de-

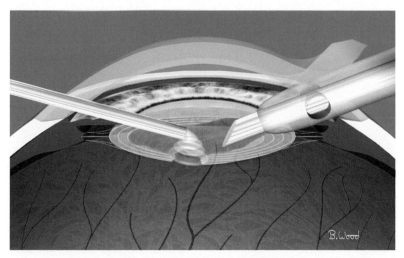

FIG. 3.11. Injection of viscoelastic into the capsular defect serves as a barrier to the anterior vitreous cortex, allowing safe completion of phakoemulsification.

fect. This discussion intentionally precedes the discussion of the management of dislocated lens material because retinal detachment prevention is the most important issue.

Vitreous Loss

As previously stated, use of the phakoemulsifier to remove vitreous is a dangerous step that should never be undertaken. Phaco probes liquefy hyaluronic acid but do not cut collagen fibers. A large-bore needle to aspirate "liquid" vitreous should not be used because of the obligate vitreoretinal traction. The theoretical "pockets" of liquid vitreous are more difficult to locate than the fountain of youth.

Cellulose sponge vitrectomy as developed by Kasner has been an obsolete and dangerous method for two decades in spite of the important role it played before machine vitrectomy. A cellulose sponge causes significant traction on the retina as the sponge is lifted to transect the adherent vitreous (Fig. 3.12). Removal of all vitreous by a vitreous cutter causes virtually no inflammation, whereas marked inflammation is the rule after sponge vitrectomy. Mechanical damage to the iris caused by contact with the sponge as it swells and is lifted appears to be the cause of this inflammation. The principal author has also observed cellulose material on the anterior vitreous cortex after sponge vitrectomy has been performed. One can speculate that this retained material causes inflammation in addition to that caused by iris trauma. Testing for vitreous can be accomplished by injecting air into the anterior chamber via the sideport incision and looking for fragmentation of the bubble. Alternatively, a single drop of sterile fluoroscein from a newly opened ampule can be used to stain the vitreous.

Vitrectomy with a high-quality vitreous cutter is the preferred method of managing vitreous that presents in the anterior chamber. Alcon builds high-quality cutters for use with their phako systems such as the Legacy. These cutters should be operated at the highest possible cutting rate and very low vacuum/flow (Fig. 3.13). Posterior vitreous surgeons use vacuum control in addition to flow control to reduce vitreoretinal traction. The anterior

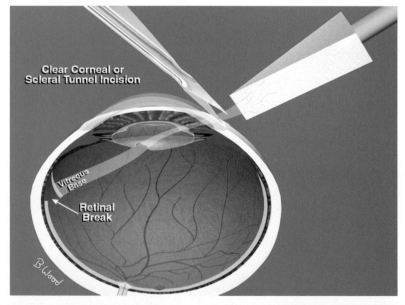

FIG. 3.12. Cellulose sponge vitrectomy engenders dangerous retinal traction as the sponge is lifted to transect the adherent vitreous.

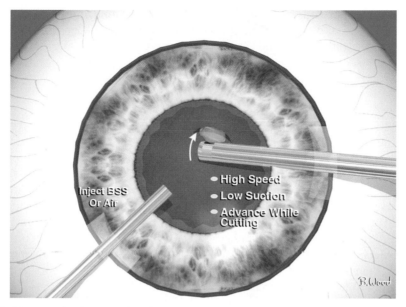

FIG. 3.13. Vitreous in the anterior chamber should be removed with a high-quality vitreous cutter operated at the maximum cutting rate and low vacuum/flow.

segment machines frequently utilize peristaltic pumps, which do not directly control the vacuum. The best procedure is to use a very low flow rate and vacuum settings to reduce traction on the retina. The cutter should be advanced or held stationary during vitrectomy, never retracted. Pulling the cutter back while vacuum is applied dramatically increases vitreoretinal traction (Fig. 3.14). Sideport infusion is preferable to "dry" vitrectomy because it prevents hypotony and therefore reduces the chance of choroidal hemorrhage. Air

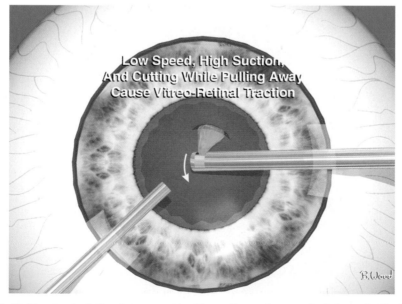

FIG. 3.14. Pulling back during low-speed cutting with suction applied dramatically increases vitreoretinal traction.

can be used instead of infusion fluid to keep the vitreous from hydrating and coming forward. The air helps to delineate the surface of the vitreous and keep it confined by surface tension. Sweeping the wound for vitreous is dangerous because of the vitreoretinal traction it causes.

Dislocated Lens Material

Phakoemulsifiers, lens loops, and irrigation should *never* be utilized to try to extract lens material from the vitreous cavity. If lens material falls posteriorly, there is a natural tendency for the surgeon to chase it with the phako probe. The phaco probe gives the appearance of vitreous emulsification but does not sever the collagen fibers (Fig. 3.15). The surgeon must consciously stop, relax, and plan before performing any further maneuvers. The best plan is usually to let the material fall posteriorly and focus on vitreous cleanup and intraocular lens implantation. Lens loops can put significant traction on the retina and cause retinal breaks and detachments (Fig. 3.16). Foulds and subsequently Machemer used a saline stream directed at the retina to create experimental retinal detachments. There is significant risk of retinal breaks if saline irrigation is used in an attempt to move the lens material anteriorly (Fig. 3.17).

If the pupil is large, the cornea clear, and the surgeon and available staff are optimum for posterior vitrectomy, immediate intervention may be undertaken. In most instances, it is preferable to perform posterior vitrectomy and removal of lens material at a second procedure. This procedure should be performed when the cornea is clear, the wound is sealed, and the pupil is well dilated. The timing can be from several days to weeks later. If there is a moderate amount of cortex, no inflammation, no glaucoma, and no lens-corneal touch, a vitrectomy may not be necessary.

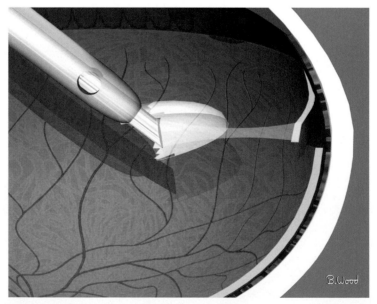

FIG. 3.15. Phakoemulsifiers do not sever collagen fibers, resulting in vitreous traction if the lens is chased.

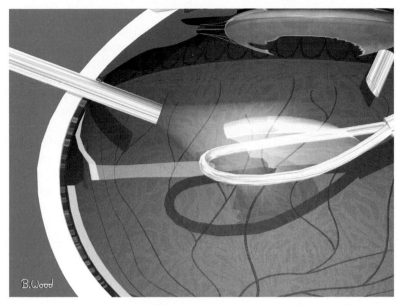

FIG. 3.16. Lens loops can cause significant vitreous traction and retinal detachments if used in the vitreous.

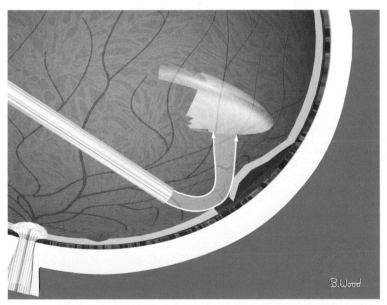

FIG. 3.17. Saline irrigation streams of sufficient force to move lens material anteriorly can also cause retinal breaks.

Posterior vitrectomy requires a surgeon specifically trained in posterior vitrectomy techniques and a sophisticated vitrectomy system. A sew-on infusion cannula placed through the pars plana is essential. An assistant-supported, fundus contact lens (Machemer) is easier and faster to use than a sutured-on contact lens. Wide-angle visualization systems increase cost, complexity, and the learning curve, although they provide an excellent view. A fiberoptic endoilluminator is essential for all cases. Light reflexes from the cornea prevent the surgeon from having an optimal view if coaxial illumination is used. Iris retractors increase inflammation and cost, and may cause a distorted pupil after surgery. Some surgeons have advocated indirect ophthalmoscopic visualization, but an inverted view and the need to support the lens with one hand make this approach dangerous.

All vitreous should be removed before removing any dislocated lens material. Many surgeons have the misconception that lens material can damage the retina if it falls posteriorly. Inappropriate techniques, not the lens, damage the retina. It is dangerous and unnecessary to leave a layer of vitreous under the lens material until it is removed. Some cortex may be removed with the vitreous cutter, but nuclear material requires the phakofragmenter. Fragmenters are 20-gauge-like vitreous cutters that eliminate the need for the larger wounds required for phakoemulsifier probes. The Alcon four-crystal fragmenter utilizes the same drive electronics and piezo driver as the Legacy phako probe and, similarly, is able to handle most nuclear sclerosis cases.

After removal of the vitreous, the fragmenter is introduced and moved to the surface of the lens material. Linear (proportional) suction is increased gradually until the lens material is picked up. The lens material is then moved away from the retina and the foot pedal is used to activate sonification in mid-vitreous. Proportional fragmentation power is used to adjust the power until sufficient sculpting occurs without bouncing of the lens material. If the fragmenter drills into the lens, the endoilluminator is used to push the lens material off the tip. Alternatively, the endoilluminator can be used to crush or "chop" the fragment that is speared on the fragmenter tip. This process is continued until all lens fragments are removed.

Perfluorocarbon (PFC) liquids (Chang) were introduced to vitreoretinal surgery for unfolding giant breaks, draining subretinal fluid, and stabilizing the retina during dissection of epiretinal membranes. PFC liquids can also be used to float the lens material away from the retina allowing aspiration-fragmentation or phakoemulsification to be performed anteriorly (Fig. 3.18). This method increases cost and may require a subsequent procedure to remove residual PFC liquids. The PFC liquid method is safe but unnecessary unless there is extremely dense nuclear sclerosis that should not have been managed with phako in the first place. It may be useful for surgeons with limited posterior vitrectomy experience.

Hard Dislocated Lens Material

Hard dislocated nuclei can usually be crushed between the endoilluminator and the aspirating 20-gauge ultrasonic fragmenter (14). After the pieces are made smaller, they can be removed with the fragmenter. If the fragmenter becomes plugged, it can be removed from the eye and back-flushed with sonification as often as required.

If the bimanual crush technique is not effective because of a dense, black nucleus, internal simultaneous fluid/gas exchange can be performed if PFC liquids are not available. The endoilluminator should then be removed and the sclerotomy plugged with a scleral plug. The surgeon's other hand can then make a razor blade/scissors limbal incision of 90° to 110° to remove the nucleus. The iris will prolapse unless the infusion is turned off after the section is made. An assistant can elevate the cornea and the lens removed with

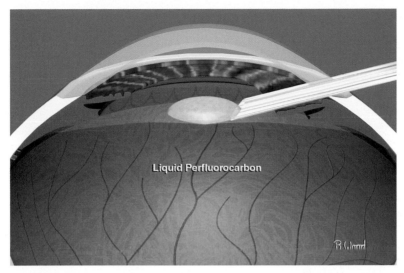

FIG. 3.18. PFC liquids can be utilized to float lens material anteriorly for removal away from the retinal surface.

a 1-mm cryoprobe without touching the endothelium or iris. PFC liquids can be used to eliminate the need for a cryoprobe. The wound is then closed with a running shoelace or X-type 8-0 or 9-0 monofilament nylon sutures.

Intraocular Lens Implantation

Some retinal surgeons are opposed to lens implantation in cases of posterior dislocation of lens material. The authors recommend lens implantation if certain conditions are met. If the capsule can support an IOL, it can be placed in the bag with the haptics rotated away from the capsular defect. If the posterior capsule will not support an IOL, the IOL can be implanted in the ciliary sulcus anterior to the anterior lens capsule.

If the capsule is not sufficient to support the IOL, an anterior chamber lens can be used. Anterior chamber lenses are contraindicated if there is a low endothelial cell count, open-angle glaucoma, or uveitis. Judgment is required to set the level of cell counts and severity of glaucoma that represent contraindications.

If there is insufficient capsular support for a posterior chamber lens *and* low corneal endothelial cell counts or significant glaucoma prevent use of an anterior chamber lens, a sutured lens can be used. This technique requires practice and can result in significant intra- and postoperative complications, including suprachoroidal hemorrhage.

CONGENITAL AND PEDIATRIC CATARACTS

Pars plana lensectomy is suitable for cataracts occurring in infants and young children. Extracapsular cataract extraction technique in this age group uniformly results in capsular clouding requiring discission or YAG capsulotomy (15–18). Limbal anterior vitrectomy (16) reduces late vitreoretinal traction and detachment. A pars plana approach has less corneal problems and permits removal of all peripheral cortex and capsule. The principal author has operated on many pediatric cataracts since 1975 and has never had a postoperative retinal detachment. The conventional I/A approach results in a fibrous ring often including iris, neocortex, ciliary body, pars plana, and peripheral vitreoretinal traction. This configuration can lead to retinal detachment with even minor trauma. Phako and IOL implantation often with primary posterior capsulorhexis and anterior vitrectomy can be used in children, if there is a normal-sized eye and no glaucoma or vitreoretinal problems (19–22).

TRAUMATIC CATARACTS

Most traumatic cataracts either are subluxated or have had interruption of the anterior vitreous cortex. Vitrectomy instruments should be used to remove all vitreous and soft lens material using pars plana techniques. A 20-gauge, 30° angulated cannula or sew-on infusion cannula should be used for infusion. After vitrectomy, the fragmenter can be utilized if denser lens material is present.

PUPILLARY MEMBRANES

Multiple tissues contribute to the formation of pupillary membranes. There is a wide range in density from an opaque hyaloid to extremely dense calcified membranes. These membranes may be postsurgical or posttraumatic, or they may occur spontaneously. A range of approaches to these problems, depending on density, is required (23). Neodymium YAG laser capsulectomy can be utilized for thin or moderately dense pupillary membranes. The extravagant term *anterior segment reconstruction* is inappropriate. As discussed earlier, the pars plana approach is preferable to the limbal approach in managing most pupillary membranes.

Membranotomy (Discission)

Simple membranotomy (discission) or neodymium YAG laser techniques will suffice for a thin membrane such as lens capsule. The MVR blade can be utilized translimbally or through the pars plana for the task. If membranectomy is required, pars plana membranotomy serves as the initial stage to provide an edge on which the vitrectomy instrument can imbricate and cut. Double-edged blades with round shanks (MVR) or Sutherland scissors are advantageous because the wound is predictable in location and size.

Membranectomy

After an edge is made with the MVR blade, the vitrectomy instrument can be used to remove a moderately dense lens, iris, or fibrous material. The infusion cannula should be placed only if the pars plana is visible through the membrane to verify infusion at the correct location. The best approach if the infusion site cannot be visualized is bimanual, using a 20-gauge, 30° angulated, blunt infusion cannula, through the superonasal pars plana.

Dense Membranectomy

If the vitrectomy cutter using moderate suction levels cannot cut a dense membrane, scissors should be utilized. The membrane is cut into many small triangular pieces that can be removed with the vitrectomy instrument, using the bimanual 20-gauge angulated needle for infusion. Bipolar bimanual diathermy (see Chapter 4) can be used to control bleeding from these membranes. Care should be taken to avoid excessive tissue removal;

a 4- to 5-mm opening is usually sufficient if the iris is incorporated into the membrane. Off-center opening can be used to avoid areas of corneal astigmatism or opacity. All tissue adherent to the ciliary body can be removed to reduce hypotony and phthisis.

While an 8-mm opening resembles a dilated pupil, it causes glare, discomfort, reduced vision, and cosmetic problems postoperatively. Occasionally, a calcified membrane will be resectable outside the calcified zone or crushable with a posterior lip sclerectomy punch. Limited anterior vitrectomy should then follow to prevent subsequent pupillary block or corneal touch.

ANTERIOR VITRECTOMY

Anterior vitrectomy is useful for a wide variety of anterior segment problems: aphakic pupillary block, vitreous touch, CME with vitreous to the wound, vitreous loss at cataract surgery, aphakic keratoplasty, secondary IOL implantation, and aphakic trabeculectomy. Each of these will be discussed individually, but the methodology is similar and will be discussed later.

Translimbal Anterior Vitrectomy

The simplest and most frequent form of anterior vitrectomy is that required for vitreous loss at cataract surgery or aphakic keratoplasty. The vitrectomy probe is placed in the central anterior vitreous space and used with minimal movement. The iris, endothelium, and especially the peripheral vitreous are avoided. Slight increased suction is required, compared with closed vitrectomy, because there is no infusion to contribute to transorifice pressure. Care should be taken to avoid air into the cutter port, as it increases vacuum requirements and thereby decreases safety. A rapid cutting rate is to be used to avoid pulsatile traction and increase safe removal rates. The approach in penetrating keratoplasty is similar, but more extensive vitrectomy is usually required to prevent postoperative corneal vitreous touch. Closure on an air bubble is usually best to avoid residual strands to the wound.

Infusion Sources for Closed Anterior Vitrectomy

Unless prior removal of hyphema, cataract, or pupillary membranes dictates use of the bimanual, angulated cannula approach, the sew-on infusion cannula is the best method for elective anterior vitrectomy. If more extensive vitrectomy is required, the sew-on infusion cannula should be placed after the initial bimanual infusion technique and removal of anterior opacities have been used to view the pars plana.

Vitreocorneal Touch

Anterior vitrectomy can cause complete clearing of corneal edema due to vitreous contact, if rigid case selection is utilized (24). It is essential to obtain a history showing that the cornea was once clear after lens removal, subluxation, or dislocation (25), and that endothelial cell counts are reasonable. In this way, surgery for corneal edema primarily due to endothelial trauma, which will not respond to subsequent vitrectomy, can be avoided. Long-term touch with retrocorneal membrane formation is equally unresponsive to anterior vitrectomy. The pars plana approach reduces further endothelial trauma, in contrast to a limbal approach. Vitrectomies should be completed behind the iris and using the sew-on infusion cannula to minimize anterior chamber turbulence and reduce endothelial damage.

Aphakic Pupillary Block

While simple slashing of the anterior vitreous cortex or YAG laser vitreolysis will suffice in some cases of pupillary block, more frequently an anterior vitrectomy is required (26). The pars plana approach decreases iris and endothelial damage in these shallow-chamber cases.

Ciliary Block Glaucoma

Trans–pars plana lensectomy (TPPL) and vitrectomy (TPPV) will alleviate ciliary block (malignant, aqueous misdirection) glaucoma in every case. It is not known whether vitrectomy without lens removal is sufficient.

Aphakic Trabeculectomy

Most aphakic filtering procedures fail because of closure of the filtration site by episcleral tissue proliferation. Occasionally, vitreous can plug a filtration site internally. On occasion, this can be recognized at the time of aphakic trabeculectomy and managed with the vitrectomy instrument. The sleeve is quite useful in these cases because the incision is already large and the eye too soft to place the infusion cannula or make a second incision. Vitrectomy plays a role in the management of other glaucoma problems such as phakolytic glaucoma, as discussed elsewhere.

Vitreous Loss at Cataract Surgery

If vitreous presents in the anterior chamber during cataract surgery, the vitrectomy instrument can be used with sideport air infusion for anterior vitrectomy. So-called dry vitrectomy is not advised because of unavoidable hypotony and risk of suprachoroidal hemorrhage. Hypotony also causes striate keratopathy and miosis. Air can be used instead of BSS to eliminate hydration of the vitreous as well as to prevent vitreous to the wound. If a sideport is present, infusion should be used through this site to reduce turbulence. If "one-handed" technique was used without a sideport, a sleeve (Charles) can be slipped over the vitreous cutter for infusion, although sideport infusion is preferable.

Cystoid Macular Edema

There is no need to perform anterior vitrectomy if vitreous is in the cataract wound and there is no CME. If CME is present without vitreous in the wound, vitrectomy is highly unlikely to improve the edema (27,28). Leakage of the perifoveal capillary bed persists after vitrectomy, and the visual improvement is usually modest. It is probable that the visual improvement results primarily from clearing the media. It appears that vitrectomy can rarely cause CME, and an occasional successful case will develop recurrent CME in spite of having the vitreous removed. Because of the modest differences between vitrectomized and nonvitrectomized eyes in the national collaborative study (29), confusion about its pathogenesis, and risk of aphakic retinal detachment and endothelial damage, caution must be applied in the utilization of vitrectomy for CME (30–32).

Some physicians have suggested that the positive steroid response test is an indication for anterior vitrectomy. Conversely, subconjunctival or topical steroids and topical or systemic NSAIDs should be used instead of surgery if they are shown to be effective.

If surgery is undertaken, the infusion cannula can be used superotemporally and the vitrectomy instrument, inferotemporally. In this way, the fibers from iris border to cataract wound can be removed without dangerous sweeping techniques. All vitreous adherence to the iris should be eliminated because this may play a role in inflammation and CME. Low suction force should be used to reduce postoperative aphakic retinal detachment. Vitreous scissors can be used to sever iris-to-wound vitreous fibers. Subconjunctival steroids are essential at the end of surgery unless the patient is a steroid glaucoma responder. Retrobulbar steroids injected with a flexible cannula at the end of the case maximize the dose to the posterior segment while reducing the risk of steroid glaucoma compared with subconjunctival or peribulbar steroids.

Aphakic Keratoplasty

Successful aphakic keratoplasty can be threatened by vitreous touch, pupillary block, and iris touch to the host/donor interface. Anterior, open-sky vitrectomy can be used without infusion in these cases. Care should be taken to avoid pulling the probe back during cutting to avoid vitreoretinal traction and air ingestion. Chamber deepening by pressing on the mid-iris with a small iris spatula through the pars plana wound can deepen the chamber without placing an instrument in the angle.

PHAKOLYTIC GLAUCOMA

Macrophages laden with ingested lens material clogging the trabecular meshwork are best managed with vitrectomy. Gentle suction with a small, blunt cannula near the trabecular meshwork can enhance the removal process. Careful irrigation of the angle can be utilized as well. Frequently, cortex is entrapped in the peripheral cortical vitreous, usually inferiorly. Care should be taken to remove this material without vitreoretinal traction.

UVEITIS

Cataracts secondary to uveitis are usually best removed by a trans–pars plana lensectomy and vitrectomy approach. Vitrectomy without lens removal for uveitis usually results in deposition of inflammation on the posterior lens capsule and little, if any, improvement in cystoid macular edema (CME) and therefore should be avoided. Cataract surgery without vitrectomy may result in pupillary or cyclitic membranes and pupillary block. It is not necessary to "quiet" eyes with steroids before vitrectomy and lensectomy. Vitrectomy and lensectomy reduces, rather than increases, inflammation and the risk of phthisis.

Iris contact should be avoided to reduce inflammation. Scleral depression can be used to remove all peripheral lens material without iridectomy. Because of the well-known medical risk factors, the authors *never* use systemic steroids.

The authors strongly urge surgeons to avoid phacoemulsification in moderate to severe uveitis cases. Capsule retention and the IOL result in a two-compartment eye with increased retention of prostaglandins, complement, cells, and other components of the inflammatory process in the vitreous cavity, thereby increasing CME.

The lens capsule should be removed after lensectomy using diamond-coated, end-opening forceps to reduce lens-related inflammation and prevent retro-iris membranes, which increase hypotony, phthisis, and vitreoretinal traction.

Retrobulbar steroids injected with a flexible cannula at the end of the case maximize the dose to the posterior segment while reducing the risk of steroid glaucoma compared with subconjunctival or peribulbar steroids.

INTRAOCULAR LENSES

Many IOL problems can be managed effectively with a vitrectomy. At times, a normal-functioning IOL must be removed in the context of posterior vitreoretinal surgery. It is essential that the implant surgeon be familiar with the vitrectomy-based management of postoperative problems.

Retrolental Intraocular Lens Membranes

The YAG laser can manage most posterior capsula opacification. Trans–pars plana or limbal membranotomy (discission) is infrequently indicated. Denser membranes require trans–pars plana membranectomy with the vitrectomy instrument. Although the infusion sleeve can be utilized, it increases probe diameter and reduces access to the membrane. The 20-gauge, 30° angulated, blunt infusion cannula should be used if the pars plana cannot be visualized, but the sew-on infusion cannula is preferred if visibility permits. Membranotomy with the scissors or MVR blade must precede membranectomy to provide an edge. Occasionally, dense membranes will require scissors to radially segment and circumferentially dissect the membrane away from the ciliary body and iris.

Dislocated Intraocular Lens Repositioning

Posterior chamber lens implants occasionally dislocate into the vitreous cavity. On rare occasion, positioning and miotics can return the implant to proper position without surgery. If this approach is unsuccessful, vitrectomy is required.

Complete vitrectomy with the infusion cannula, vitrectomy probe, contact lens (wide-angle system), and endoilluminator should precede IOL repositioning to avoid vitreoretinal traction (Fig. 3.19). Twenty-gauge forceps (33) should be used to grasp the IOL optic, with the endoilluminator providing illumination and additional support for the lens. The implant can be placed in the intact portion of the capsule, the ciliary sulcus, or the anterior chamber (Fig. 3.20). Rotation of the lens in the capsular bag away from the defect that caused the dislocation can be effective in certain cases (Fig. 3.21). Ciliary sulcus placement can be used if the anterior and posterior capsules are fused together and there is sufficient capsular support (Fig. 3.22). Anterior chamber relocation of three-piece polymethyl methacrylate (PMMA) lenses can be utilized if there is no glaucoma and the endothelial cell counts are good. Vaulting of single-piece PMMA, plate IOLs, silicone IOLs, and Acrysoft limit the value of this method. A peripheral iridectomy with the vitreous cutter should be used in all cases to prevent pupillary block. Ciliary sulcus suturing through positioning holes was reported by the principal author, but is seldom possible or indicated today. Sutures can be passed around the haptics for ciliary sulcus suturing. This method is complex and requires experience and careful planning.

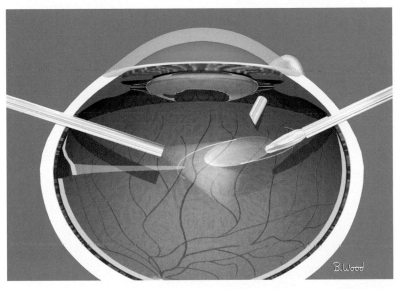

FIG. 3.19. Complete vitrectomy should precede IOL repositioning to avoid vitreoretinal traction.

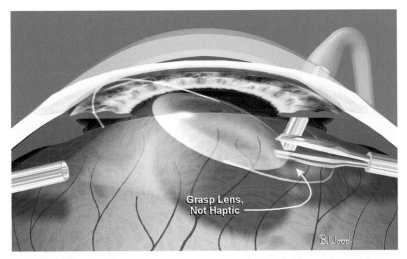

FIG. 3.20. The IOL can be implanted in the intact portion of the capsule, the ciliary sulcus, or the anterior chamber.

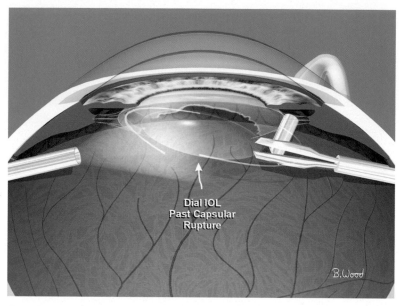

FIG. 3.21. Rotation of the lens into the capsular bag away from the rupture site can be effective.

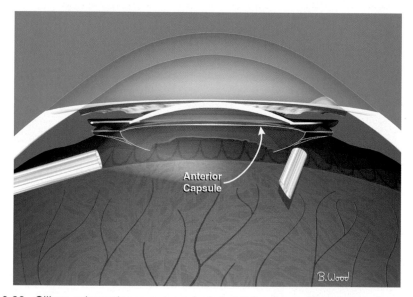

FIG. 3.22. Ciliary sulcus placement can be used if there is sufficient capsular support.

Dislocated Intraocular Lens Removal

On occasion, marked inflammation or retinal problems necessitate removal of a dislocated IOL. A total vitrectomy should be performed as described earlier and the lens optic grasped with 20-gauge diamond-coated forceps. The IOL should be brought anteriorly and a scleral plug placed in the endoilluminator opening. A limbal or clear corneal section of appropriate size should be made with the surgeon's other hand using the diamond knife/scissors technique also used for very dense nuclei and large intraocular foreign bodies. After the IOL is removed, the limbal wound is closed with a running shoelace or X-type 8-0, 9-0, or 10-0 monofilament nylon suture. Smaller-diameter sutures cause less astigmatism but may result in wound leaks during the vitrectomy.

Intraocular Lens Removal Before Trans–Pars Plana Vitrectomy

Occasionally, IOLs should be removed because of fibrovascular membranes from diabetic anterior vitreous cortex Fibro vascular proliferation (AVCFVP), trauma, or uveitis. The haptics should be cut with scissors with viscoelastics used to maintain the anterior chamber. The haptics can be left in the eye, if they are surrounded by a fibrous capsule and cannot be rotated out with forceps. A running shoelace 8-0 or 9-0 monofilament nylon suture facilitates tight wound closure.

Epithelial Ingrowth

Vitrectomy instruments can permit removal of the fibrous tissue, anterior vitreous cortex, and lens remnants in the treatment of epithelial ingrowth (34). Pretreatment of the iris with argon laser photocoagulation aids in identification of the tissue and its removal. It does not kill all abnormal cells but can be advantageous in defining the extent of involvement. The wound should be explored and the edges excised. An iridectomy with a 1- to 2-mm margin should then be performed with Vannas scissors. The wound should be closed tightly with a running shoelace, 8-0 monofilament nylon suture. Internal fluid/air exchange (see Chapter 4) should be performed by injecting air through the infusion system while allowing fluid egress with the vitrectomy instrument. Transcorneal and transscleral cryopexy are then applied over affected areas with a 2-mm margin. The thermal insulating effect of the air bubble causes more uniform destruction of abnormal tissue with less scleral damage.

The cytotoxin 5-fluorouracil has been used in conjunction with the surgical approach by some investigators in the hope of inhibiting regrowth of epithelial cells. Its long-term efficacy is uncertain. Fortunately, ingrowth through cataract wounds is extremely rare because of small incision techniques and advanced wound construction.

REFERENCES

1. Michels RG. Anterior segment and vitreoretinal surgery through the pars plana, Part I. *Ann Ophthalmol* 1976;8: 1353.
2. Michels RG. Anterior segment and vitreoretinal surgery through the pars plana, Part V. *Ann Ophthalmol* 1976;8: 1497.
3. Michels RG, Stark WJ. Vitrectomy technique in anterior segment surgery. *Trans Am Acad Ophthalmol Otolaryngol* 1976;81:382.
4. Taylor HR, Michels RG, Stark WJ. Vitrectomy methods in anterior segment surgery. *Ophthalmic Surg* 1979;10:25.
5. Michels RG: Anterior segment applications of vitrectomy techniques. *Trans Ophthalmol Soc UK* 1978;98:458.

6. Stark WJ, Michels RG. Anterior segment surgery using instruments designed for pars plana vitrectomy. *Trans Penn Acad Ophthalmol Otolaryngol* 1981;34:27.
7. Michels RG, Paton D. Results of radical anterior vitrectomy-a preliminary report of 26 cases. *Ophthalmic Surg* 1970;1:33.
8. Charles S. Anterior segment vitrectomy. In: D. Carroll, ed. *Surgery of the eye.* New York: Churchill Livingstone, 1987.
9. Charles S. The Charles anterior segment infusion sleeve. *Ocutome Fragmatome Newsletter* 1978;3:6.
10. May D. Closed vitrectomy for vitreous prolapse during cataract extraction. *Ocutome Fragmatome Newsletter* 1979;4:2.
11. Girard LJ, Hawkins RS. Cataract extraction by ultrasonic aspiration, vitrectomy by ultrasonic aspiration. *Trans Am Acad Ophthalmol Otolaryngol* 1974;78:50.
12. Charles S. Trans–pars plana and posterior chamber lensectomy with the Girard phakofragmenter and automated suction. In: Emery J, ed. *Current concepts in cataract surgery, Selected Proceedings of the Fifth Biennial Cataract Surgical Congress.* St. Louis: CV Mosby, 1978.
13. Charles S. Trans–pars plana lensectomy update. *Ocutome Fragmatome Newsletter* 1980;5.
14. Michels RG, Shockett DE. Vitrectomy techniques for removal of cataract lens material. *Arch Ophthalmol* 1977;95:1767.
15. Parks MM, Hiles DA. Management of infantile cataracts. *Am J Ophthalmol* 1967;63:10.
16. Parks MM. Posterior lens capsulectomy during primary cataract surgery in children. *Ophthalmology* 1983; 90:344.
17. Calhoun JH. Cutting-aspiration instruments. *Int Ophthalmol Clin* 1977;17:103.
18. Chrousos GA, Parks MM, O'Neill JF. Incidence of chronic glaucoma, retinal detachment and secondary membrane surgery in pediatric aphakic patients. *Ophthalmology* 1984;91:1238.
19. Hamill MB, Koch DD. Pediatric cataracts. *Curr Opin Ophthalmol* 1999;10:4–9.
20. Malukiewicz-Wisniewska G, Kaluzny J, Lesiewska-Junk H, et al. Intraocular lens implantation in children and youth. *J Pediatr Ophthalmol Strabismus* 1999;36:129–133.
21. Simons BD, Siatkowski RM, Schiffman JC, et al. Surgical technique, visual outcome, and complications of pediatric intraocular lens implantation. *J Pediatr Ophthalmol Strabismus* 199;36:118–124.
22. Zwaan J, Mullaney PB, Awad A, et al. Pediatric intraocular lens implantation: surgical results and complications in more than 300 patients. *Ophthalmology* 1998;105:112–128.
23. Treister G, Machemer R. Pars plana approach for pupillary membranes. *Arch Ophthalmol* 1978;96:1014.
24. Wilkinson CP, Ramsey JJ. Closed vitrectomy for the vitreous touch syndrome. *Am J Ophthalmol* 1980;90:304.
25. Snip RC, Kenyon KR, Green WR. Retrocorneal fibrous membrane in the vitreous touch syndrome. *Am J Ophthalmol* 1975;79:233.
26. Irvine A. Pars plana vitrectomy for malignant and aphakic pupillary block glaucoma. *Trans Pac Coast Otoophthalmol Soc* 1977;58:189.
27. Orth DH, Henry MD. Management of Irvine Gass syndrome using argon laser photocoagulation and pars plana vitrectomy. Presented at the Bicentennial Cataract Surgical Congress, Miami Beach, Florida, February 1977.
28. Rice TA, Michels RG. Vitreous wick syndrome-current surgical management. *Am J Ophthalmol* 1978;85:656.
29. Fung WE. Vitrectomy for chronic aphakic cystoid macular edema. *Ophthalmology* 1985;92:1102.
30. Pendergast SD, Margherio RR, Williams GA, et al. Vitrectomy for chronic pseudophakic cystoid macular edema. *Am J Ophthalmol* 1999;128:317–323.
31. Ikeda T, Sato K, Katano T, et al. Vitrectomy for cystoid macular edema with attached posterior hyaloid membrane in patients with diabetes. *Br J Ophthalmol* 1999;83:12–14.
32. Holekamp NM. Treatment of pseudophakic CME. *Ocul Immunol Inflamm* 1998;6:121–123.
33. Wilson DL. A new intraocular foreign body retriever. *Ophthal Surg* 1975;6:64.
34. Stark WJ, Michels RG, Maumenee AE, et al. Surgical management of epithelial ingrowth. *Am J Ophthalmol* 1978;85:772.

4

General Posterior Segment Techniques

STRATEGIES

All surgery requires a prior strategy, game plan, or algorithm. The complexity of high-technology vitreoretinal surgery requires extensive preoperative planning. The surgical algorithm must include an expected series of events but must contain branches to allow for the contingencies and discoveries that occur in the course of surgery. The main branches of the algorithm are determined by the expected techniques, such as lens removal, endophotocoagulation, silicone oil, gas, scleral buckling, and so on. Equipment, disposables, gas, oil, buckles, and so on, must be available for any possible additional techniques driven by the individual case and any intraoperative findings or complications.

SPECULUM

A heavy wire speculum is an effective means of retracting the eyelids. Larger specula that lift the lids may interfere with the contact lens and infusion cannula. A lateral canthotomy is never necessary. The drape should not have a precut hole; it should be placed with the lids open and cut so the flaps completely cover both lid margins, using the speculum to hold them in place. Covering the lashes and lid margins is done to reduce the chance of endophthalmitis and to prevent cilia from being entrapped in tissue. Aspirating speculums may reduce fluid runoff under the drape or unto the foot pedals, surgeon's feet, and floor.

CONJUNCTIVAL INCISIONS

Posterior segment vitreous surgery is usually best performed through the pars plana; thus some conjunctival incision will have to be made. For surgery not requiring scleral buckling, two or three conjunctival incisions are needed. Care should be taken to avoid highly scarred or vascular areas, filtering blebs, setons, and flaps for sutured intraocular lenses (IOLs). A temporal incision is made for the cutter, scissors, forceps, fragmenter, laser, and the infusion cannula and should be 120°, limbus-parallel, 1 mm posterior to the limbus, and centered at the lateral rectus. The nasal incision is for the endoilluminator and should be limbus-parallel, 60°, 1 mm posterior to the limbus, and centered at the upper border of the medial rectus. If there is conjunctival scarring at the lateral rectus, two small incisions can be used temporally. A small radial extension of the limbus parallel incisions at one or both ends facilitates better exposure and one suture closure.

For any vitreous surgery in which scleral buckling is anticipated, it is best to make a continuous incision in each quadrant requiring buckling, which should be placed 1 mm posterior to the limbus. A limbal peritomy tends to bleed under the contact lens, causes conjunctival retraction and redundancy problems in the postoperative course, and makes postoperative contact lens fitting difficult. Incisions more than 1 mm behind the limbus increase risk of exposure of scleral sutures and make visualization of the sclerotomies difficult because of the anterior flap.

TRACTION SUTURES

Traction sutures under the muscles are of no value in vitrectomy because the endosurgical instruments move the eye. Transconjunctival sutures not only are unnecessary but have several disadvantages: (a) the sclera can be perforated by the needle, (b) the muscle can be torn, (c) the suture must be removed if buckling is to be performed, and (d) the holes in the conjunctiva can allow bacteria access to a buckle postoperatively. Only if scleral buckling is anticipated should traction sutures be used, and then they should be placed beneath the muscles directly, using a short-handled fenestrated muscle hook with chamfered hole. Large sutures (0 to 2-0 silk or cotton) do not cut the muscle tendons and provide a good grip for the assistant. Only the muscles absolutely required for access to the sclera should be trapped to reduce postoperative pain, ptosis, and strabismus. The superior rectus should be avoided if possible to reduce vertical strabismus and ptosis. In the authors' experience, it is never necessary to remove muscles for scleral buckling or trauma repair.

BUCKLING ANTICIPATED OR PREVIOUS BUCKLE PRESENT

The operating microscope is useful for all scleral buckling procedures, even if vitrectomy is not planned. Better visualization reduces inadvertent scleral perforation, decreases damage to the muscles and ocular blood supply, and improves conjunctival closure and patient comfort. Practice with the microscope improves surgical skills. If an existing buckle is to be revised or removed, it should be exposed under the microscope by dissection with a hockey stick–type blade. A small suction cannula can be used to aspirate routine bleeding, which usually subsides with minimal diathermy. Bipolar diathermy coagulation should be used only for major bleeding, as these techniques increase conjunctival and episcleral scarring. Bipolar forceps seem to produce more focused diathermy than the "eraser."

Excellent exposure can be obtained by using a "microretinal" retractor without a slot. The slot on the Schepens retractor allows prolapse of orbital tissues into the surgical field. The assistant's hand is kept out of the surgical field because of the right angle part of the handle and can exert a lateral pull rather than a twisting force, resulting in reduced hand fatigue. If scleral buckling elements are to be removed, it is best to place the infusion cannula, verify placement, and turn it on before buckle removal to prevent hypotony. Care must be taken when rotating the eye temporally so as not to rotate the interior portion of the infusion cannula posteriorly into the peripheral retina as the cannula strikes the lids.

SCLERAL INCISIONS

Sclerotomies for the endosurgical instruments will be focal points for the remainder of the operation (1). If they are incorrectly placed or constructed, the entire course of the operation can be adversely influenced. The incisions should be placed in the anterior pars plana to reduce the risk of damage to the peripheral retina. Contrary to customary teaching, bleeding of the ciliary body is infrequent and rarely serious when it does occur. Except in children, patients with an abnormal pars plana, and microphthalmic patients, the sclerotomies should be placed 3 mm posterior to the limbus if the lens is absent or to be removed and 4 mm posterior if the lens is to be saved (Fig. 4.1). Some surgeons compromise and use 3.5 mm for all cases.

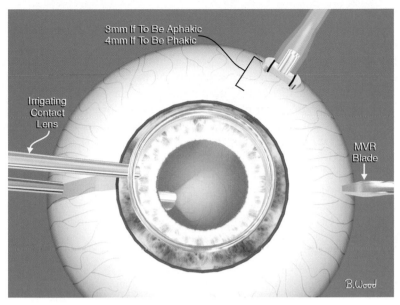

FIG. 4.1. All sclerotomies are made with the MVR blade, 3 mm posterior to the limbus if the lens is absent or to be removed, 4 mm posterior if the lens is to be saved.

The disposable microvitreoretinal (MVR) blade is ideal for making sclerotomies. The blade is lancet-shaped to ensure that the incision is centered at the initial entry point (Fig. 4.2). The blade is 1.4 mm in width, which makes a linear incision that becomes 0.89 mm (20-gauge) in diameter when deformed to a circular shape by the instruments. The non-tapered, 20-gauge shank and 25-mm length correspond to the dimensions of the other endo-surgical instruments. Stilettos, myringotomy blades, illuminated stab needles, 20-gauge needles, and transilluminators are unnecessary with this method. Prefirming before use

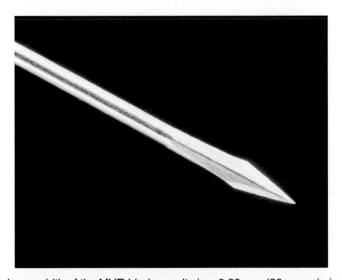

FIG. 4.2. The 1.4-mm width of the MVR blade results in a 0.89 mm (20 gauge) circular sclerotomy.

of the MVR blade is unnecessary because the tip of a high-quality MVR blade is typically sharper than a 30-gauge needle and provides a correct size incision if a subsequent fluid injection is required.

The sharpness of a new MVR blade point usually prevents the ciliary epithelium from being pushed ahead of it. The possibility of penetrating the sclera but not the choroid/ciliary epithelium should be a reminder to use these blades for one case only. To verify proper penetration, the blade should be seen through the operating microscope. Under no circumstances should the naked eye be used to check the cannula, nor should the cannula be used for infusion without inspection. If the eye is soft, a 20-gauge needle should be placed through the initial MVR incision and infusion fluid should be injected with the needle tip visible. This step will decrease the incidence of suprachoroidal and subretinal infusion. If excessive bleeding through the sclerotomy occurs, it can be treated by external/internal bipolar diathermy with the aid of a scleral plug or by placing one blade of the bipolar in the sclerotomy and the other on the adjacent scleral surface.

INFUSION CANNULA PLACEMENT

Unless there is severe fibrovascular proliferation or some other obstruction discussed earlier at this region of the pars plana, the infusion cannula is placed near the inferior border of the lateral rectus. In this position it does not hit the nose, lids, or speculum, or interfere with the surgical instruments.

Because it decreases the incidence of choroidal infusion and directs infusion fluid further away from the lens than does the 2-mm cannula, the 4-mm cannula should be used in all cases. Unless it is carelessly directed anteriorly, the 4-mm cannula will not damage the lens. A 6-mm cannula can be used for thick choroid cases but can bump the lens.

The authors make the sclerotomy for the infusion cannula before placing the cannula retention suture. By placing the incision before the suture, each edge of the wound can be grasped with 0.12 forceps. The tension applied to the sclera makes possible a deep suture bite. The suture bites should be at least 3/4 scleral deep and 1 mm long so that they will not fall off the tabs of the infusion cannula. They should be widely spaced to ensure imbrication of the cannula into the sclera, similar to a buckle. A braided, flexible suture (6-0 silk) is easier to place over the cannula footplates than is a springy nylon or polypropylene suture. Some surgeons use the cannula retention suture for wound closure. The authors are opposed to this method because it compromises imbrication of the cannula into the sclera as well as tight wound closure.

After insertion, the cannula should always be inspected with the operating microscope *before* the infusion is turned on. If the pupil is very small, the indirect ophthalmoscope can be used for visualization. To see the cannula, it is usually necessary to push it gently toward the center of the eye, being careful to avoid the lens, if it is a phakic eye. If the tip appears shiny and clear of overlying tissue, then infusion may be turned on. Observing the cannula with the unaided eye and endoilluminator has insufficient magnification and can result in inadvertent suprachoroidal or subretinal infusion.

If tissue is seen over the cannula, the corrective action depends on the status of the lens (Fig. 4.3). If the eye is aphakic or will be at the end of the operation, the MVR blade is inserted from the opposite side of the eye to incise the tissue over the cannula internally, so that it will retract down over the entire interior portion of the cannula. This technique is also effective if a choroidal infusion is present from previous problems or occurs during surgery from dislocation of the cannula. If the eye is to remain phakic, the cannula should be removed and a 20-gauge needle should be inserted to repressurize the globe and compress the choroid back against the sclera before reinserting the cannula.

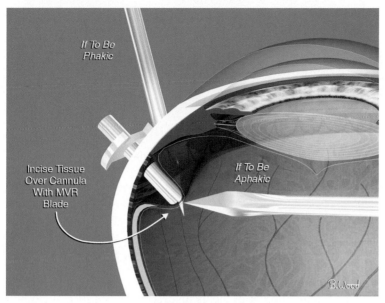

FIG. 4.3. If tissue is seen over the infusion cannula, it can be incised with the MVR blade. The blade is inserted from the opposite side if the eye is to be aphakic, and from the same side if the eye is to be phakic.

If the pars plana is not visible preoperatively, the sew-on infusion cannula cannot be turned on at this point. Infusion should begin using an angulated 30°, 20-gauge blunt infusion cannula placed through the supranasal sclerotomy (Fig. 4.4). If the lens is absent or to be removed, the cannula can be visualized by indenting the cannula toward the pupil. When the anterior segment opacity has been removed, facilitating view of the cannula, the surgeon can turn on the infusion cannula before proceeding with the rest of the vitrectomy.

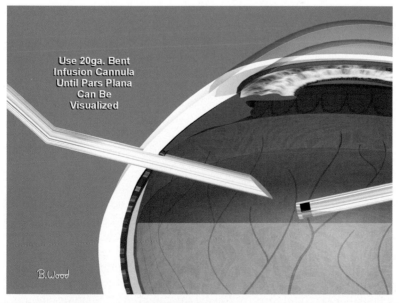

FIG. 4.4. If the pars plana cannot be visualized, infusion is initiated with the long, 30° bent infusion cannula. The sew-in cannula is used after anterior opacities are removed.

Basics of Cannula Use

The infusion cannula should be placed as soon as the sclera is exposed. The infusion should remain until just before conjunctival closure. Any infusion system should be visualized before use. This first-in, last-out approach is essential to prevent hypotony leading to intraocular or suprachoroidal choroidal hemorrhage as well as miosis.

INSTRUMENT SCLEROTOMIES

After the infusion cannula is inspected, the infusion is turned on with the infusion set at 45 mm Hg in adults or 35 mm Hg in children or patients with extremely low perfusion (blood) pressure. Use of the Alcon VGFI or even GFI systems is better than placing the bottle a certain distance above the eye because it gives a direct digital readout of the infusion pressure. Starting the infusion before the second and third incisions are made inflates the uvea against the sclera, permitting the other sclerotomies to be made through the choroid, and nonpigmented ciliary epithelium. This approach also prevents the miosis and bleeding that accompany hypotony.

The second scleral incision, usually for the endoilluminator, is made superonasally. It is best made near the upper border of the medial rectus, 4 mm from the limbus in eyes to remain phakic and 3 mm for aphakic eyes. This incision is plugged with the endoilluminator as the MVR blade is removed to maintain intraocular pressure (IOP) rather than the unnecessary step of placing a scleral plug.

The third scleral incision is primarily for the vitreous cutter, fragmenter, scissors, forceps, endophotocoagulator, and so on. It is placed even with the upper border of the lateral rectus and at the usual distance from the limbus. Vitreoretinal instruments bump the brow or nose and have difficulty reaching the anterior chamber if entered superiorly or nasally. By using the active instruments in the hand corresponding to the eye being operated on (right eye/right hand; left eye/left hand) and having the pair of instruments about 170° apart, access to all portions of the globe, precise positioning, and comfort are maximized. Many surgeons limit their capabilities by always using the active instruments in their dominant hand. There are certain maneuvers that involve exchanging the active instrument to the opposite hand for better access to the pathology. This is frequently the case with endophotocoagulation, scissors delamination, submacular surgery, and drainage of subretinal fluid through peripheral breaks.

In all cases, the placement of sclerotomies should avoid previous incisions, areas of known fibrovascular proliferation on the pars plana, and dense vascularity. Most attempts to use previous sclerotomies result in wound leaks, tearing of the sclera, excessive bleeding, and possible fibrovascular proliferation.

INFUSION FLUID

High-quality infusion fluid containing dextrose, glutathione, and a bicarbonate buffer should be used for all cases (see Chapter 2). This should be freshly prepared just before the operation. High-quality commercial solutions (Balanced Salt Solution, BSS Plus, Alcon Laboratories) should be utilized in all cases, if available. Use of BSS Plus reduces corneal endothelial cell loss and trabecular meshwork damage compared with other solutions. The authors do not add glucose, epinephrine, or antibiotics to the fluid to reduce the chances of using incorrect agents or concentrations as well as to reduce the risk of corneal, lenticular, and retinal toxicity. Plastic infusion fluid containers should be avoided because air diffuses through the plastic during storage causing bubbles. Two-component infusate systems should be designed so the substance in the actual infusion container is safe if the second component is inadvertently omitted; this is the case only with BSS Plus at this time.

IMPORTANCE OF VISUALIZATION

Optimal visualization is essential to safe vitrectomy. While it is obviously desirable to preserve the corneal epithelium and the lens, neither one is as important as the ability to perform a safe vitrectomy. This simple principle is often overlooked with adverse consequences. Similarly, IOL implantation should not become more important than optimal vitreoretinal management.

Fundus Contact Lens

A glass, irrigating type contact lens with a handle for the assistant is usually the best visualization system. Unlike nonirrigating lenses, it washes away bleeding, maintains a clear view, requires no viscoelastics, and helps preserve the epithelium. Unlike lenses without handles, it does not decenter when the eye is rotated to visualize the periphery. The fluid meniscus eliminates astigmatism and allows prism effects, so that the periphery may be viewed with less ocular rotation. In all cases, the holder of the contact lens must visualize the eye through a beam splitter on the surgeon's operating microscope. Sew-on lenses take more time, cause more bleeding under the contact, cost more money because of viscoelastics and sutures, but can be used if a steady-handed assistant is not available. Technicians and nurses frequently do a superior job of holding the lens, and therefore an assistant surgeon is not required to hold the lens.

Wide-angle, noninverted, 105 degrees contact lenses (Peyman) have recently been found to be very useful in peripheral dissection, fluid air/gas exchange, and internal drainage of subretinal fluid. This approach has none of the cost, complexity, and geometry problems associated with microscope and inverted solutions. This lens can often replace the conventional Landers lens for phakic and pseudophakic fluid air/gas exchange and internal drainage of subretinal fluid.

The highest-quality irrigating solution available (BSS Plus) should be used with the contact lens if possible. If the epithelium becomes cloudy, it should be removed with a rounded end-cutting disposable blade. Under no circumstances should the blade touch an area from which the epithelium has already been removed. Scraping of deepithelialized areas, use of cotton tip applicator sticks, and chemical removal are all traumatic to the basement membrane and retard postoperative healing and epithelial adherence. The authors remove the corneal epithelium in 1% to 2% of cases.

Pupillary Dilation

The preoperative administration of topical adrenergic (phenylepherine 2.5% to 10%) and anticholinergic (tropicamide, 1%; cyclopentolate, 1%; hyoscine, 0.25%; or homatropine, 2.5 %) dilating drops is critical to safe vitrectomy. Minimization of hypotony and mechanical iris trauma usually allow the preoperative dilation to be sustained throughout the case. If pupillary constriction occurs, a small pulse of intraocular epinephrine can redilate the pupil. This epinephrine should be labeled "for injection," contain minimal amounts of sodium bisulfite antioxidant, and be diluted to 1:10,000 (2). Intracardiac injection preparations, although labeled as containing no preservative, contain too much sodium bisulfite and are potentially toxic to the corneal endothelium. Iris surgery should be avoided unless the preceding steps fail and the fundus cannot be seen adequately for safe surgery. Iris surgery leads to postoperative glare, photophobia, and cosmetic problems, as well as increased postoperative inflammation. Iris retractors and sutures cause iris trauma, inflammation, longer operating time, and increased cost.

Lens Removal

If lens removal is necessary, it should be performed before proceeding with vitrectomy, unless the lens is subluxated or dislocated. Relative miosis may occur as the vitrectomy progresses, and early lens removal permits better access to the peripheral capsule and cortex, and prevents unnecessary iris surgery. The view is always better in aphakic eyes, and safe vitrectomy should never be compromised to preserve the lens, even if it is relatively clear. Saving the anterior lens capsule until the end of the operation hinders the view and is necessary only if a ciliary sulcus IOL is to be implanted at the end of the case. Forceps removal of the lens capsule facilitates total capsule removal without iris touch and resultant miosis.

VITRECTOMY OBJECTIVES

Vitreous removal requires a thorough understanding of surgical anatomy and must proceed in a systematic fashion. The vitreous body should be thought of in terms of discrete surfaces that are removed in a specific order. The goals should not be band cutting, obtaining a view on the posterior pole, or core vitrectomy only; instead, the aim should be to manage the underlying vitreoretinal disease. When vitrectomy was performed using rotating cutters with syringe-controlled suction, the surgeon was able to remove much of the vitreous without moving the instrument from the center of the vitreous cavity. This occurred because of excessive traction, which drew the vitreous inward; however, such traction is now recognized to be dangerous. From this traction-induced central relocation of the vitreous arose the erroneous concept of "core vitrectomy." In fact, many eyes with sufficient vitreoretinal disease to require vitrectomy do not even have a vitreous "core." Recent trauma, recent retinal detachments, and macular hole cases may have relatively normal vitreous requiring core vitrectomy.

Better cutters, combined with higher cutting rates and proportional (linear) suction control, facilitate cutting the vitreous without moving it from its original position. The surgeon accustomed to low-performance systems may at first be confused by the better systems' lack of traction and may feel that they are not working.

If the eye is aphakic at the commencement of vitrectomy, the anterior vitreous cortex (AVC) should be removed first, starting centrally and progressing peripherally. Any attachments to anterior segment wounds or the iris should be removed before proceeding posteriorly. In phakic eyes, the AVC is frequently adherent to the posterior lens capsule, making removal difficult without lens damage. A clear AVC not causing traction should be avoided in eyes without retinal detachment to reduce lens damage. Sew-on infusion cannulas permit the surgeon to change sides between the vitrectomy instrument and the endoilluminator, thereby gaining access to the whole posterior curve of the lens. Removal of the AVC in a phakic eye requires direct microscope viewing and coaxial plus endoillumination without a contact or wide-angle system to avoid lens damage. Eyes with retinal detachment involving the periphery, fibrovascular prolifera-

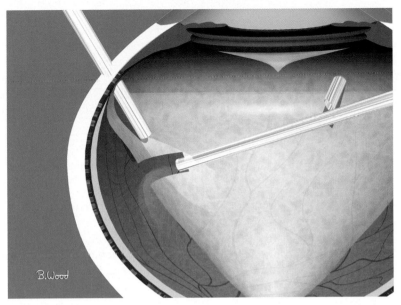

FIG. 4.5. Entry into the PVC should be made nasally, or into an area know to have PVD by ultrasound or ophthalmoscopy.

tion on or near the pars plana, or a significant inflammatory component should have lens removal as a precaution against the formation of a cyclitic membrane at the lens/AVC interface.

After removal of the AVC, the second objective is usually the removal of the posterior vitreous cortex (PVC). Eyes requiring trans–pars plana vitrectomy usually have either total vitreoretinal contact, partial posterior vitreous detachment (PVD) with a conical vitreous configuration, or total PVD with a frontal plane configuration. Entry into the PVC should be made in an area nasally (Fig. 4.5) or preferably known to have a PVD by ophthalmoscopy or ultrasound. The portions of PVC extending between areas of vitreoretinal adherence are known as bridging or tangential traction. All portions of the PVC not in contact with the retina, that is, both cone and bridging portions, must be removed to relieve traction. However, the vitreous "skirt," which is the anterior edge of the truncated cone, must be treated differently. Because retinal breaks can be caused by surgically induced traction on the skirt, only enough skirt should be removed to allow satisfactory surgical visualization and to prevent the superior skirt from covering any portion of the view when the patient is upright. If blood products are incorporated in the skirt, they should be carefully debulked to diminish postoperative hemolytic and erythroclastic glaucoma.

EPIRETINAL MEMBRANES

The PVC may include new cellular elements and collagen along its surface at sites of vitreoretinal adherence in addition to hypocellular contraction of preexisting vitreous collagen. This type of pathoanatomy is usually referred to as an epiretinal membrane (ERM). The treatment of ERM is a challenging and essential component of management or vitreoretinal cases. The approach to ERM varies with the disease; specific techniques will be discussed with the specific diseases.

Forceps membrane peeling, scissors segmentation, and scissors delamination, are all useful approaches to ERM. The goal of ERM surgery is to reattach the retina while minimizing recurrences and complications. If the membrane is loosely adherent and can be removed without internal limiting membrane (ILM) damage, retinal break, or bleeding, forceps membrane peeling is the best approach. In diabetes, retinopathy of prematurity (ROP), and some trauma and proliferative vitreoretinopathy (PVR) cases the membrane is quite adherent, requiring scissors segmentation or delamination. Excellent visualization is necessary for ERM dissection.

Simplified Epiretinal Membrane Dissection

Current approaches to vitreoretinal surgery utilize a wide variety of techniques and technologies. The techniques for PVR, proliferative diabetic retinopathy (PDR), ROP, epimacular membranes, macular holes, and other causes of vitreoretinal traction typically vary considerably with the diagnosis. It is likely that fibrin syndrome, corneal problems, cataract, photo toxicity, postanesthesia complications, postoperative pain, lid and conjunctival hyperemia, and edema are more frequent after longer procedures. Postoperative atelectasis, infection, pulmonary embolism, and increased length of stay have been associated with longer operating times in the surgical literature. The principal author has observed a relationship between number of tools used, longer operating times, and worse surgical outcomes. A unified, all-disease approach to tools, techniques, and algorithms could theoretically reduce costs associated with longer operating times, staff training time, setup time, and instrument acquisition and maintenance. Advancements in manufacturing technology generally decrease the cost while increasing the quality of the product by reducing the number of steps or processes. A central theme of this book is to present a simplified, faster, less-step, less-tool approach to vitreoretinal surgery.

At present, the authors use end-opening forceps for *all* epiretinal and subretinal membrane peeling, the MVR blade for submacular surgery, and curved, fine scissors for *all* segmentation and delamination. These three instruments, one of which was already used to make the sclerotomies, are the only dissection tools used by the authors for virtually all vitreoretinal surgery. The following section describes a unified approach to tool and technique selection for vitreoretinal surgery that was developed for use by novice and advanced surgeons alike.

Dissection Methods

Machemer developed membrane peeling (stripping) in 1972 and it has continued to serve the vitreoretinal surgeon well in appropriate cases. The original implementation of this method involved passing a bent needle under the outer margin of the membrane into the potential space between the ERM and the retina in order to apply a lifting force. O'Malley modified this method by developing a blunt device known as the pic. In either instance, the central notion was to enter the potential space and break the membrane/retinal adhesions by applying an elongation force. The principal author developed forceps membrane peeling in order to remove the ERM without entering this potential space or contacting the retina (Fig. 4.6). The principal author developed the diamond-coated, end-opening forceps with Hans Grieshaber to facilitate grasping the membrane en face. This method, termed *forceps membrane peeling,* has many advantages over needles, pics, or forceps, that are designed to have one blade in the aforementioned potential space between the membrane and the retina. The authors use the inside-out, forceps membrane

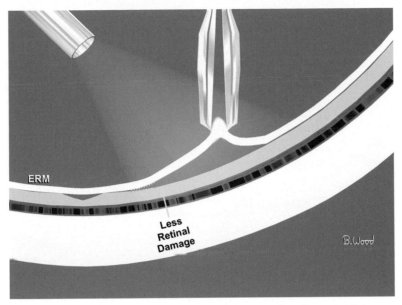

FIG. 4.6. Forceps membrane peeling does not require entering the potential space between membrane and retina or contacting the retina, resulting in less retinal damage.

peeling method for all epimacular membranes and most PVR cases. A variant of this technique is used for macular hole cortex/ILM/ERM peeling.

Scissors segmentation of epiretinal membranes was developed by the principal author in 1974 to address the problem of excessive adherence between the ERM and the retina, which prevented safe membrane peeling. Vertical scissors were used to segment the epiretinal membrane into smaller zones (epicenters), thereby reducing tangential force on the retina (Fig. 4.7). This method, like membrane peeling, continues to have a place in our technique library, although the author usually prefers scissors delamination in PDR cases. Scissors segmentation does not culminate in ERM removal in contrast to peeling and delamination. In short, *segmentation* means "cut up the membrane," whereas *delamination* means "cut it off."

Scissors delamination of epiretinal membranes was developed by the principal author in 1978 to address the issue of glial proliferation on fibrin surfaces caused by bleeding from the cut edge of segmented epiretinal membranes. In addition, late, rhegmatogenous retinal detachment secondary to atrophic retinal breaks from persistent elevation of the retina can occur after segmentation. With the delamination method, fine, curved scissors are used to shear the attachments between the ERM and the retina, removing most or all of the ERM (Fig. 4.8). The scissors are used with blades in the potential space between the retina and the ERM. If the scissors are inserted and then opened, the retina is torn as the blades push the attachment points outward. If the scissors are opened fully and then closed as they enter the potential space between ERM and retina, the retina will be torn before the shear point of the scissors moves forward to shear the attachments. The scissors should be advanced into the potential space while making frequent, small, cutting motions of the scissors with the blades barely opened to admit the tissue to be sheared (Fig. 4.9). The scissors are moved side to side to enable scrolling of the ERM as attachment points are sheared. Using this technique, all cutting will occur at the tips of the scissors.

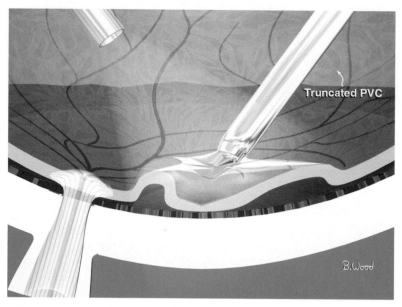

FIG. 4.7. Scissors segmentation of epiretinal membranes divides the membrane into smaller pieces, reducing tangential traction in cases where the membrane is too adherent to peel safely.

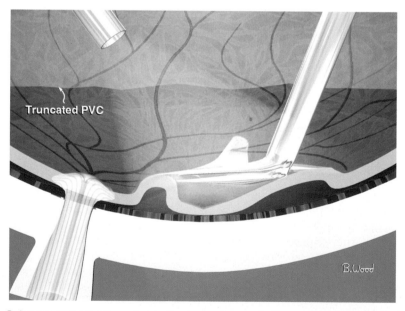

FIG. 4.8. Scissors delamination of epiretinal membranes is the preferred method of removing highly adherent membranes, as it allows complete membrane removal.

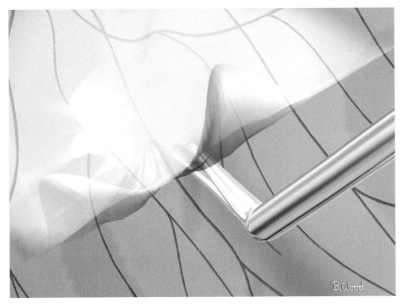

FIG. 4.9. While making frequent small cutting motions with the tips, the scissors are moved from side to side, enabling scrolling of the ERM while attachment points are sheared.

Retinal Stabilization

Retina has approximately 1/100 the tensile strength of ERM. This property, in conjunction with strong vitreoretinal adherence, results in retinal movement during ERM dissection. Chang developed perfluorocarbon liquid-assisted ERM dissection to stabilize the retina during ERM dissection, as well as to float the subretinal fluid out through peripheral retinal breaks into the vitreous cavity (Fig. 4.10) (3–6). Perfluorocarbon liquids work very well but are relatively expensive and somewhat difficult to remove. The authors use liquid PFC for giant breaks and selected retinal detachments but believe that it is not required for most retinal detachment, PVR and PDR/TRD cases.

The authors often perform fluid/air exchange to stabilize a mobile retina, which facilitates completion of the dissection. Air has no cost and is easy to obtain, nontoxic, and easy to remove. Forceps membrane peeling, scissors segmentation, scissors delamination, further vitrectomy, or retinectomy can be easily performed under air. Air can, however, cause cataracts with prolonged lens contact, a flat chamber or miosis, fogging with IOLs, and a very bad view in an aphakic eye with striate keratopathy. Perfluorocarbon liquids are preferred in these instances.

Scissors Mechanics

All scissors shear at a single contact point between the two blades. This shear point moves forward as the scissors close, creating an exclusion force. This push-out force can tear or displace the retina (Fig. 4.11). Machemer and Parel developed the membrane peeler cutter (MPC) to use high-speed cutting with near parallel blades to reduce the exclusive shear (squeeze-out) problem of conventional scissors. The vitreous cutter is a parallel blade shear but requires vacuum imbrication of the tissue into the port to accomplish shearing.

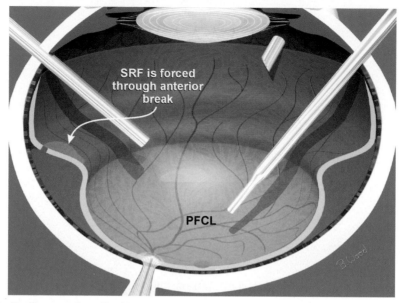

FIG. 4.10. Perfluorocarbon liquid stabilizes mobile retina during dissection, while floating out subretinal fluid through peripheral breaks.

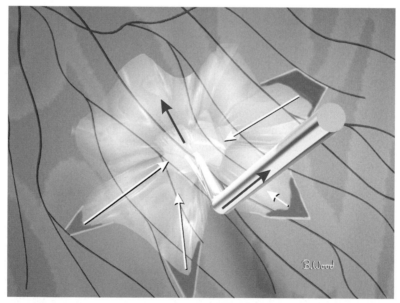

FIG. 4.11. The shear point of scissors moves forward as the scissors close, creating an exclusion force that can tear or displace the retina.

Bimanual Surgery

While at Duke University, Dyson Hickingbotham developed "bimanual surgery." Some surgeons use this method to lift the ERM before cutting the attachment points. The authors believe that the lift-and-cut approach increases iatrogenic breaks and bleeding. Others use the technique because of an interest in understanding patho-anatomy. Although greater understanding is noble, it should not come at the expense of greater complications. The authors recommend bimanual surgery, better termed *forceps membrane stabilization* (Fig. 4.12), if it is needed to counteract the exclusive (push-out) force of scissors and forces on the retina caused by membrane peeling. Fiberoptic forceps developed by Hickingbotham with Grieshaber facilitate bimanual surgery by freeing up the hand normally holding the endoilluminator. Glare is a problem with many fiberoptic instruments.

Outside-In Versus Inside-Out ERM Dissection

Classic membrane peeling as introduced by Machemer is based on the concept of searching for the outer margin (edge) of the ERM and dissecting inward from this margin. The principal author developed the concept termed *inside-out* membrane peeling to address the problem of thin membranes with virtually invisible outer margins. The authors believe that inside-out membrane peeling has many advantages over the more traditional outside-in approach. Inside-out dissection is advantageous because the retina is thicker, stronger, and more redundant centrally; the ERM is thicker and more visible centrally; and the view is better centrally (Fig. 4.13). The inside-out direction is used by the authors and recommended for most peeling, segmentation, and delamination.

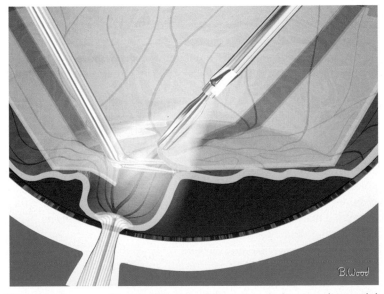

FIG. 4.12. Fiberoptic forceps allow stabilization of the retina during membrane delamination or peeling.

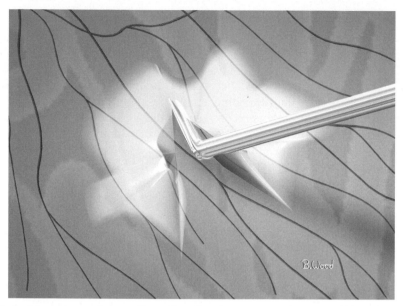

FIG. 4.13. Inside-out membrane dissection is advantageous because the retina is thicker, stronger and more redundant centrally, the ERM is thicker and more visible centrally, and the view is better centrally.

ERM Dissection Flowchart

Removal of all apparent vitreoretinal traction should precede ERM dissection unless there is limited separation of the posterior cortical vitreous from the retina. The principal author developed the concept of inside-out membrane delamination preceding removal of the posterior cortical vitreous for cases without apparent PVD. Abrams et al. subsequently recommended an outside-in approach for delamination before the cortex is removed, which they termed *en bloc* (7). In this paper they recommended using traction on the vitreous to lift up the ERM. This approach may create peripheral retinal breaks because of countertraction and is not recommended by the authors. Many now call the inside-out delamination before posterior cortical vitreous separation method "en bloc" even though that is not how it was originally described.

The first stage of ERM dissection is to carefully test the adherence of the ERM to the retina. In general, EMM, macular hole, and PVR have less adherence than PDR or ROP. If the adherence is low, inside-out forceps membrane peeling is the best approach. If the adherence is high, inside-out delamination is the next step. Segmentation can be used to facilitate access for delamination. In general, almost all ERM is delaminated using an inside-out orientation in PDR and ROP cases. The procedure is halted at the segmentation step if it is thought that excessive retinal surface damage or bleeding will result if delamination is used. This is sometimes the case with peripheral regions of long-standing diabetic traction retinal detachments.

If the retina is pushed away by the scissors or if peeling is causing excessive retinal movement, forceps stabilization of the epiretinal membrane can be used. If the retinal mobility is excessive, PFC liquid or air stabilization of the retina can be used; this is typically required in retinal detachment and PVR cases.

After all vitreoretinal traction and all apparent ERM-induced retinal foreshortening have been managed, internal or direct needle drainage of subretinal fluid should be initiated in cases with a rhegmatogenous component. After retinal movement in the direction of attachment ceases, internal fluid/air exchange should be started while continuing to drain subretinal fluid (SRF). If the retina does not completely reattach or subretinal air appears, the remaining traction should be managed by further vitrectomy, peeling, segmentation, delamination, subretinal traction removal, or lastly, retinectomy.

Suction Forceps Membrane Peeling

If a loose edge of a flexible ERM or PVC requires peeling, it can be held in the port of the vitrectomy instrument, a soft-tip cannula, or the aspiration port of a manipulator using the suction-only mode of the foot pedal. The tool can then be moved, lifting the membrane or vitreous away from the retina (8). The suction force can, however, cause retinal traction, and certain membranes are difficult to imbricate into a port. Forceps peeling is preferable in most instances except for PVD creation.

"Chopsticks" Membrane Peeling

If a flexible ERM has been partially lifted from the retina surface by peeling, removal can be completed by holding the membrane between the endoilluminator and the vitrectomy probe (9). However, if excessive pressure is utilized with this bimanual method, the instruments may slip past one another. Outward spreading of a pair of blunt tools such as the probe and the endoilluminator can be used to separate the posterior vitreous cortex or an ERM from the retina by blunt dissection. This method is very useful in PVR cases.

Power Scissors

Power scissors have been developed to reduce hand fatigue as well as inadvertent movement of the blades caused by finger actuation (10–13). Electrically operated scissors are heavier and have larger handles than pneumatic scissors. Some power scissors vibrate in operation, decreasing proprioception and precise control. There is no proprioceptive feedback from the physical properties of the tissue with current power scissors. Although proportional control systems (first developed for electric scissors by S. Charles and H. Grieshaber) for power scissors (pneumatic power scissors developed by Charles, Wang) are available, the authors usually prefer manual scissors. Power scissors prevent inadvertent scissors movement caused by finger actuation but are slower because of foot control and require precise engineering of the driver because scissors blades are manufactured by hand with resultant variability in dimensional tolerances.

Vacuum Cleaning/Extrusion

When an opening is made in the PVC, nonclotted blood, hemoglobin products, and erythroclasts tend to flow out the opening into the vitreous cavity. This is often falsely perceived as active bleeding and should be removed by vacuum cleaning/extrusion (Fig. 4.14) before continuing with PVC truncation, to ensure excellent visualization and avoid the flow of blood products to the lens, cornea, and trabecular meshwork.

The vacuum-cleaning method utilizes a blunt, end-opening cannula and a nonpulsatile, controlled pressure gradient across the needle port. Keeping the cannula away from the infusion port minimizes turbulence. If console controlled, this method has been referred to as "extrusion" (O'Malley). The key to understanding extrusion is to remember these features: (a) relatively high flow; (b) low, precisely controlled pressure gradient; (c) nonpulsatile; and (d) end-opening. The original and now obsolete form of vacuum cleaning

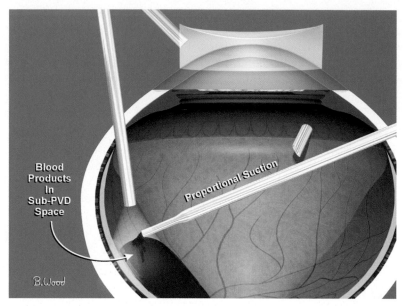

FIG. 4.14. After making an opening in the PVC, sub-PVD blood products should be removed with vacuum cleaning/extrusion before continuing with PVC truncation.

utilized the flute needle (Charles), in which egress is controlled by the surgeon's forefinger over the exit port on the side of the handle (14). This has been incorrectly termed *passive egress*. Whether these techniques are considered "active" or "passive" is irrelevant; precise control of transorifice pressure is the key concept. The extrusion method utilizes a 20-gauge, end-opening cannula, vitreous cutter, or end-aspirating laser probe connected to the console-based suction system, with foot control by the surgeon (15–17). Proportional (linear) suction control allows greater control over the extrusion process and has supplanted flute needle vacuum cleaning. Proportional suction applied to a cannula is very effective for removing blood products, substances to be exchanged, and subretinal fluid. Extrusion allows for reflux using the Accurus foot pedal.

Vacuum cleaning/extrusion should be utilized only when there is a region of nonclotted blood in the vitreous cavity, in the sub-PVD space, or on the retinal surface. The cannula should never touch the vitreous or retinal surface but may be held very close to the retina if the transorifice pressure is kept low. Intentionally lowered IOP can be used to induce bleeding, so that the source of the hemorrhage can be located and treated.

The Chang end-aspirating endolaser probe is ideal for removal of preretinal blood and active bleeding while treating surface bleeders in diabetic cases.

FLUID/AIR EXCHANGE

Before vitrectomy, air/gas surface tension management consisted of the injection of a relatively small intravitreal air/gas bubble. With the advent of vitreous removal, it became possible to exchange the entire intraocular fluid component for air/gas. Although the word *tamponade* implies "plugging," many surgeons mistakenly believe that the main role of intraocular air/gas is to push the retina into contact with the retinal pigment epithelium (RPE). The pushing effect of a bubble, due to buoyancy, is relatively insignificant compared with its retinal break sealing effect from interfacial (surface) tension. Intraocular air/gas is usually of little use if there are no retinal breaks. In cases of traction detachment or epimacular membrane, gas neither "flattens out" retinal folds nor causes more rapid disappearance of SRF. The phrase "no tear, no air" can be a helpful in remembering this concept.

Rhegmatogenous detachment can be defined as the elimination of the normal transretinal pressure gradient because of transbreak fluid flow. The immediate goal in rhegmatogenous detachment repair is to arrest transbreak flow; this is accomplished by either utilizing surface tension management via air/gas, perfluorocarbon liquids (PFCL), or silicone or by bringing about retina/RPE near contact through direct relief of traction or indirectly by scleral buckling.

Air Versus Other Gases

Intraoperatively, air has the same properties as any other gas; the differences become apparent only in the postoperative course. If sulfur hexafluoride (SF_6) (18–23) is used in a concentration exceeding 25%, it will cause postoperative expansion of the bubble. Expansion is of value in certain cases of scleral buckling without vitrectomy and in pneumatic retinopexy when only a small volume of gas can be injected. Expansion is both unnecessary and unsafe, however, with the total fill accomplished using internal fluid/gas exchange. SF_6 concentrations greater than 25% used in a total fill can result in expansion-induced central retinal artery occlusion. The peak expansion of SF_6 occurs 6 to 12 hours after injection (24–26). Therefore an IOP check cannot be put off until the morning after surgery; vascular occlusion and blindness will already have occurred. The same concepts apply to C_3F_8 except that the isoexpansive concentration is approximately 18%.

If nitrous oxide is used for inhalation anesthesia, it must be turned off at least 10 minutes before air or gas injection and remain off for the duration of the operation. If a bubble equilibrates with the gas dissolved in blood when there is nitrous oxide in the blood, the bubble will undergo considerable size reduction and therefore hypotony when the gas is turned off. Conversely, if nitrous oxide enters the blood when a bubble is already present, it will induce significant bubble expansion, causing significant and potentially dangerous increased IOP.

LONGER-ACTING GASES

Perfluorocarbon gases have been used for durations of 2 to 6 weeks (27–33). Three weeks (C_3F_8) appears ideal because this coincides with the maximum tensile strength of retinopexy scars. Inflammatory capsules have developed around bubbles, especially with the longer-acting gases and postoperative reinjections. Durations longer than 3 weeks are extremely difficult for the patient because of positioning requirements.

Methods of Fluid/Air Exchange

Sequential (External)

Sequential fluid/air/gas exchange (also called "single needle" or "external") was the original method (34), but it is almost never used now. This method started with removal of intraocular fluid using a needle and syringe, followed by turning a stopcock attached to the syringe to allow the injection of air/gas. Disadvantages include incomplete exchange, hypotony, bubbles, poor visualization during injection, and the dangerous combination of ocular collapse, a sharp intraocular needle, and inadvertent syringe movement while turning the stopcock.

Simultaneous (Internal) Fluid/Air Exchange

With simultaneous or internal fluid/air exchange, air is injected into the eye through one opening (infusion cannula or "up" needle in the office) while fluid is removed through another opening such as the soft-tip cannula in the operating room or a second "down" needle in the office. A total air or air/gas fill is thus possible, and hypotony and ocular collapse are avoided. The elimination of ocular collapse reduces bleeding and permits better visualization and safety. Equally important is the ability to produce an isoexpansive total fill without the impossibility of guessing the correct volume of gas to inject if expansion is anticipated.

Full-Function Probe

Internal fluid/air/gas exchange was developed while using full-function probes (S. Charles developed, unpublished data, 1973). The air was injected through the infusion port while allowing the fluid to leave the eye through the suction system, which was left open to the atmosphere. Because full-function probes are obsolete, this fluid/gas exchange method is no longer used.

Coaxial Cannula

While using the preceding method, it was noted that the incoming gas was breaking into small bubbles, which collected under the lens or cornea and hindered visualization. To correct this, a coaxial cannula was designed (35), matching the probe in size but with the infusion port separated from the egress port and located near the pars plana. A single bubble would be formed initially, into which all subsequent injection would occur. This method has also become outdated with the obsolescence of full-function probes and the use of sew-on infusion cannulas.

Two-Needle Method

After a vitrectomy has been performed it is possible to perform fluid/air/gas exchange using two-needle technique. This method is utilized primarily in the office environment with the patient positioned on his or her side. The "up" needle is used for injection and the "down" needle for egress. The needles are inserted just through the eye wall, not deep into the eye, in order to eliminate multiple small bubbles.

Infusion Cannula Method

The sew-on infusion cannula system permits injection of air anteriorly in the supine patient so that a subsequent injection occurs into the original bubble (36). Multiple small bubbles that limit visualization are avoided. The fluid is removed through a cannula (S. Charles, 1976) controlled by the proportional (linear) suction system and placed behind the fluid/gas interface (Fig. 4.15). The flute needle is obsolete because of poor IOP control and inadvertent movement while controlling the fluid egress port with a fingertip. Injection should be continued until the fluid/gas interface reaches the infusion cannula. Placing the cannula in the angle recess to momentarily drain the chamber early in the exchange can often prevent a flat chamber. Small bubbles can be removed with the cannula so that a single bubble fills the eye. If the anterior chamber becomes flat it should usually be allowed to remain flat; immediate postoperative facedown repositioning will almost always correct the problem.

The air can be injected into the eye by a syringe operated by the assistant, but an air pump is preferred (37). Air pumps should be used rather than syringes because they handle large-volume wound leaks, allow accurate control of IOP, and eliminate syringe refill

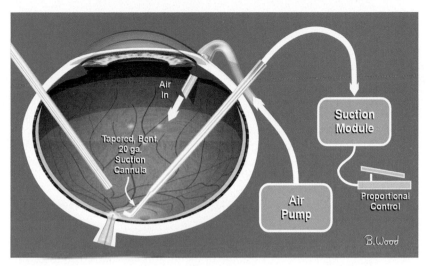

FIG. 4.15. Simultaneous fluid/air exchange should utilize the infusion cannula and a tapered, bent cannula attached to proportional suction. Multiple small bubbles that limit visualization are avoided, and a total air/gas fill can be achieved.

delays and soft eyes (38). Advanced vitrectomy systems such as the Alcon Accurus integrate the air pump into the system.

Air/Gas Exchange

At the end of the procedure, air/gas exchange should be used if long-acting gases are required (Fig. 4.16). Air/gas exchange is better than injecting small aliquots of gas into

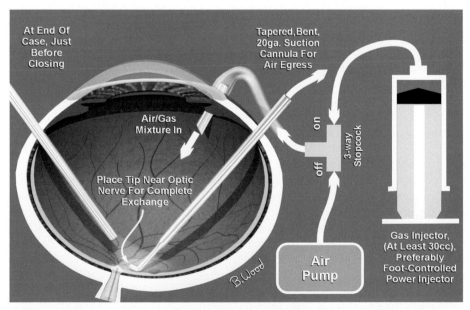

FIG. 4.16. Air/gas exchange produces a precise concentration of the long-acting gases, reducing postoperative variations in bubble size and IOP.

an air bubble because it produces a precise concentration of gas, preventing postoperative variance in bubble size and IOP. Air/gas exchange allows complete exchange of air for a precise air/gas mixture. The assistant preferably should observe the fundus through an observer tube on the operating microscope to inject gas safely.

A foot-controlled, reversible, variable-speed, motorized gas injector (Charles, Wang) offers much better control than the manual syringe drive (39), but it is not commercially available. This device offers the benefits of controlled pressure injection and allows control by the surgeon instead of the assistant. Pressure transducers and a solenoid pinch valve limit the maximum injection pressure and vacuum. The Alcon Accurus Viscous Fluid Controller (VFC) may be adapted to the injection of air/gas mixtures in the future.

The Use of the Infusion System for Pressure Control

When fluid/air exchange has been completed, the infusion cannula and air-filled tubing are left connected to the air pump. If leaks occur or as SRF is drained, IOP and volume are stabilized by air infusion. Leakage or aspiration is required to lower the IOP as a buckle is tightened because air pumps do not permit retrograde flow. A sew-on infusion cannula in conjunction with an air pump permits an accuracy of IOP control not possible without vitrectomy and makes possible the use of large scleral buckles without consequent high IOP. The cannula should be put in at the beginning of the procedure and removed only to permit closure of the conjunctiva at the end of the operation. The phrase "first in, last out" may serve as a reminder of correct infusion cannula practice. It should only be turned off if there is concern that it has become subretinal or suprachoroidal or is causing retinal, vitreous, or iris prolapse.

Phakic Versus Aphakic

The lens should be removed in many vitrectomies for PVR, giant breaks, and trauma. On occasion it is necessary to utilize air/gas in a phakic eye. Optically, the air/lens interface requires a convex, minifying contact lens (Landers) to view the fundus with the operating microscope. Gas/lens contact for a few days will cause a transient posterior subcapsular cataract; contact for a longer period will cause a permanent cataract. Postoperative facedown positioning is particularly critical in gas cases.

If fluid/air exchange is necessary in phakic or pseudophakic eyes, the extrusion cannula should be positioned about just above the optic nerve and away from mobile retina. Air is then injected with the air pump through the infusion cannula until it begins coming through the extrusion cannula. A minus 90D or equivalent, concave/concave contact lens (40) is then used to visualize the fundus in conjunction with the operating microscope while completing the exchange.

If the contact lens is not available due to breakage or contamination, indirect ophthalmoscopy must be utilized. The endoilluminator is then removed from the eye and the wound plugged with a scleral plug. Although the apparent reverse motion makes this procedure difficult, it permits total fluid/gas exchange and internal drainage of SRF in the phakic eye. When used with proportional suction, air pump infusion, and the surgeon seated on a stable stool, it is reasonably safe.

Air/gas exchange should be performed just before wound closure, with the gas syringe operated by the assistant and a cannula or vitreous cutter connected to proportional suction for air removal. This permits complete exchange of air with an accurate concentration of long-acting gas, thus avoiding the possibility of small bubbles or increased intraocular pressure postoperatively. An isoexpansive total fill is routinely achieved with this approach.

Vitrectomy Under Air

Certain portions of the vitreous surgery procedure can be completed after fluid/air exchange (see Chapter 7) (S. Charles, unpublished data, 1974). At times, continuous severe bleeding cannot be controlled with combined extrusion and bipolar diathermy or endophotocoagulation. If internal fluid/air exchange is performed in such an instance, the bubble will confine the blood to a small space so that visualization and diathermy or endophotocoagulation of the vessel can be completed.

Forceps membrane peeling, scissors segmentation and delamination, subretinal surgery, retinectomy, laser endophotocoagulation, and foreign-body removal can be performed under air if it is not an aphakic eye with striate keratopathy. Fogging of intraocular lenses is a serious limitation of this method. The authors refrigerate the BSS Plus before all vitrectomies except those with intraocular lenses because hypothermia reduces inflammation, ischemic damage, endothelial damage, pupil constriction, and light toxicity. Silicone lenses fog much more than acrylic or PMMA lenses. Prior YAG capsulectomy and intraoperative removal of the AVC creates the fogging problem. Intraocular lenses fog because they have significant thermal inertia, they are cooled by room temperature infusion fluid, and the air in the eye is saturated with water vapor. Viscoelastics can be injected against the posterior surface of the lens to reduce fogging, but this creates a morphed image, increases cost, and increases silicone emulsification. The authors use a soft-tip cannula as a windshield wiper until the procedure is completed or the fogging abates. PFC liquids can eliminate this problem by facilitating removal of SRF and performing endophotocoagulation without an air exchange.

Because prolonged contact with air is damaging to the cornea and lens, operating under air should be reserved for situations that cannot be handled in a more conventional manner. Air in contact with a cornea with striate keratopathy results in a very poor view.

Postoperative Positioning

In all cases in which air/gas injection has been performed, the patient must remain face down until the bubble has decreased to approximately 10% of the ocular volume. It is crucial that the patient be in a prone seated position; face down on pillows on a bedside table. In cases of inferior retinal tears, prone positioning is essential but it can lead to greater lid swelling, chemosis, and possibly a small hyphema on the central corneal endothelium. Patients with temporal or nasal breaks only can lie on their side with the break side up.

Making an analogy to a "cast on a broken arm" can enhance patient acceptance. Phrases like "put the bubble on the trouble" and "longer-duration bubbles cause higher success rates" help the patient gain understanding. Numerous pillows facilitate comfortable positioning. A comparison can be made to sleeping with crossed arms on a school desk and a table at home used with a pillow for padding. Wingback chairs and sofas are similar to the car, bus, or airplane seating position and can be used to explain the required position. Some doctors recommend expensive special chairs or support systems, which the authors believe to be unnecessary in most cases. These devices require immobility, which increases muscle cramping and psychologic stress.

The reduced atmospheric pressures intrinsic to air travel or ground travel to higher altitudes dictate marked caution when a bubble is present. Bubble expansion from air travel causes a severe increase in IOP and can cause vascular occlusion (41,42). Air travel is best prohibited in all gas cases, although clinically it has been stated that a bubble less than 10% of ocular volume can be tolerated. Ocular hypotensive drugs such as carbonic anhydrase inhibitors may be used prophylactically or given to the patient to take if pain occurs. Ground travel should be used to prevent this severe problem. Patients should be cautioned to avoid rapid ground travel from low to high altitudes.

Air/Silicone Exchange

Because silicone has much less interfacial tension than gas (air), internal drainage of SRF, then fluid/air exchange, then completion of internal drainage of SRF should always precede air/silicone exchange. Fluid/silicone exchange is unnecessary and more difficult to visualize. Because high viscosity causes very high injection forces, a Leveen screw-driven syringe or power injector (Wang and others, Accurus VFC) should be used. An air pump is ideal to control the IOP during silicone injection. An extrusion cannula in the anterior chamber just behind the IOL allows air removal and pressure control. Preferably a short, blunt 18- to 20-gauge cannula or alternatively a special sew-on cannula with a short tubing segment built to withstand high pressure can be used to infuse the oil (Fig. 4.17). Injection forces are higher with 5,000-cs oil than 1,000-cs oil.

Nomenclature for Exchanges

The authors suggest that exchanges be named by first stating the current material in the eye, followed by the substance to be injected. For example, fluid/air exchange means injecting air while aspirating fluid. The authors always perform fluid/air exchange before

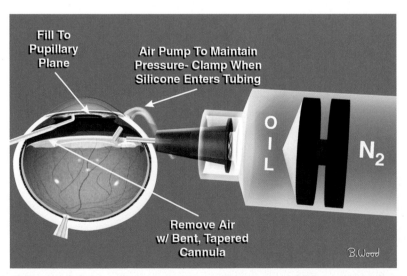

FIG. 4.17. Following fluid/air exchange and internal drainage of SRF, special high-pressure injection systems are used to infuse silicone oil. IOP is controlled via an air pump connected to the air infusion cannula, and by varying the proportional vacuum on the bent, tapered suction cannula for air egress.

air/gas or air/silicone exchange. A typical procedure can be described as fluid/air/gas or fluid/air/silicone exchange. An exchange does not imply drainage of subretinal fluid; thus this step must be described separately.

Subretinal Fluid Removal

Indications for Drainage of Subretinal Fluid

The debate over the necessity of drainage of subretinal fluid has raged for years and will not be settled by this book. Drainage of subretinal fluid is essential in difficult retinal detachment cases because it instantaneously determines the need for subsequent surgical steps. It is not always possible for even the most experienced surgeons to correctly determine the exact steps to accomplish retinal reattachment from the preoperative examination. The author (SC) refers to subretinal fluid drainage with fluid/air exchange as the "reattachment experiment" because it frequently helps determine the need for further vitreous removal, peeling, segmentation, delamination, retinectomy, or scleral buckling.

Removal of virtually all subretinal fluid before fluid/air/gas or fluid/air/silicone exchange increases the likelihood of injection of the correct volume of isoexpansive gas mixtures or silicone oil. It is virtually impossible for the surgeon to accurately estimate the volume of the subretinal space or vitreous cavity. Expanding gas mixtures should not be used with total fluid/gas exchange because of the risk of central retinal artery occlusion due to high pressure. Similarly, if the volume of isoexpansive gas or silicone oil required is overestimated, central retinal artery occlusion can result. If the volume of gas or oil is underestimated, the area of contact with the surface tension management agent may be insufficient, causing the procedure to fail.

The principal author introduced the concept of internal (transretinal) drainage of subretinal fluid and post reattachment retinopexy in 1973. Before that time, retinopexy was performed before the vitrectomy, and expanding gas bubbles were used to slowly reattach the retina postoperatively. Post reattachment retinopexy probably reduces dispersion of retinal and RPE cells, potentially reducing PVR recurrences. Post reattachment retinopexy allows accurately placed, controlled-intensity retinopexy to the retina as well as the RPE. Overtreatment is a significant factor in PVR recurrences and fibrin syndrome.

Internal drainage methods and exchanges allow the benefits of post reattachment retinopexy, accurate air, gas and silicone volumes, and the reattachment experiment to be used on a routine basis.

External Versus Internal Drainage

External drainage of subretinal fluid requires an opening through the sclera, choroid, and RPE. In contrast, internal or transretinal drainage requires no eye wall incision if used in the context of vitrectomy. Internal drainage enables total drainage of the SRF, prevents incarceration of retina in the sclera, prevents choroidal bleeding, reduces RPE damage, and is faster and easier during vitrectomy.

Direct Needle Transscleral Drainage of Subretinal Fluid

The principal author developed direct (transscleral) needle drainage of subretinal fluid to reduce the complications of the scleral cutdown method. Direct needle drainage has been shown in a randomized trail (Cairns) to eliminate the problem of retinal incarceration in the drain site (greater than 3% with the scleral cutdown method), allow more complete drainage, and reduce hypotony; without adding any complications. Direct needle drainage of subretinal fluid can be performed through the conjunctiva, a buckle, or a choroidal detachment (edema). This method is performed using a 25- to 27-gauge, 0.5-inch, disposable needle on a tuberculin syringe with the plunger removed. A transparent needle hub (such as Monoject) is preferred because it allows early visualization of fluid egress (43). A site is selected that has the highest retinal detachment by viewing through the operating microscope using the endoilluminator and contact lens. Indirect ophthalmoscopy can be used if an operating microscope is not being utilized. The bevel of the needle is always oriented away from the retina to prevent retinal entrapment. The tip of the needle is kept away from the sclera by intentional "shanking" until the entry point is located. The needle is then oriented in a more tangential manner and advanced slowly through the sclera until a slight proprioceptive "pop" is felt (Fig. 4.18). At this point a brown pencil point–like structure may be seen in the subretinal space, which is the RPE stretched over the needle tip. The needle is then advanced slightly under direct visualization through the RPE until the silvery sheen of the needle is seen under the retina (Fig. 4.19). At this point the retina begins to tremble due to turbulence in the needle lumen. The needle cannot be visualized if the subretinal fluid is turbid, but the trembling of the retina will indicate fluid egress. The needle should be angulated slightly to place it tangential to the retina after the initial placement. The needle should be held immobile until all the subretinal fluid is gone (Fig. 4.20). Pigment typically comes through the needle hub as the last fluid drains.

Conventional Transscleral Drainage of Subretinal Fluid

The customary method of draining SRF is to make a cutdown incision through the sclera and then puncture the choroid and RPE. This method can result in intraocular hemorrhage or retinal incarceration. If fluid/air exchange precedes SRF drainage, the bubble causes lateral displacement of the retina with posterior displacement of the SRF. It is

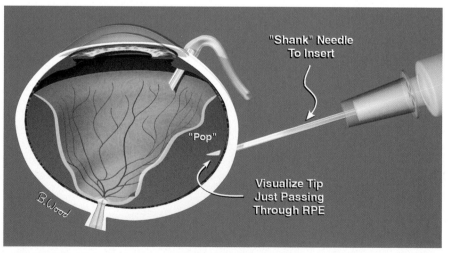

FIG. 4.18. Direct needle drainage of subretinal fluid is initiated by inserting a 27-gauge 0.5-in. needle (attached to a tuberculin syringe with the plunger removed) through the sclera at the highest point of retinal detachment, until a "pop" is felt.

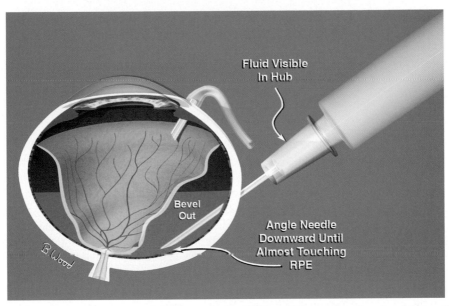

FIG. 4.19. The needle is advanced through the RPE until it can be visualized beneath the retina and SRF appears in the needle hub. This is accompanied by undulations of the retina, due to turbulence in the needle lumen.

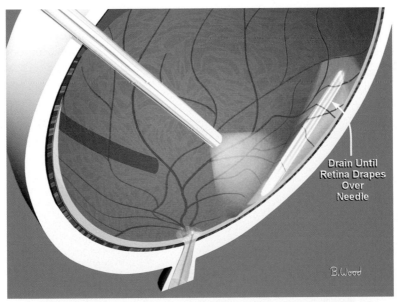

FIG. 4.20. The needle should be held immobile until all SRF is drained, and the retina drapes over the needle. Pigment typically presents in the hub when this is accomplished.

therefore quite easy to incarcerate retina when the customary equatorial external drainage site is used. Using very posterior drainage sites, rotating the eye to place the fluid in the dependent position, and using scleral depression to shift the posterior fluid to the drainage site may prevent incarceration. If retinal breaks are not present, external drainage can precede fluid/gas exchange.

Internal Drainage of Subretinal Fluid

The first internal aspiration of subretinal fluid was performed by Cibis (44) during scleral buckling for giant break cases and was followed by reinjection in front of the retina. The principal author used the vitreous cutter to drain subretinal fluid through a retinal break in 1973 but soon developed a tapered cannula with a 20-gauge shank and a 25-gauge tip. It was found that bending the tip to approximately a 135° angle facilitated entry through small breaks into the subretinal space. In 1981 the principal author developed a cannulated extrusion needle but felt that it increased complications by accidentally incarcerating retina or RPE. This work was not reported and Blumenkranz and Flynn later independently developed a cannulated extrusion needle with Grieshaber (Fig. 4.21), which has become popular. Grizzard subsequently developed soft-tipped needles (cannulas) (Fig. 4.22). The author (SC) has repeatedly evaluated and compared these alternatives to the tapered, angulated cannula and now prefers soft-tip cannulas. The advantages of soft-tip cannulas are reduced choroidal bleeding if inadvertent contact is made and the ability to cannulate the subretinal space and reduce incarceration of the retina in the port. Flexible cannulas are much safer in the context of patient movement with local anesthesia. The Chang end-aspirating laser probe is ideal for removal of subretinal fluid that shifts posteriorly during laser photocoagulation of retinal breaks or drainage retinotomy sites (Fig. 4.23).

The principal author developed the flute needle to control fluid egress in 1974. This concept is based on using the pressure gradient that exists between the intraocular pressure and atmospheric pressure to cause fluid egress. The resultant flow was modulated by

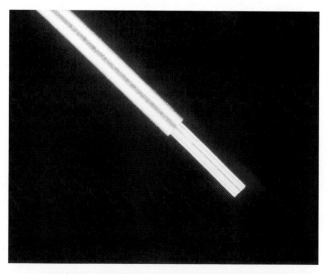

FIG. 4.21. Straight soft-tip extrusion cannula.

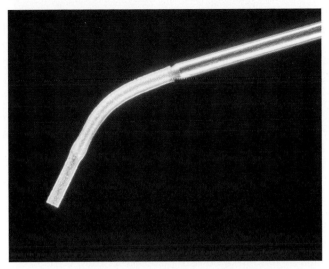

FIG. 4.22. Angulated soft-tip extrusion cannula.

the surgeon's fingertip partially covering a side port in the handle; hence the term *flute* (often incorrectly stated as *fluted*). Many incorrectly term this "passive egress" and incorrectly believe that it is somehow better than "active suction." The (SC) author developed this concept to avoid the pulsatile pressure gradient that is caused by the opening and closing of the vitreous cutter. The author also desired a low, constant pressure gradient, which could not be accomplished by an assistant-controlled syringe or early automated suction systems. O'Malley developed the concept of foot-controlled suction (extrusion) to replace the fingertip control of the flute needle. The advantage of foot control is that it provides a more constant pressure gradient and prevents inadvertent movement of the needle by the action of modulating the sideport with the fingertip. This later notion is similar to one of the primary reasons for use of powered scissors. The principal author

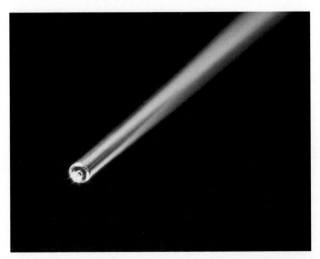

FIG. 4.23. Chang end-aspirating endophotocoagulation probe.

abandoned the flute needle in favor of the "extrusion method" soon after it was reported. The term *extrusion* is inappropriate because it means deforming a plastic material through an opening under pressure. This concept is better termed *foot-controlled suction,* but the term *extrusion* nevertheless enjoys widespread usage.

Drainage Retinotomy

Although one of the authors (SC) developed internal drainage of subretinal fluid and independently co-developed "relaxing" retinotomy/retinectomy, drainage retinotomies were infrequently used for many years. More recently, small drainage retinotomies have been utilized safely and effectively when the tear could not be adequately visualized because of miosis, posterior capsular opacification, lens remnants, or cataract. A small spot of diathermy can be made using the Two-Function Manipulator or disposable bipolar endoilluminator before making a small, round retinotomy with a single cut of the vitreous cutter. The hole should be made rather posterior, away from retinal vessels but outside the temporal arcades. The soft-tip cannula followed by the Chang End-Aspirating laser probe can then be used to drain all the subretinal fluid through the retinotomy.

Perfluorocarbon Liquids

Chang developed the use of perfluorocarbon liquids for use in vitreoretinal surgery. PFC liquids work because they are immiscible in water and their specific gravity is higher than water. The subretinal fluid simply floats out of the subretinal space through anterior retinal breaks or retinectomies. Occasionally some SRF may be forced anterior to the retinal breaks with this method. This method is essential for modern giant break repair, but it is unnecessary for many vitreoretinal cases. Perfluorocarbon liquids add cost to the procedure but are very helpful in certain situations. PFC liquids are somewhat difficult to remove, may end up in the subretinal space if the retina is stiff, and are toxic to the photoreceptors if allowed to remain in the subretinal space. Small droplets left behind after surgical removal usually cause no problems, but it is possible to remove PFC liquids at the slit lamp with a small needle through the inferior limbus. PFC liquids stabilize the retina, decreasing the anxiety that occurs when the retina moves during epiretinal membrane dissection. PFC liquids float the retina upward if a giant break or large retinectomy is present because the retina is less dense than PFC liquids. PFC is being utilized more frequently by the authors for short-term (7 to 10 days) treatment of recurrent, inferior retinal detachments and giant breaks.

Drainage of Subretinal Fluid Through Peripheral Breaks

The conventional algorithm for vitreoretinal surgery for retinal detachment begins with vitrectomy, then fluid/air exchange, then internal drainage of subretinal fluid, followed by retinopexy. The authors (and the late Ron Michels) strongly advocate performing internal drainage of SRF before fluid/air exchange. The highly viscous subretinal fluid will then be diluted and a drainage pathway will be established for posterior fluid to drain through small, peripheral breaks. Typically the retina will become much more concave but fluid will flow through retinal breaks until air is introduced for surface tension management. It is always necessary to perform further drainage of subretinal fluid during and after fluid/air exchange. If fluid/air exchange precedes internal drainage of SRF, SRF will be forced posteriorly, which may cause an otherwise unnecessary drainage retinotomy.

Internal drainage is performed by placing the soft-tip cannula through the retinal break until it is near, but not touching, the RPE. The internal drainage is continued and the infusion is switched from fluid to air after the retina stops becoming more concave. Bubbles may impair visualization of the cannula briefly during the early phase of fluid/air exchange, making it essential to hold the cannula immobile. As the air level moves posteriorly, the bubbles will coalesce, improving the view.

The Reattachment Experiment

Internal (simultaneous) fluid/air exchange combined with internal drainage of SRF is an excellent test for relief of traction on the retina. This can be thought of as the reattachment experiment. If after this procedure the retina does not completely attach, further vitreous removal, forceps membrane peeling, scissors segmentation, scissors delamination, subretinal surgery, retinectomy, or scleral buckling is necessary. Surface tension stabilizes the retina and allows visualization of mechanical factors preventing reattachment. If all these techniques fail, this test serves to indicate inoperability.

If subretinal air appears, it is indicative of residual traction that must be treated as outlined earlier. Direct needle drainage of SRF posterior to a just imbricated scleral buckle will also remove subretinal air.

Total intraoperative reattachment eliminates postoperative questions concerning leakage through the tear or rate of RPE pumping of SRF. In addition, retinopexy performed after reattachment allows for more precise localization, less risk of RPE migration, and treatment of the retina as well as the RPE, ensuring better adherence. The guesswork method of using a small expanding bubble without completion of SRF drainage leaves many questions unanswered at the time of vitrectomy and consequently lowers the success rate.

ENDODIATHERMY

Although neovascularization is frequently encountered in diabetic vitrectomy, intraoperative bleeding is seldom of great consequence. Because endodiatherms can cause tissue shrinkage, retinal breaks, nerve fiber layer damage, and optic atrophy, it should be reserved for vessels that are to be transected or that actually bleed during surgery. When extensive networks of neovascularization are associated with ERM, it is best to control bleeding during the dissection by using transient elevation of IOP. Vascular attachment points can then be treated as needed with endodiatherms. Frequently, those networks have only a few connections to the retinal arterial system, which are only recognized and treated after delamination of the ERM.

Every attempt should be made to prevent and control bleeding; blood can form a substrate and stimulus for postoperative cellular proliferation. As it is not always possible to safely control bleeding, it is fortunate that the aphakic, vitrectomized eye rapidly clears postoperative hemorrhage.

Elevated new vessels are best coagulated with diathermy. Unipolar diathermy, which was used originally, has been supplanted by bipolar diathermy because of the latter's greater safety (45,46). If unipolar diathermy is applied near the optic nerve, radio frequency energy can travel through the optic nerve, causing optic atrophy and permanent blindness. Unimanual bipolar diathermy (UBD) functions well if care is taken to maintain at least 1 mm distance from the optic nerve. By controlling bleeding with transient increases in IOP, UBD can be very effective in treating vascular attachment points.

Bimanual bipolar diathermy (BBD) (47) can function through any two intraocular instruments or one intraocular and one extraocular instrument by the simple attachment of unshielded wires and clips. Insulated microclips or connectors in the instrument handles (Charles, Grieshaber) can be used. This method has been largely supplanted by the multi-function manipulators. The Alcon/Grieshaber Two or Three Function Manipulators or Alcon/Infinitec disposable bipolar endoilluminator combine diathermy with the endoilluminator and, optionally, a lumen. This device is ideal for coagulating vascular attachment points during delamination as well as segmentation of ERM. Bipolar diathermy on a multifunction manipulator is typically utilized in conjunction with the vitreous cutter or extrusion. It is unnecessary to interrupt the procedure in order to place a specialized instrument in the eye, and bleeding can be washed away continuously to permit excellent visualization of the bleeding vessel during dissection. By intentionally allowing the IOP to become very low, bleeding can be stimulated so that its source can be identified and coagulated. Although bipolar diathermy can be used for retinopexy, there is little effect at the RPE level. Endophotocoagulation is better suited to retinopexy than is endodiathermy.

Laser Endophotocoagulation

Xenon arc light energy can be delivered to the retinal surface with the endophotocoagulator (Charles et al.). The prototype was an adaptor to the Zeiss xenon photocoagulator. The first commercial endophotocoagulator was an adapter to the Clinitex Log III portable xenon arc photocoagulator (48). A xenon endophotocoagulator has high beam divergence and reliability problems and is no longer used by most surgeons.

Laser endophotocoagulation was developed later (Peyman, Fleischman, Charles, and Landers, independently) and is preferable to xenon because of less beam divergence, better reliability, and more rapid firing. Virtually all compact, laser photocoagulator systems can be utilized for endophotocoagulation.

Near IR (infrared) diode lasers (Tano) are 20% to 30% efficient in converting electrical to light energy in contrast to ion lasers (argon) at 0.0001% or less. For this reason they use standard electrical power instead of high-current, three-phase power. Because of their efficiency, they are far more reliable, are more compact, and do not require water cooling. The near IR wavelength is the major disadvantage of these lasers because it is much more difficult to judge the correct power threshold and the lesion is deeper.

Diode-pumped, frequency YAG up-converted, continuous, 532-nm lasers are ideal for all operating room and most office photocoagulation. They have all the previously described advantages of diode laser but use an ideal wavelength for hemoglobin absorption and xanthophyll avoidance.

The endophotocoagulator is used primarily for the treatment of bleeding from surface neovascularization, retinopexy, and panretinal photocoagulation (PRP). Endophotocoagulation should only be used for surface bleeding from specific sites, usually after scissors delamination of ERMs. When using the endophotocoagulator, the endoilluminator is usually held in the opposite hand to provide diffuse illumination. Illuminating laser probes (Chang) have been developed to solve this problem. When there is acute bleeding, it is recommended that the suction cannula or vitreous cutter be alternated with the laser probe to remove blood and facilitate precise coagulation. The aspirating endophotocoagulator probe (Chang) can be used to aspirate subretinal fluid and blood during endophotocoagulation.

The endophotocoagulator is well suited for PRP concomitant with vitreous surgery for diabetic retinopathy, venous occlusive disease, hemoglobinopathies, and teleangectasia. As discussed in the chapter on diabetic retinopathy (see Chapter 5), endo-PRP can bring about a decreased incidence of neovascular glaucoma and anterior vitreous cortex fibrovascular proliferation. The only limitation of endophotocoagulation is that elevated retina cannot be treated.

In contrast to endocryopexy, endophotocoagulation is a noncontact method. Therefore dispersion of RPE cells, choroidal bleeding, retinal tears, and the increased wound size associated with endocryopexy are avoided. Endophotocoagulation lesions are between 600 and 1,000 μm in diameter, depending on the distance from the tip of the probe to the retinal surface, the beam divergence, and the power setting. If the retina is detached, endophotocoagulation must be preceded by fluid/air exchange and internal drainage of SRF, which bring the retina and RPE into contact to permit energy absorption. For focal treatment of retinal breaks, the continuous mode is utilized to treat in a confluent manner ("painting") around the breaks. This technique minimizes the possibility of undertreatment or overtreatment, which frequently occurs with the placement of discrete photocoagulation spots in rows. Periodically during treatment, small amounts of SRF will shift posteriorly, making repeated internal drainage necessary to permit retinopexy. Chang has developed a probe with end aspiration to facilitate removal of reaccumulating SRF simultaneously or alternately with application of laser energy. The principal author uses the Chang probe for all retinopexy in the presence of retinal breaks and retinal detachment.

The endophotocoagulator should never be utilized in air/gas when there is blood on its tip, or damage to the probe may result. Pan-retinal photocoagulation under air to areas of retina that had been detached before surgery is a common cause of fibrin syndrome.

A microscope filter attenuates the laser energy in the optic path of the operating microscope during endophotocoagulation and ensures continued dark adaptation and safety. The fovea and optic nerve must be avoided, and all treatment must be initiated at low energy with stepwise increases until the desired effect is achieved.

The endophotocoagulator can be used to dilate the pupil by treating the posterior surface of the iris sphincter. Endophotocorepexy is of special use when iris neovascularization prohibits sphincterotomy with the vitrectomy instrument. The ciliary processes can be endophotocoagulated in glaucoma cases, with subsequent decrease in pressure.

The principal author first reported endocyclophotocoagulation but is concerned that it is significantly overutilized by cataract surgeons in conjunction with phakoemulsification. Many glaucoma experts share this concern based on the observation that the apparent benefits are short term and CME increases.

RETINOPEXY

All retinal breaks, except macular holes, peripapillary breaks, and retinotomies for submacular surgery, should be treated with some form of retinopexy. This policy is necessary because of the impossibility of predicting which retinal break will result in detachment, and it is justified because of the relative safety of retinopexy.

Although it may be contrary to the tendency of the scleral buckling surgeon, retinopexy should be used only after vitrectomy, surgical dissection, and internal drainage of SRF, fluid/air exchange, and completion of SRF drainage have reattached the retina. Performed at the beginning of the operation, retinopexy may cause choroidal hemorrhage due to the combination of engorged choroidal vessels. Post reattachment retinopexy will ensure better visualization, so that all breaks can be identified and iatrogenic breaks can be treated simultaneously. Completion of internal fluid/gas exchange and internal drainage of SRF will confine any RPE cells mobilized by retinopexy to the area of the break and possibly decrease the incidence of PVR.

Transscleral cryopexy in vitrectomy has long been replaced by transscleral diathermy, transscleral diode laser retinopexy, and more typically, laser endophotocoagulation. Cryopexy disperses live RPE and glial cells and causes more inflammation and PVR.

Endocryopexy is an unsafe, contact-based method that requires an enlarged opening and is fortunately no longer used by most surgeons. This method causes increased cellular proliferation and choroidal hemorrhages. As discussed previously, endophotocoagulation now performs the tasks formerly handled by endocryopexy. Endophotocoagulation is used far more commonly than transscleral retinopexy. Transscleral retinopexy is used primarily for scleral buckling without vitrectomy.

Diathermy

Transscleral diathermy probably creates less proliferation than cryopexy but causes more scleral damage. It can be used with fiberoptic transillumination to find and treat any breaks, except in the macular and peripapillary area. The small probe fits under buckles more easily than a cryoprobe.

Because of the thermal and electrical insulating properties of an air/gas bubble, diathermy causes larger retinal lesions and less scleral damage in an air/gas-filled eye than in a fluid-filled eye. Endophotocoagulation is preferred in almost all instances.

INTRAOPERATIVE FLUORESCEIN ANGIOSCOPY

Intravenous sodium fluorescein dye (3.0 mL of 25%) can be administered during vitreous surgery after the retina is visualized (Charles, unpublished data, 1974). The dye can then be made to fluoresce by putting a fluorescent interference-type exciter filter in the path of the endoilluminator light source. The sources of bleeding, especially in reoperation, can be readily identified. Many vitrectomy consoles have such filters in the light sources, which can be readily moved into the light path.

WOUND CLOSURE AND POSTOPERATIVE MEDICATION

Wound Closure

Cryopexy, diathermy, or thermal cautery should not be applied to pars plana incisions. These modalities damage the sclera and predispose it to poor healing, poor closure, and tissue ingrowth. Any form of retinopexy is inappropriate at pars plana sites because the sites are anterior to the retina. If there is excessive bleeding, minimal bipolar diathermy can be applied, but an instrument through the wound or closure by the suture will stop most bleeding. Absorbable sutures are not used in the sclera by the authors because their inelasticity facilitates wound leakage during the operation, postoperatively, and during reoperations. The principal author has observed many filtering blebs from the use of absorbable sutures by other surgeons. Wound leaks may cause hypotony and predispose to tissue ingrowth. The tightest closure is achieved with running shoelace 8-0 monofilament nylon sutures (Fig. 4.24). A running suture can be placed more rapidly than interrupted sutures, equalizes the tensions between loops, and has fewer ends to protrude through the

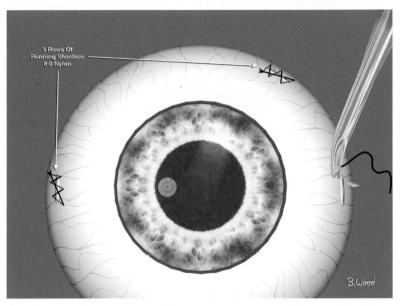

FIG. 4.24. Running shoelace 8-0 monofilament nylon sutures achieve rapid closure with even tension, fewer filtering blebs, and fewer ends to protrude through the conjunctiva.

conjunctiva. The ends should be cut right on the knot with a disposable small blade under operating microscope visualization by moving the suture toward the blade. The ends can be buried in the wound to prevent conjunctival erosion, but this makes a watertight wound more difficult to attain.

CONJUNCTIVA AND TENON'S CAPSULE

The conjunctiva and Tenon's capsule are closed with interrupted 6-0 plain gut or equivalent sutures trimmed on the knot in a single layer. The Tenon's capsule should not be sutured to the muscle insertions because this decreases the lid fissure, limits ocular motility postoperatively, and makes reoperation more difficult. Longer-lasting sutures are very irritating to the patient and are unnecessary. Conjunctival closure with bipolar diathermy can cause conjunctival shrinkage and fistulas, and is less secure than suturing.

Injection of Antibiotics and Steroids

Before conjunctival closure, antibiotics and repository steroid are injected near the sclera, posteriorly using a flexible cannula. Use of a retrobulbar cannula eliminates the chance of scleral perforation, increases the dose to the posterior segment, reduces steroid glaucoma, reduces pain, and prevents runoff from the conjunctival perforation. Antibiotics effective against Gram-positive penicillinase producers and Gram-negative organisms are used (Ancef and ceftriaxone [Rocephin 100 mg in 0.3 mL]). This use of antibiotics is necessary with the extensive amount of tubing connections, instrumentation, and irrigating fluid utilized in vitreous surgery. It is thought, however, that the myelinolytic effect of aminoglycoside antibiotics may contribute to an occasional transient neuritis-like facial pain after surgery. This lasts several weeks, can be managed medically, and always disappears. Most "scleral buckle pain" is probably caused by this mechanism.

A subconjunctival repository steroid (triamcinolone acetonide 40 mg in 0.5 mL or Celestone 8 mg) is injected in every case unless the patient is an infant, has a macular hole, or is known to be a steroid glaucoma responder. Retrobulbar injections are more effective than systemic or topical steroids and are medically safer than systemic steroids.

SUMMARY

This chapter provides a discussion of the basic building blocks of successful posterior vitrectomy. Each step must be understood and the proper equipment must be available so that complications or unexpected findings can be managed safely, rapidly, and effectively. Even the infrequent vitreous surgeon who tries to limit himself or herself to "easier" cases can find the unexpected and is obliged to use these "advanced" techniques to safely complete the surgery. Implicit in understanding the building blocks is using them in the appropriate sequence.

REFERENCES

1. O'Malley C, Heintz RM. Vitrectomy via the pars plana, a new instrument system. *Trans Pac Coast Otoophthalmol Soc* 1972;53:121.
2. Edelhauser HF, Hyndiuk RA, Zeeb A, et al. Corneal edema and the use of epinephrine. *Am J Ophthalmol* 1982;93:327–333.
3. Chang S, Ozmert E, Zimmerman NJ, et al. Intraoperative perfluorocarbon liquids in the management of proliferative vitreoretinopathy. *Am J Ophthalmol* 1988;15;106:668–674.
4. Chang S, Lincoff H, Zimmerman NJ, et al. Giant retinal tears: surgical techniques and results using perfluorocarbon liquids. *Arch Ophthalmol* 1989;107:761–766.
5. Chang S, Reppucci V, Zimmerman NJ, et al. Perfluorocarbon liquids in the management of traumatic retinal detachments. *Ophthalmology* 1989;96:785–791.
6. Chang S. Perfluorocarbon liquids in vitreoretinal surgery. *Int Ophthalmol Clin* 1992;32:153–163.
7. Abrams GW, Williams GA. "En bloc" excision of diabetic membranes. *Am J Ophthalmol* 1987;15;103:302–308.
8. Charles S (Developer). Suction forceps membrane peeling. Presented at Wilmer Vitrectomy Course, The Johns Hopkins School of Medicine, Baltimore, May 1976.
9. Charles S (Developer). Chopsticks membrane peeling. Presented at Wilmer Vitrectomy Course, The Johns Hopkins School of Medicine, Baltimore, May 1976.
10. Sutherland G. Anterior chamber microsurgery. *Trans Aust Coll Ophthalmol* 1967;1:33.
11. Federman J. Automated microsurgical scissors. Presented at the Vitrectomy Study Club, Vail, CO, March 1980.
12. Machemer R, Parel JM, Hickingbotham D, et al. Membrane peeler cutter: automated vitreous scissors and hooked needle. *Arch Ophthalmol* 1981;99:152.
13. Charles S, Wang C. Pneumatic intraocular microscissors. *Arch Ophthalmol* 1981;99:1251.
14. Wang CT, Charles S. Microsurgical instrumentation for vitrectomy, Part 1. *J Clin Eng* 1983;8:321.
15. Charles S (Developer, March 1974): Vacuum cleaning. *Ocutome Newsletter* 1977;2:2.
16. O'Malley C (Developer). Extrusion method. *Ocutome Fragmatome Newsletter* 1978;3:3.
17. Landers MB. Removal of blood from the retinal surface in pars plana vitrectomy. *Am J Ophthalmol* 1978;86:427.
18. Norton EWD. Intraocular gas in the management of selected retinal detachments. *Trans Am Acad Ophthalmol Otolaryngol* 1973;77:85.
19. Fineberg E, Machemer R, Sullivan P. SF_6 for retinal detachment surgery: a preliminary report. *Mod Probl Ophthalmol* 1974;12:173.
20. Fineberg E, Machemer R, Sullivan P, et al. Sulfur hexafluoride in owl monkey vitreous cavity. *Am J Ophthalmol* 1975;79:67.
21. Machemer R. Intravitreal injection of sulfur hexafluoride gas (SF_6). In: Freeman HM, Hirose T, Schepens CL, eds. *Vitreous surgery and advances in fundus diagnosis and treatment.* New York: Appleton-Century-Crofts, 1977:421–422.
22. Bourgeois JE, Machemer R. Results of sulfur hexafluoride gas in vitreous surgery. *Am J Ophthalmol* 1983; 96:405.
23. Aaberg TM, Abrams GW, Edelhauser HF. Intraocular sulfur hexafluoride: experimental and clinical correlation. In: *International Symposium on New and Controversial Aspects of Vitreoretinal Surgery, Texas Medical Center, Houston, Texas.* St. Louis: CV Mosby, 1977:393–397.

24. Abrams GW, Edelhauser HF, Aaberg TM, et al. Dynamics of intravitreal sulfur hexafluoride gas. *Invest Ophthalmol* 1974;13:863.
25. Killey F, Edelhauser H, Aaberg TM. The effects of intraocular sulfur hexafluoride and freon gas on intraocular pressure and vitreous volume. *Arch Ophthalmol* 1978;96:521.
26. Miller B, Lean JS, Miller H, et al. Intravitreal expanding gas bubble: a morphologic study in the rabbit eye. *Arch Ophthalmol* 1984;102:1708.
27. Lincoff A, Lincoff H, Iwamoto T, et al. Perfluoro-n-butane. A gas for a maximum duration retinal tamponade. *Arch Ophthalmol* 1983;101:460.
28. Lincoff H, Coleman J, Kreissig J, et al. The perfluorocarbon gases in the treatment of retinal detachment. *Am Acad Ophthalmol* 1983;90:546.
29. Lincoff H, Mardirossian J, Lincoff A, et al. Intravitreal longevity of three perfluorocarbon gases. *Arch Ophthalmol* 1980;98:1610.
30. Lincoff A, Haft D, Liggett P, et al. Intravitreal expansion of perfluorocarbon bubbles. *Arch Ophthalmol* 1980;98:1646.
31. Lincoff A, Kreissig I. Intravitreal behavior of perfluorocarbons. *Surv Ophthalmol* 1981;2:17.
32. Lincoff H, Kreissig J. Intravitreal behaviour of perfluorocarbons. *Dev Ophthalmol* 1981;2:17.
33. Chang S, Lincoff H, Coleman J, et al. Perfluorocarbon gases in vitreous surgery. *Ophthalmology* 1985;92:651.
34. Machemer R, Aaberg T (Developers). *Vitrectomy, 2nd ed.* New York: Grune & Stratton, 1979:132.
35. Charles S (Developer, August 1974). In: McPherson A, ed. *New and controversial aspects of vitreoretinal surgery.* St. Louis: CV Mosby, 1977:196–197.
36. Charles S (Developer, March 1976). Fluid/gas exchange in the vitreous cavity. *Ocutome Newsletter* 1977;2:1.
37. Charles S, McCarthy C, Eichenbaum D. A mechanical syringe drive for vitreous surgery. *Am J Ophthalmol* 1975;79:879.
38. McCuen BW, Bessler M, Hickingbotham D, et al. Automated fluid-gas exchange. *Am J Ophthalmol* 1983;95:717.
39. Charles S, Wang C. A motorized gas injector for vitreous surgery. *Arch Ophthalmol* 1981;99:1398.
40. Landers MB, Stefansson E, Wolbarsht ML. The optics of vitreous surgery. *Am J Ophthalmol* 1981;91:611.
41. Fuller D. Flying and intraocular gas bubbles (letter). *Am J Ophthalmol* 1981;91:276.
42. Dieckert JP, O'Connor PS, Schacklett DE, et al. The effects of air travel on eyes with intraocular gas. Presented at the Annual Meeting, American Academy of Ophthalmology, Atlanta, GA, October 2, 1985.
43. Charles S. Controlled drainage of subretinal and choroidal fluid. *Retina* 1985;5:233.
44. Cibis PA. *Vitreoretinal pathology and surgery in retinal detachment.* St. Louis: CV Mosby, 1965.
45. Machemer R. Letter to the editor. *Am J Ophthalmol* 1977;83:282.
46. Schepens C: Letter to the editor. *Am J Ophthalmol* 1978;85:574.
47. Charles S, White J, Dennison C, et al. Bipolar bimanual intraocular diathermy. *Am J Ophthalmol* 1976;81:101.
48. O'Malley P. Portable xenon arc light coagulator. *Br J Ophthalmol* 197357:935–944.

5

Diabetic Retinopathy

MEDICAL ISSUES

Diabetes is increasing in prevalence in the American population for many reasons (1,2). Diabetics are living longer because of dialysis, kidney and pancreas transplants, improved cardiovascular management, and new medications. The availability of high-calorie and high-carbohydrate, -fat, and -sugar foods; fast-food restaurants; cultural attitudes toward eating; poor role models; large serving sizes; and many other factors contribute to the problem (3). Joslin observed that in 1912 there was no diabetes in the Pima Indian population. The incidence is now almost 70%. Friedman and others have attributed this to the "thrifty gene," which enabled survival of man with "occasional" eating rather the three square meals that many believe we should eat. It is of interest that beef, pork, egg, fast food, and dairy business interests support the nutrition community and make very large political donations. If dieticians, teachers, parents, doctors, nurses, ministers, and coaches eat improperly, there is no positive role model for the diet of our youth. The author (SC) never consumes egg yolks, beef, pork, lamb, or dairy products with any fat. The author eats only vegetables, fruit, whole grains, skinned fish, skinned poultry white meat, and nonfat dairy products. All fish and poultry are grilled, baked, steamed, or poached but never fried. The author stresses that the diabetic, antiatherosclerosis, anticancer, weight-loss, longevity, feel-good, look-good, and fitness diets are virtually the same. If the doctor eats properly, exercises, and educates the family and staff to do the same, a positive model is created for all. Everyone who comes into contact with the patient and family can support better health habits.

FLUORESCEIN ANGIOGRAPHY

Fluorescein angiography was very useful for understanding the stages in the pathogenesis of diabetic retinopathy and remains a valuable management tool for focal treatment of macular edema. The confocal, laser scanning, digital imager provides better contrast and resolution (Fig. 5.1); eliminates the bright strobe, which increases patient comfort; and has a faster frame rate when compared with digital or film-based angiography systems. Better image quality is achieved because confocal imaging increases the image-to-background ratio via rejection of light scattered by the cornea, lens, and vitreous. In addition, lasers are more efficient in stimulating the fluorescein fluorophore than filtered noncoherent light, allowing use of smaller doses of dye.

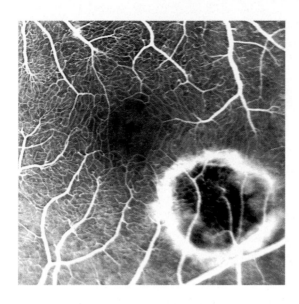

FIG. 5.1. Macular fluorescein angiogram demonstrates the superior contrast and resolution of the confocal scanning laser ophthalmoscope.

SCREENING

Up to 70% of the known diabetic population in America does not have an annual eye examination. Many studies have utilized various methods to screen this population as well as monitor patients with no retinopathy or before clinically significant macular edema (CSME) nonproliferative diabetic retinopathy (NPDR) at their last examination. It appears that color images are somewhat more sensitive than monochrome and that Polaroid images are adequate for screening purposes. Digital cameras are decreasing in cost and increasing in quality, and may compete on a quality-versus-cost basis with Polaroid images in the near future. Nonmydriatic fundus cameras have proven to be very useful for diabetic screening. Screeners, optometrists, general ophthalmologists, and retinal specialists can evaluate the captured images, if properly trained.

RETINAL THICKNESS MEASUREMENT

The ocular coherence tomography (Zeiss-Humphrey OCT) and slit-based retinal thickness analyzer (Talia RTA) have been used in pilot studies to evaluate retinal thickness in patients with nonproliferative diabetic retinopathy. Although the studies demonstrated excellent sensitivity to macular edema, the real issue is whether it is beneficial to perform focal laser before clinically significant macular edema (CSME) is present. This issue will be addressed in the next section.

NONPROLIFERATIVE RETINOPATHY

The Early Treatment of Diabetic Retinopathy Study (ETDRS) has contributed greatly to our management of patients with NPDR (4,5). The principal author performed a fax survey of the Macula Society members in April–May 1998 to determine if they laser before the ETDRS criteria referred to as CSME are reached. The ETDRS defined CSME as (a) thickening of the retina at or within 500 μm of the center of the macula, (b) hard

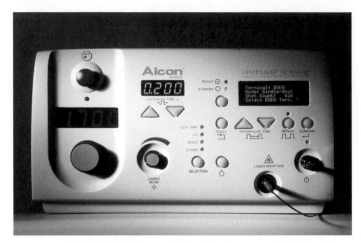

FIG. 5.2. Alcon 532 Eyelite laser console.

exudates at or within 500 μm of the center of the macula if associated with thickening of adjacent retina, or (c) an area of retinal thickening one disk diameter or larger, part of which is within one disk diameter of the center of the macula. Most respondents (57.3%) indicated they do not treat pre-CSME patients. Those who treated pre-CSME patients (28.1%) and those who rarely treated this group (12.4%) did so based on upcoming cataract surgery, poor result in the other eye, marked peripheral capillary nonperfusion (CNP), upcoming panretinal photocoagulation (PRP), or an estimation that the patient was unlikely to return for follow-up visits. Most surgeons used the Goldmann (flat) contact lens and started with a 100-μm, 100-mW, and 100-msec spot. Many believe that there is a tendency toward lighter treatment. Some surgeons primarily treat microaneurysms and microangiopathy noted to leak on angiography, others primarily used a light grid in the thickened, leaking area, but most treated both. Preferred lasers include argon green (514 nm), diode or flash tube pumped diode lasers (532 nm), krypton yellow (577 nm), but few preferred near infrared (IR) diode (>800 nm) lasers. The authors prefer a 532-nm, diode pumped, frequency up-converted continuous wave YAG laser (Fig. 5.2).

Macular edema is apparently caused by vascular endothelial growth factor (VEGF), the same agent that causes neovascularization. Ischemia leading to VEGF production may be a factor in certain macular edema cases. For this reason, patients with macular edema not responding to direct focal treatment of leaking microaneurysms, or areas of leakage on fluorescein angiography, may respond to treating areas of ischemia. Heavy grid photocoagulation probably has little effect in reducing neovascularization but significantly reduces reading speeds and causes patients with excellent Snellen acuity to complain that they cannot see.

PROLIFERATIVE RETINOPATHY

The DRS randomized, multicenter clinical trial proved that pan-retinal photocoagulation is effective for patients with proliferative diabetic retinopathy (6–8). Many surgeons now treat before the DRS treatment criteria are reached, in part because of the subsequent ETDRS study data. The DRS criteria are based on high-risk characteristics as compared with standard photographs. The authors use light treatment with small spot size (100 to

200 μm) with the spots placed one spot size apart. Many surgeons treat using a very large number of spots and see the patient in follow-up in 3 months. Some of this behavior is unfortunately driven by the so-called global period for Medicare payment. It is probably better to use a moderate number of spots and reexamine the patients in 1 month. Some surgeons have a protocol mindset with respect to PRP treatment. This approach may result in inappropriate therapy when the "protocol has been completed" and active neovascularization (NV) is present. It is safer to perform PRP fill-in, if there is any neovascularization (ANV) and the patient is greater than 1 month after treatment. The authors believe that this titration approach reduces treatment-related complications and discomfort.

The authors never use a retrobulbar block for laser treatment. Red and IR lasers cause more pain than green-yellow lasers. Durations greater than 100 msec cause more pain because of thermal diffusion. Larger spot sizes and higher powers cause more pain, light scattering, and potentially more nuclear sclerosis and occult macular damage.

VITRECTOMY

Better medical management and laser photocoagulation should significantly reduce the need for vitrectomy for the complications of proliferative diabetic retinopathy (PDR). Vitrectomy, when indicated, has an excellent prognosis when appropriate patient selection and techniques are utilized (9).

CASE SELECTION

It is useful to divide blindness from diabetic retinopathy into two subgroups: those cases requiring immediate surgery and those in which surgery is elective. Traction retinal detachment involving the macula (MTRD), neovascular glaucoma (NVG), and anterior vitreous cortex fibrovascular proliferation (AVCVP, retrolenticular neovascularization [RLNV]) are permanently blinding if left untreated. In contrast, the visual potential probably does not change in the treatment of vitreous or preretinal hemorrhage if there is substantial delay before surgery is performed.

Vitreous Hemorrhage

Early experimental work incorrectly concluded that vitreous hemorrhage caused neovascularization via organization of the blood clot. Vitreous hemorrhage is a *result* of neovascularization rather than the cause. Although longstanding vitreous hemorrhage can deposit iron on many intraocular structures, there is usually no retinal damage from a vitreous hemorrhage. Retinal detachment, macular damage, ischemia, and optic nerve function will determine the ultimate visual outcome when longstanding vitreous hemorrhages are removed, not the hemorrhage per se.

If the other eye has good vision, a unilateral hemorrhage can be followed indefinitely with ultrasound, unless retinal detachment, anterior vitreous cortex neovascularization, or iris neovascularization occurs. An eye without prior PRP is at greater risk for the development of neovascular complications and must be watched more closely. B-scan ultrasonography should be repeated at each visit, preferably at 1-month intervals, until the blood clears or surgery is performed. Ultrasonic evidence of posterior pole detachment requires immediate vitrectomy. The usual question of duration of a vitreous hemorrhage plays a less important role in the surgical decision-making process than other factors. If it does not appear that near-term clearing will occur, bilateral hemorrhage requires surgery on the eye with the best visual prognosis. Vitreous hemorrhage in a patient with only one eye as well as the better eye of bilateral cases should be operated on to improve visual function. Those patients with shortened lifespan and multisystem disease need immediate visual rehabilitation for emotional and social reasons. Subposterior vitreous detachment and preretinal hemorrhages clear more rapidly than does hemorrhage in the vitreous cortex. For this reason patients with bilateral or only-eye sub-PVD or preretinal hemorrhage can be followed for as long as the patient's emotional and social needs permit. If one eye has macular ischemia and the other, better, eye develops a vitreous hemorrhage, vitrectomy may be indicated to improve the patient's overall visual function.

Traction Retinal Detachment

Traction retinal detachment (TRD) can be diagnosed by ophthalmoscopic or ultrasonic means. If the macula is detached, vitreous surgery should be performed within 2 weeks, in most cases. If there is active neovascularization, it is better to perform panretinal photocoagulation (PRP) before vitrectomy if possible. Because of extensive exudation and fibrous proliferation, panretinal cryopexy should not be utilized. If vitrectomy indications are present, endo-PRP can be combined with vitrectomy. If vitrectomy is postponed until PRP-induced or spontaneous involution of neovascularization occurs, the incidence of postoperative neovascular glaucoma (NVG) and anterior vitreous cortex fibrovascular proliferation is dramatically reduced.

Because of the relatively high rate of biologic complications and medical risk factors, vitrectomy is not indicated in extramacular TRD. This is true even if progression toward the macula or a similar condition in the other eye seems to "threaten" the macula. It is safer to operate on actual, rather than predicted, visual loss. The rate of progression of extramacular TRD to include the macula is about 15% per year (10,11). After several years, progression to MTRD stabilizes at a cumulative rate of about 30%, and there are many patients with 5 to 10 year duration extramacular TRDs surrounding the macula with good vision that never required surgery.

Cataract surgery can result in anterior movement of the vitreous with progression of extramacular TRD to macular involvement. Once again, vitreous surgery should only be performed if the macula actually becomes elevated (12).

MACULAR EDEMA

Hilel Lewis first reported vitrectomy with peeling of taut posterior vitreous cortex from diffuse macula edema not responsive to focal laser photocoagulation. D'Amico, Blumenkranz, and others have also reported success in these cases as well. Evidence of prior PVD would appear to be a contraindication to this procedure. Some also advocate peeling of the internal limiting membrane (ILM) for macula edema, but this has not been shown to be either safe or effective. Charles has postulated that separation of the posterior vitreous cortex could allow greater egress of VEGF, known to cause macular edema. It has not been shown that tangential traction on ILM causes macular edema. It is more likely that taut posterior vitreous cortex (PVC) causes elevation of the macula, pulling the macula away from the dehydrating effects of the retinal pigment epithelium (RPE) pump. Some surgeons have reported removal of submacular exudates or puncturing macular cysts, but there is no scientific evidence of efficacy at this time, and there is great concern about retinal damage caused by the procedure.

CONTRAINDICATIONS

The absence of light perception indicates glaucomatous optic atrophy, ischemic optic neuropathy, or extensive retinal vascular occlusive disease and contraindicates vitreous surgery. Corneal changes; corneal, lid, or conjunctival infection; or inability to withstand local anesthesia are obvious contraindications.

Iris neovascularization can be an indication for surgery in diabetic TRDs (13–15). Vitrectomy for retinal reattachment and PRP are the only treatments for neovascularization of disk (NVD), neovascularization elsewhere (NVE), iris NV, AVCFVP, and trabecular meshwork neovascularization. Vitrectomy in an aphakic eye with active iris neovascularization will result in rapid progression to postoperative NVG unless extensive PRP or retinal reattachment can be performed intraoperatively.

Cases of several years' duration may exhibit extensive white vessels and retinal atrophy. If the temporal arcades are not perfusing the macula, there is no need for vitreous surgery because visual improvement will not occur. If the retina is extremely atrophic but PRP has not previously been performed, this is an indication that limited visual improvement will occur from reattachment. There are, however, cases of 3 or 4 years' duration that have improved to ambulatory vision levels after vitrectomy. As a rule, these late atrophic cases have a lesser incidence of NVG and anterior vitreous cortex fibrovascular proliferation.

SURGICAL SEQUENCE AND TECHNIQUES

Vitreous surgery for hemorrhage or TRD requires a planned sequence of surgical steps, with multiple branches, depending on different intraoperative scenarios. As in all vitreous surgery, a full complement of sterile tools and materials must be immediately available.

Anesthesia

The frequency of cardiovascular and renal disease in the diabetic patient requires especially careful preoperative medical evaluation. The anesthesiologist should take part in the medical evaluation. Local anesthesia with monitoring by an anesthesiologist should be used in all cases. An intravenous line, EKG, pulse oximetry, blood pressure monitoring, and oxygen mask and a suction line to prevent hypercapnia must be utilized in all cases. The anesthesiologist or anesthetist should make liberal use of intraoperative blood sugar testing.

Incisions

Limbus-based conjunctival flaps 1 mm wide are preferable to a fornix-based flap or 4- to 5-mm flaps. The 4-mm infusion cannula is placed 3 mm posterior to the limbus if the eye is to be aphakic, or 4 mm back if the intent is to spare the lens. The incision for the endoilluminator is made nasally just above the center of the medial rectus, and the active instrument incision is made temporally just above the center of the lateral rectus. Radial extensions at the ends of the circumferential incision facilitate exposure and one-suture closure. The microvitreoretinal blade is used to make all sclerotomies. The sew-on infusion cannula should be inspected with the operating microscope before initiating infusion.

Management of the Lens

Lens removal correlates with an increased incidence of postoperative NVG (16–20) but prevents anterior vitreous cortex fibrovascular proliferation. The anterior vitreous cortex (AVC) and lens apparently act as barriers to the anterior diffusion of VEGF; therefore their presence reduces the incidence of NVG. A specific attempt should be made to leave the

AVC, if the lens is retained during vitrectomy in an effort to reduce development of posterior subcapsular cataract. Blankenship and Kokame reported saving the anterior lens capsule when performing lensectomy enabling sulcus implantation of a posterior chamber lens after the vitrectomy is complete. Endocapsular lensectomy was developed by the principal author to facilitate anterior capsular retention and eliminate iris damage. This method starts with an anterior vitrectomy, then posterior capsular rhexis with the vitreous cutter, then cortical cleaving hydrodissection, followed by sculpting of the nucleus with the fragmenter and finally aspiration-cutting of the cortex with the vitrectomy cutter.

Contact lenses should be utilized judiciously because of decreased corneal sensitivity but are effective in a surprising number of patients. Spectacle correction is surprisingly well tolerated in these patients. Implantation of posterior chamber lenses (PCLs) after endocapsular lensectomy or phakoemulsification surgery tends to keep the AVC and posterior capsule intact and probably decrease NVG. Endocapsular lensectomy (ECL) with an aspiration-type 20-gauge ultrasonic fragmenter is preferable to phakoemulsification combined with vitrectomy. ECL uses the same 20-gauge wounds, and the anterior chamber is not entered until the vitrectomy is complete, and then only if a PCL is to be implanted. A judgment should be made preoperatively as to whether the cataract will interfere with surgical visualization, and endocapsular lensectomy should then be performed accordingly. Endo-PRP should be performed in all cases with active retinal or iris neovascularization or no prior PRP.

Vitrectomy

The continuity of the PVC is a critical concept in the understanding and planning for the vitrectomy process. The PVC will either be completely adherent to the retina, partially detached, or completely detached from the retina. The "core" vitrectomy misconception stems from the tendency of rotating full-function probes with syringe-operated suction to pull vitreous into the central portion of the eye. Complete sectioning or truncation of the PVC (Fig. 5.3), rather than "band cutting" or "core vitrectomy," must be understood before surgical success is possible. These concepts apply whether the vitreous is opaque, semiopaque, or clear.

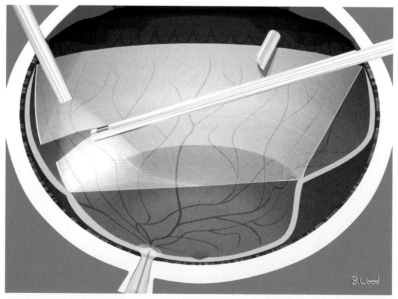

FIG. 5.3. Truncation of posterior vitreous cortex relieves perpendicular forces on the retina.

Procedure with Posterior Vitreous Detachment

If the posterior vitreous cortex is detached from the retina, a central opening in the vitreous should be created and linear extrusion with a straight 20-gauge cannula should be performed if any subvitreous erythroclastic or hemolytic material is present. This step is also known as vacuum cleaning or extrusion. When a clear effluent is obtained from this fenestration, the opening should be enlarged with the cutter until only a small "skirt" at the confluence of the anterior and posterior vitreous cortex remains. Particular care must be taken to trim the superior "skirt" if it is opaque, because it can hang down postoperatively and obscure the seated patient's view. Linear suction with a straight 20-gauge cannula should be performed to remove all preretinal blood products and permit better visualization, less postoperative erythroclastic glaucoma, and photocoagulation without damaging the retina. If a complete PVD is present, there is no perpendicular force on the retina, and tangential force from epiretinal membranes (ERM) can cause TRD. Vascular attachment points of the ERM to the retina should be treated with the bipolar diathermy or endophotocoagulator only if they bleed intraoperatively or appear active. The combined diathermy and endoilluminator instruments are ideal for this technique.

Procedure with Partial Posterior Vitreous Detachment

If only a partial PVD has occurred, the vitreous will be adherent to the retina at one or more epicenters. Typically, the optic nerve and vessels serve as attachment points because of glial proliferation. As the vitreous contracts, these attachment points become the apex (apices) of the now-conical PVC. This is the most common vitreous configuration encountered in PDR. It is critical in these patients to section or truncate the posterior vitreous cortex to completely eliminate any anteroposterior traction. Vitreous bands do not exist as such but are actually more visible portions of the PVC continuum. The posterior vitreous cortex penetration is initiated in an area indicated by preoperative ultrasound or indirect ophthalmoscopy to have attached retina (Fig. 5.4).

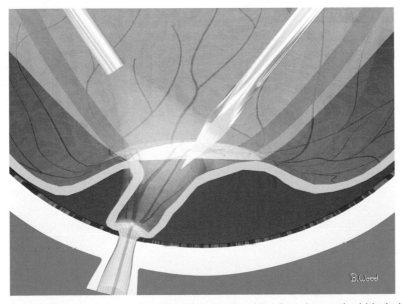

FIG. 5.4. Posterior vitreous cortex is entered centrally with microvitreoretinal blade in an area of attached retina.

In the absence of this information, the first opening should be made nasally in the mid-periphery to avoid the macula and be easily treatable if a retinal break occurs. After an opening is made, extrusion (vacuum cleaning) through the opening must be continued until a clear effluent is obtained. At this time the novice vitreous surgeon could mistake voluminous old blood trapped behind the vitreous for active bleeding. When the retina is visualized through the opening, a safe circumferential truncation of the posterior vitreous cortex can proceed from this point and extend for 360°. It is unnecessary to make multiple openings in the posterior vitreous cortex or to dissect the layers of the posterior vitreous cortex in "onion skin" fashion. The "skirt" must be trimmed as described earlier and the portion connected to the retina trimmed down to near the retinal surface. Any areas of PVC connected to two or more retinal points should be sectioned with the vitrectomy instrument if there is sufficient clearance for the tip, or with the 20-gauge, delamination scissors. If these bridging areas of PVC are vascularized, they should be precoagulated using a disposable combined endoilluminator and bipolar diathermy.

Procedure with No Posterior Vitreous Detachment

In some diabetics the entire PVC is adherent to the retina. In the unlikely event that the PVC is only slightly adherent, membrane peeling can be performed. Caution must be exercised in attempting to peel the PVC in a single sheet because retinal breaks can occur in sites remote from the grasp site (Fig. 5.5). Areas of photocoagulation can bind the PVC to the retina and even to the choroid and sclera. If strongly adherent zones are present, the PVC should be allowed to remain in these locations, and the scissors or vitrectomy instruments should be used to sever all tangential traction. Posterior vitreous cortex truncation must be completed in every case (Fig. 5.6) but can be performed with scissors in

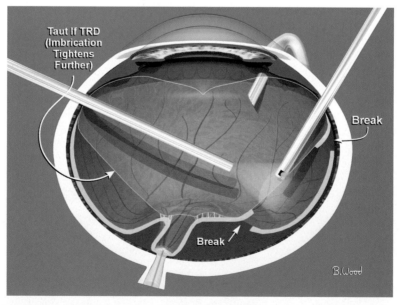

FIG. 5.5. Imbrication of taut posterior vitreous cortex into vitreous cutter port can cause remote retinal breaks.

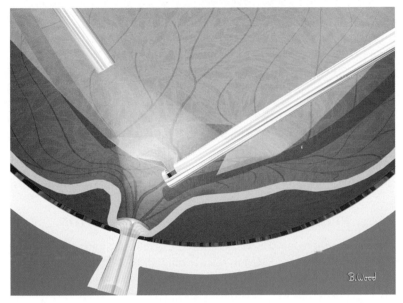

FIG. 5.6. Completion of posterior vitreous cortex truncation after delamination with curved scissors.

the case of shallow PVDs or following inside-out delamination if a TRD is present (Fig. 5.7). This latter method, developed by the principal author, was later termed *en bloc* when described by others using a less safe, outside-in direction of dissection. Even worse, the advocates of en-bloc dissection, as originally described, suggest that intentional traction on the vitreous can facilitate dissection. Using the vitreous to lift the ERM has substantial risk of causing peripheral retinal breaks from countertraction.

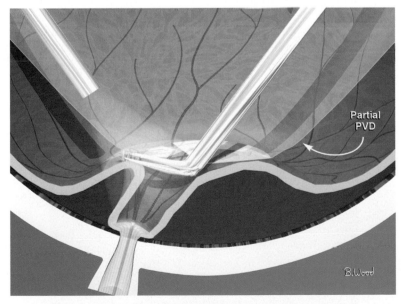

FIG. 5.7. Inside-out delamination of posterior vitreous cortex.

TRACTION RETINAL DETACHMENT

Traction retinal detachments result from posterior vitreous cortex (anteroposterior) as well as surface (tangential) traction. Although less apparent in cases with clear media, adherence of the posterior vitreous cortex to the retina is virtually always present when TRD exists. Clear media and excellent endoillumination are essential for visualization of the clear posterior vitreous cortex. The posterior vitreous cortex apices may be single or multiple, and the adherence zones may be small to large. The least complex TRDs involve single-point posterior vitreous cortex attachment with a small zone of adherence on the temporal arcades elevating the macula. Posterior vitreous cortex truncation alone is sufficient to reattach the retina in this situation. If multiple apices with small adherent zones are present, again, posterior vitreous cortex truncation alone is sufficient to cause retinal reattachment.

EPIRETINAL MEMBRANE DELAMINATION

Broader zones of adherence (ERMs) are more difficult to manage and require inside-out scissors delamination of the ERM to release tangential traction. Delamination was developed by the principal author to allow more complete removal of epiretinal membranes with less trauma to the retina. ERMs are attached to the retinal surface at individual points where glial and vascular proliferation has penetrated the ILM. Although ERMs may appear to be incorporated into the retina, they are always extrinsic to the retina. Horizontal, 20-gauge, curved scissors are utilized for delamination (Fig. 5.8). It is better to avoid any traction on the ERM caused by the use of forceps or pics. The ERM can be gently reflected back without traction on the retina using the endoilluminator or multifunction manipulator (Fig. 5.9). The membranes are usually delaminated from the retinal surface in a single sheet or a small number of pieces in an inside-out direction. As previously stated, inside-out delamination is safer than outside-in because the central retina is stronger, the retina is redundant centrally, and the view is better. On occasion, access segmentation can assist with visualization of the surfaces for delamination. Delamination should usually begin centrally and proceed in inside out (Fig. 5.10). The ultimate goal in scissors delamination is to remove most or all ERM. At times the membrane is extremely vascular, or the retina very atrophic, making this goal unachievable. Scissors segmentation of ERM is utilized when the membrane is markedly adherent to atrophic retina. At

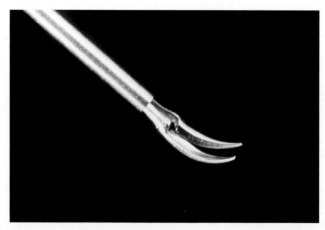

FIG. 5.8. Horizontal, 20-gauge curved scissors used for delamination.

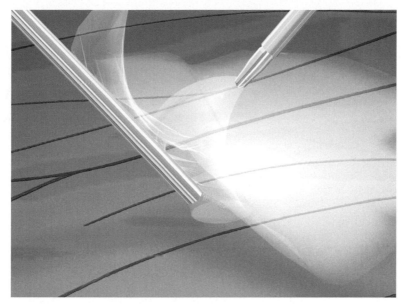

FIG. 5.9. Blunt dissection of epiretinal membrane using endoilluminator and end-opening forceps.

the very least, the goal is to convert all angulated retinal contours to gently rounded contours (Fig. 5.11). Scissors segmentation has been largely supplanted by scissors delamination because delamination allows for complete removal of virtually all ERM. Eliminating the cut edges of ERM is advantageous because edges serve as a source of fibrin that is a substrate for glial reproliferation. Delamination prevents persistent small areas of retinal elevation from causing late rhegmatogenous detachment. Complete reattachment probably decreases VEGF production.

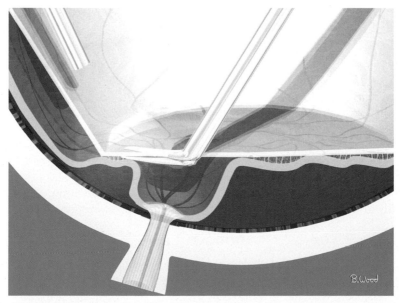

FIG. 5.10. Delamination of epiretinal membranes should begin centrally and proceed in an inside-out direction.

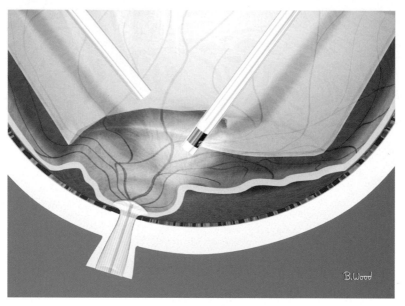

FIG. 5.11. Epiretinal membrane is removed with the vitreous cutter after delamination has converted angulated retinal contours to gently rounded contours.

MEMBRANE PEELING

On occasion membranes are minimally adherent to the retinal surface, but much more frequently they are tightly adherent to extensive glial attachment points. If peeling occurs spontaneously during scissors delamination-segmentation, it can be utilized to the surgeon's advantage. Peeling often causes bleeding, retinal breaks, and defects in the ILM that may lead to recurrent glial proliferation. Inappropriate peeling of the ILM can be recognized by the many tiny white fibers stretching from the membrane to the peeled surface. For these reasons, scissors delamination is preferred to membrane peeling in almost all situations.

RETINECTOMY

When extensive retinal foreshortening, especially from glial recurrences, prevents a delamination approach, retinectomy should be used. If internal drainage of SRF followed by internal fluid/air exchange demonstrates nonconformation of the retina to the RPE, as signified by subretinal air, and scissors delamination has already been completed to its maximum safe level, retinectomy is indicated. Large retinectomies are best managed by the use of long-term silicone oil for rhegmatogenous confinement. The silicone can also serve in the role of retinopexy avoidance to reduce glial reproliferation. Retinectomy can also be utilized for undissectable glial proliferation or reproliferation.

ENDODIATHERMY

Endodiathermy causes tissue shrinkage and retinal necrosis. Prophylactic coagulation of vessels that are not to be transected is unsafe and unnecessary. As blood can function as a matrix for postoperative glial proliferation, bleeding should be minimized. The two- or three-function manipulators (Fig. 5.11) as developed by Grieshaber and Brooks McCuen

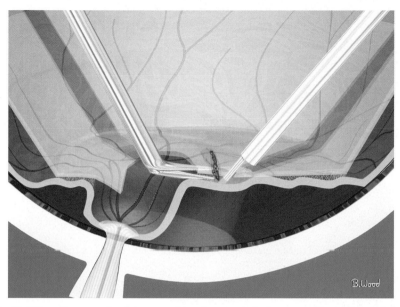

FIG. 5.12. Multifunction manipulator provides focused diathermy with minimal delay and reduced bleeding.

are excellent second instruments during delamination and segmentation. When combined with the Accurus foot-controlled tamponade, troublesome intraoperative blood clots on the retinal surface can be significantly reduced (Fig. 5.12). The endophotocoagulator can be used for bleeding, nonelevated, glial attachment points. The design of the manipulators and disposable bipolar endoilluminator create a more focused coagulation pattern than the standard bipolar probe.

INTERNAL FLUID/GAS EXCHANGE

Intraocular air/gas is only utilized if a retinal break is suspected or seen. The only role of air/gas is to restore the transretinal pressure gradient via surface tension. Air/gas surface tension management has no role in the treatment of traction retinal detachment without retinal breaks ("no tear, no air"). If a retinal break is seen, internal drainage of subretinal fluid with fluid/air exchange then air/gas should be used, followed by confluent, single-row photocoagulation around all breaks.

DRAINAGE OF SUBRETINAL FLUID

If a retinal break is present, internal drainage of subretinal fluid (SRF) with a soft-tip cannula (Fig. 5.13) followed by internal fluid/air exchange and then completion of internal drainage of SRF should be performed. If no retinal break is present, it is typically unnecessary to drain SRF unless the detachment is extremely high and there is concern about the ability of the retina to conform to the retinal pigment epithelium (RPE). If no retinal break is present and a decision is made to drain SRF, direct, transscleral needle drainage of subretinal fluid is a safe alternative (Fig. 5.14).

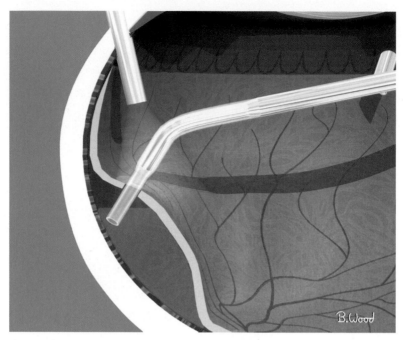

FIG. 5.13. Internal drainage of subretinal fluid with soft-tip cannula through existing retinal break.

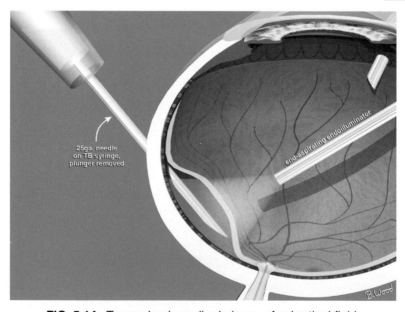

FIG. 5.14. Transscleral needle drainage of subretinal fluid.

SILICONE OIL SURFACE TENSION MANAGEMENT

Silicone should be utilized when large or multiple retinal breaks or retinectomies are present to eliminate the need for retinopexy and reduce reproliferation. Internal fluid/air exchange with the air pump and internal drainage of subretinal fluid with linear extrusion should precede air/silicone exchange.

Silicone oil acts as a barrier to the anterior diffusion of VEGF and markedly reduces anterior segment neovascularization if no inferior iridectomy is present. Because silicone recompartmentalizes the eye, fibrovascular proliferation can occur at the retina/silicone interface (Fig. 5.15). For this reason extensive PRP is our best hope for these cases. Silicone may prevent oxygen diffusion from well perfused to hypoperfused retinal areas, thus causing visual loss. The principal author used perfluorocarbon liquids in an animal model in 1976 in the hope that it could be used as a vitreous substitute in the diabetic patient. It was evaluated because it is ideal for oxygen diffusion. Unfortunately, it was discovered that it caused severe damage to the inferior cornea.

RETINOPEXY

All breaks require retinopexy unless they are macular, PM bundle, or peripapillary in location, in spite of evidence that an occasional untreated break will not result in detachment. Endocryopexy is unsafe and should never be utilized. The laser endophotocoagulator is used to treat all breaks unless they are very extensive, indicating the need for long-term silicone oil for rhegmatogenous confinement. The end-aspirating laser probe is ideal for this purpose (Fig. 5.16).

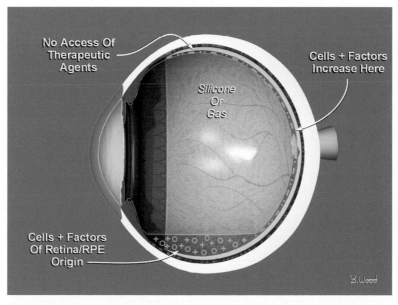

FIG. 5.15. Silicone infusion recompartmentalizes the eye, sequestering cells and factors at the retina/silicone interface.

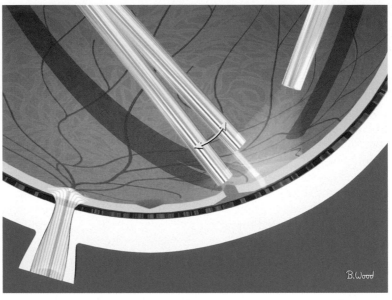

FIG. 5.16. End-aspirating laser probe enables simultaneous aspiration of SRF and retinopexy.

SCLERAL BUCKLING

A scleral buckle can support any retinal breaks that cannot reach the RPE after dissection, internal fluid/air exchange and internal drainage of SRF, but retinectomy is usually preferred. Circumferential silicone explants are used for peripheral and midperipheral breaks with unresectable traction. The principal author has not used prophylactic encircling bands and radial buckles since the early 1980s because of improved vitreous cutters, fluidics, and techniques.

ENDOPANRETINAL PHOTOCOAGULATION

Patients with active retinal neovascularization are at high risk for postoperative NVG and AVCFVP (21–23). These cases should have all nondetached, nontreated areas of retina treated with endo-PRP. Focal treatment is reserved for bleeding vessels, flat NV and is never used on the disk. Endo-PRP decreases NVG and anterior vitreous cortex fibrovascular proliferation in high-risk cases but is probably not required in cases with completely involutional neovascularization. TRD cases are at higher risk for neovascularization than are hemorrhage cases, but unfortunately endophotocoagulation cannot be safely utilized on elevated retina. PRP should not be performed on formerly detached retina because a thin layer of subretinal fluid always remains, the retina is often edematous, and overtreatment is inevitable. Overtreatment results in fibrin syndrome.

RESULTS

Greater than 80% of diabetic TRD patients managed in the preceding manner will sustain visual improvement with vision greater than 5/200 (24–26). Ninety-seven percent of the retinas of the patients are attached at the 2-week postoperative visit, but even after reoperation, 5% of the patients are blind from AVCFVP and glial recurrence with secondary retinal detachment (27–29). The incidence of glial recurrence is less with delamination than with segmentation. Glial recurrence never occurs in truncation-only cases.

Some aphakic patients with attached retinas ultimately become blind from NVG despite careful management. Neovascular glaucoma correlates with the presence of active retinal neovascularization. Anterior vitreous cortex fibrovascular proliferation causes permanent blindness in some of the phakic cases (30).

Some of the patients with attached retinas do not have improved vision because of photoreceptor damage and retinal ischemia. Some of the successfully operated cases ultimately become blind from ischemic optic neuropathy. Some become blind from open-angle glaucoma. Case selection has a large impact on success rate, but the goal is to help everyone possible, not to improve the success rate by eliminating difficult cases. Patients with good results at 6 months typically have excellent long-term success (31–35).

COMPLICATIONS

Hemorrhage

Immediate postoperative intraocular hemorrhage can occur from ERM vascular attachment points, nontreated new vessels, or sclerotomies. Approximately 50% of phakic cases develop immediate postoperative vitreous hemorrhages. In aphakic cases, this hemorrhage will typically clear in 1 to 2 weeks, but the phakic cases can take several months. If ultrasound indicates that the retina is attached, and there is excellent vision in the other eye, no reoperation is necessary. If ultrasound shows the retina to be detached, immediate reoperation is indicated. If the patient is bilaterally blind, emotional and social needs dictate the need for reoperation. It is advisable to operate on the eye with the highest visual potential whether it is a first or a reoperation.

A full vitrectomy setup with two conjunctival incisions and all three sclerotomies is better than so-called washouts in most instances. In this way, ERM and bleeding vessels can be managed and endo-PRP can be combined. Two-needle, in-office fluid/fluid exchange can be used if medical conditions do not permit surgery under monitored local anesthesia. If any neovascularization is present, focal photocoagulation and endo-PRP should be combined with the procedure.

Postoperative Cataract

If a visually significant cataract occurs in the best- or only-vision eye, it should be removed using phakoemulsification and PCL implantation. If the cataract occurs in the poorer-vision eye, the patient can be observed with ultrasound if medical status does not warrant surgery.

Erythroclastic (Hemolytic) Glaucoma

Erythroclastic (hemolytic) glaucoma is best prevented by extrusion with the blunt 20-gauge cannula, trimming of the vitreous skirt, and coagulation of all bleeding vessels. If the pressure exceeds 25 mm Hg, topical alpha-agonists, carbonic anhydrase inhibitors, and beta-blockers will usually control the pressure. On rare occasions, reoperation may be needed to control the pressure.

Neovascular Complications

Just as retinal neovascularization is the most significant complication of the unoperated PDR eye, NVG and AVCFVP [anterior hyaloidal fibrovascular proliferation (AH-

FVP), RLNV] are the most severe problems in the postvitrectomy eye. An understanding of the pathogenesis is necessary to reduce and manage neovascular complications.

Anterior segment and anterior vitreous cortex neovascularization are due to VEGF released from hypoxic but noninfarcted retina (36–40). PRP is successful in reducing VEGF by causing destruction of hypoxic retinal areas, transient release of an inhibitor substance (41), and increased choroidal oxygenation of the retina (42). Trabecular meshwork neovascularization without peripheral anterior synechia or apparent iris neovascularization can cause severe glaucoma. It is no longer thought that anterior segment NV is secondary to a circulatory disturbance or that iris neovascularization somehow migrates to the trabecular meshwork. Although vitrectomy can induce changes in the oxygen distribution in the globe, this observation does not explain the transmissibility of ocular neovascularization from human vitreous specimens to bioassay systems, which can only be explained by VEGF.

THE BARRIER CONCEPT

VEGF encounters sequential barriers in its anterior diffusion en route to ocular egress through the trabecular meshwork (Fig. 5.17). In nonoperated eyes, NVE and NVD occur along the back surface of the PVC. If vitrectomy has removed the PVC, neovascularization occurs along the back surface of the AVC. Anterior vitreous cortex fibrovascular proliferation (30), as first reported by the principal author, was previously incorrectly thought to be due to "fibrovascular ingrowth" from the sclerotomies.

In aphakic eyes or when present in high concentrations, VEGF encounters the trabecular meshwork barrier, causing neovascular glaucoma. Iris neovascularization serves to indicate the presence of VEGF in the anterior segment. Trabecular meshwork neovascularization, however, has a direct role in neovascular glaucoma. If a successful filtering procedure is performed in a diabetic, aphakic, vitrectomized eye, anterior segment neo-

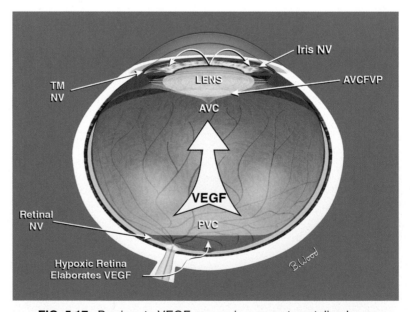

FIG. 5.17. Barriers to VEGF egress in compartmentalized eye.

vascularization will frequently disappear. This is analogous to the disappearance of NVE and NVD after removal of the PVC by vitrectomy. In these filtered cases, neovascularization occurs on the inside of the bleb, which can be thought of as the final barrier.

If any neovascularization is seen in the postoperative course, immediate laser PRP should be performed. It is not advisable to wait for pressure elevation, which may obscure the view and lead to irreversible NVG. While PRP may not affect the intraocular pressure, it decreases fibrin release and hemorrhage from the iris vessels that contribute to the phthisis process. Although on occasion iris neovascularization will disappear spontaneously or stabilize, it is better to treat all cases of iris NV with PRP.

If the eye pressure exceeds 25 mm Hg, topical timolol may be effective and can be used in combination with brimonidine, lantanoprost, and topical carbonic anhydrase inhibitors. If topical treatment cannot keep the pressure in the mid-20s, glaucoma surgery may be required. Presumably because of poor perfusion, diabetics have poor tolerance for elevated pressure. Filtering procedures are effective in some of these patients but have a tendency to cause hypotony, with resultant repeated intraocular bleeding.

Cyclocryopexy can be performed if the patient cannot tolerate an operating room procedure. Cryotherapy on bare sclera, for 6 clock hours, 4 to 5 mm posterior to the limbus to avoid the trabecular meshwork seems to have best results. The treatments are held at 80°C for 1 minute. Although this can be quite effective in controlling the pressure using a single treatment, many of these patients go on to further fibrin release, cyclitic membrane formation, fibrovascular proliferation, and phthisis bulbi. Endocyclophotocoagulation combined with PRP is better than cryotherapy, transscleral laser, and ultrasonic cyclodestructive procedures because of reduced inflammation, less pain, and better visual prognosis.

Anterior Vitreous Cortex Fibrovascular Proliferation

If anterior vitreous cortex fibrovascular proliferation develops, VEGF and other cytokines will cause cellular migration and proliferation on the AVC. The membrane causes a characteristic ring-like equatorial TRD followed by total retinal detachment. This configuration can be noted on ultrasound and must be operated on immediately. The retrolental, retro-IOL, or cyclitic membrane should be detected as early as possible by looking obliquely at the slit lamp, to ensure early treatment. Treatment requires endocapsular lensectomy, removal of the capsule and cyclitic membrane with application of the bipolar diathermy to the resected edges, internal fluid/air exchange, and long-term silicone surface tension management. Extensive PRP is necessary to reduce further neovascularization.

Rhegmatogenous Retinal Detachment

Peripheral rhegmatogenous retinal detachment is relatively infrequent in diabetic cases. If retinal detachment occurs, it is usually related to retinal breaks missed at the time of the original surgery or vitreous incarceration in the wounds. Postvitrectomy retinal detachments usually cannot be managed with scleral buckling alone. A greater success rate is usually obtained by using a vitrectomy revision approach with a search for residual traction or glial recurrence, internal drainage of SRF, internal fluid/air exchange, focal endophotocoagulation, and air/gas or air/silicone exchange.

Glial Recurrence

Epiretinal surgery, especially with peeling, can result in a recurrence of glial proliferation. Contrary to previous teaching, no vitreous substrate (often called *scaffold*) is required for a glial recurrence. Glial tissue can proliferate directly on the retinal surface, especially if it is devoid of the ILL. Fibrin from ERM epicenters can constitute a bridge-like substrate along which glial tissue can reproliferate.

Glial recurrences are managed with scissors delamination and internal drainage of SRF, internal fluid/air exchange, endophotocoagulation, and long-term silicone oil for rhegmatogenous confinement if there is a rhegmatogenous component. Frequently, retinectomy is required. These membranes are tightly adherent to the retina and cannot be treated with membrane peeling.

REFERENCES

1. Klein R, Klein BE, Moss SE, et al. The Wisconsin Epidemiologic Study of Diabetic Retinopathy. II. Prevalence and risk of diabetic retinopathy when age at diagnosis is less than 30 yrs. *Arch Ophthalmol* 1984;102:520–526.
2. Klein R, Klein BE, Moss SE, et al. The Wisconsin Epidemiologic Study of Diabetic Retinopathy. III. Prevalence and risk of diabetic retinopathy when age at diagnosis is 30 or more years. *Arch Ophthalmol* 1984;102:527–532.
3. The Diabetes Control and Complications Trial Research Group. Progression of retinopathy with intensive versus conventional treatment in the Diabetes Control and Complications Trial. *Ophthalmology* 1995;102:647–661.
4. Chew EY, Klein ML, Ferris FL, et al. Association of elevated serum lipid levels with retinal hard exudates in diabetic retinopathy: Early Rreatment of Diabetic Retinopathy Study Report 22. *Arch Ophthalmol* 1996;114: 1079–1084.
5. Early Treatment of Diabetic Retinopathy Study Research Group. Early photocoagulation for diabetic retinopathy: ETDRS report 9. *Ophthalmology* 1991;98:766–785.
6. The Diabetic Retinopathy Vitrectomy Study Research Group. Early vitrectomy for severe vitreous hemorrhage in diabetic retinopathy: two-year results of a randomized trial. DRVS Study Report 2. *Arch Ophthalmol* 1985; 103:1644–1652.
7. Diabetic Retinopathy Vitrectomy Study Research Group. Early vitrectomy for severe proliferative diabetic retinopathy in eyes with useful vision: results of a randomized trial: DRVS report 3. *Ophthalmology* 1988; 95:1307–1320.
8. Diabetic Retinopathy Study Research Group. Early vitrectomy for severe vitreous hemorrhage: four-year results of a randomized trial: DRVS report 5. *Arch Ophthalmol* 1990;108:958–964.
9. Machemer R, Buettner H, Norton EW, et al. Vitrectomy: a pars plana approach. *Trans Am Acad Ophthalmol* 1971;75:813–820.
10. Cohen HB, McMeel W, Franks EP. Diabetic traction detachment. *Arch Ophthalmol.* 1979;97:1268.
11. Flinn C, Charles S. The natural history of diabetic extramacular traction detachment. *Arch Ophthalmol* 1981;99:66.
12. Benson WE, Brown GC, Tasman W, et al. Extracapsular cataract extraction with placement of a posterior chamber lens in patients with diabetic retinopathy. *Ophthalmology* 1993;100(5):730-738.
13. Blankenship GW. Preoperative iris rubeosis and diabetic vitrectomy results. *Ophthalmology* 1980;87:176.
14. Scuderi JJ, Blumenkranz M, Blankenship G. Regression of diabetic rubeosis iridis following successful surgical reattachment of the retina by vitrectomy. *Retina* 1982;2:193.
15. Little HL. Rubeosis indis after vitrectomy for complications of diabetic retinopathy. In: Little HL, Jack RL, Patz A, et al., eds. *Diabetic retinopathy.* New York: Thieme-Stratton, 1983:315–340.
16. Blankenship G, Cortez R, Machemer R. The lens and pars plana vitrectomy for diabetic retinopathy complications. *Arch Ophthalmol* 1979;97:1263.
17. Blankenship GW. The lens influence on diabetic vitrectomy results: report of a prospective randomized study. *Arch Ophthalmol* 1980;98:2196.
18. Rice TA, Michels RG, Maguire MG, et al. The effects of lensectomy on the incidence of ins neovascularization and neovascular glaucoma after vitrectomy for diabetic retinopathy. *Am J Ophthalmol.* 1983;95:1.
19. Glaser BM. Relationship of cataract extraction and rubeosis in diabetes mellitus. *Ophthalmology* 1983;90:819.
20. Schachat AP, Oyakawa RT, Michels RG, et al. Complications of vitreous surgery for diabetic retinopathy. ll. Postoperative complications. *Ophthalmology* 1983;90:522.
21. The Diabetic Retinopathy Study Group. Preliminary report on the effects of photocoagulation therapy. *Am J Ophthalmol* 1976;81:383–396.
22. Diabetic retinopathy Study Research Group. Four risk factors for severe visual loss in diabetic retinopathy: the third report from the DRS. *Arch Ophthalmol* 1979;97:654–655.
23. Doft BH, Blankenship GW. Single versus multiple treatment sessions of argon laser panretinal photocoagulation for proliferative diabetic retinopathy. *Ophthalmology* 1982;89:772–779.
24. Blankenship GW, Machemer R. Pars plana vitrectomy for the management of severe diabetic retinopathy: an analysis of results five years after surgery. *Ophthalmology* 1978;85:553.
25. Michels RG. Vitrectomy for the complication of diabetic retinopathy. *Arch Ophthalmol* 1978;96:237.
26. Aaberg T. Clinical results in vitrectomy for diabetic traction retinal detachment. *Am J Ophthalmol.* 1979;88:246.
27. Rice TA, Michels RG. Complications of vitrectomy. In: Little HL, Jack RL, Patz A, et al., eds. *Diabetic retinopathy.* New York: Thieme-Stratton, 1983:315–340.

28. Michels RG. Vitreous surgery in proliferative diabetic retinopathy. In: Shimizu K, Oosterhuis JA, eds. *Acta XXIII Concilium Ophthalmologicurum Part 1*. Amsterdam/Oxford: Excerpta Medica, 1979:420.

29. Michels RG. Vitrectomy for complications of diabetic retinopathy. *Arch Ophthalmol.*1978;96:237.

30. Charles S. Vitreous surgery for diabetic traction detachment. Presented at Frontiers in Ophthalmology. Phoenix, AZ, February 18, 1982.

31. Rice TA, Michels RG. Long-term anatomic and functional results of initially successful vitrectomy for diabetic retinopathy. *Am J Ophthalmol* 1980;90:297.

32. Blankenship CW. Stability of pars plana vitrectomy results for diabetic retinopathy complications: a comparison of five-year and six-month postvitrectomy findings. *Arch Ophthalmol* 1981;99:1009.

33. Rice TA, Michels RG, Palmer L. Late results of initially successful vitrectomy in diabetes. *Dev Ophthalmol* 1981;2:286.

34. Blankenship GW, Machemer R. Long-term diabetic vitrectomy results: report of 10 year followup. *Ophthalmology* 1985;92:503.

35. Blankenship GW. Pars plana vitrectomy for diabetic retinopathy, a report of 8 years' experience. *Mod Probl Ophthalmol* 1979;20:376–386.

36. Glaser BM, D'Amore PA, Michels RG, et al. Demonstration of vasoproliferative activity from mammalian retina. *J Cell Biol* 1980;84:298.

37. Glaser BM, D'Amore PA, Michels RG, et al. The demonstration of angiogenic activity from ocular tissues: preliminary report. *Ophthalmology* 1980;87:440.

38. Glaser BM, D'Amore PA, Lutty GA, et al. Chemical mediators of intraocular neovascularization. *Trans Ophthalmol Soc UK* 1980;100:369.

39. Glaser BM, D'Amore PA, Michels RG. The effects of human intraocular fluid on vascular endothelial cell migration: correlation with intraocular neovascularization. *Ophthalmology* 1981;88:986.

40. Fett JW, Strydom DJ, Lobb RR, et al. Isolation and characterization of angiogenin, an angiogenic protein from human carcinoma cells. *Biochemistry* 1985;24:5480–5486.

41. Glaser BM, Campochiaro PA, Davis JL, et al. Retinal pigment epithelial cells release an inhibitor of neovascularization. *Arch Ophthalmol* 1985;103:1870.

42. Wolbarsht ML, Landers MB. The rationale of photocoagulation therapy for proliferative diabetic retinopathy—a review and a model. *Ophthalmic Surg* 1980;11:235.

6

Retinal Breaks and Detachment

PREVENTION OF RETINAL DETACHMENT

It is probable that the per capita incidence of retinal detachment has decreased over the past three decades. The replacement of intracapsular cataract surgery, first by extracapsular surgery, and then by phakoemulsification with endocapsular intraocular lenses (IOLs), has certainly contributed to the decline. The widespread use of indirect ophthalmoscopy and retinopexy for prophylaxis of retinal breaks has probably had a major impact as well. It is also likely that the increased use of protective eyewear has made a contribution.

POSSIBILITY OF EVIDENCE-BASED TREATMENT FOR RETINAL DETACHMENT

The increasing number of retinal specialists per capita, coupled with fewer detachments per patient year, variable pathology, and significantly more treatment options, has virtually guaranteed that the treatment of retinal detachment will never move to an evidence-based paradigm because of the statistical complexity. Therapeutic options include scleral buckling, primary vitrectomy, pneumatic retinopexy, and the Lincoff balloon. Gas choices include air, C_3F_8, and SF_6. Buckle options include sponges versus "hard" silicone, drainage versus nondrainage, encircling versus segmental, radial versus circumferential, and so on. Retinopexy choices include cryo- versus transscleral laser versus diathermy. Many of these therapies are used in combination, making the analysis even more complex.

PROPHYLACTIC RETINOPEXY

Laser is preferred to cryotherapy for prophylactic retinopexy because there is less pain and potentially less PVR. The authors prefer low- to moderate-intensity confluent lesions with fewer rows over the very common method of using many rows of heavy, spaced-out lesions. Many authors recommend treatment only if the retinal breaks are symptomatic (1–10). Relying on the patient can be effective in a population of highly educated people but is less reliable in patients having less education and more socioeconomic problems. Large breaks are typically more significant than small breaks. Retinal detachment in the other eye or another location in the same eye, or a family history of detachment is a relative indication for treatment. Patients for whom cataract surgery is planned, athletes, or those in certain careers may need prophylactic treatment as well. Retinal breaks outside lattice are more significant than breaks inside lattice. Superior breaks are probably more significant than inferior breaks. Pigment around breaks does not indicate adherence to the retinal pigment epithelium but does indicate chronicity.

Laser can be used to "wall off" a small retinal detachment. On occasion, walled-off detachments will spontaneously reattach. Laser confinement of relatively small retinal detachments has remarkably good long-term results and is almost certainly underutilized because of habit and economics.

PRIMARY VITRECTOMY

Indications

The use of so-called primary vitrectomy is increasing because of economic incentives and the fact that more surgeons are trained in vitrectomy, better methods for drainage of subretinal fluid (SRF) and retinopexy are available, and fewer surgeons learn scleral buckling. When vitrectomy alone, scleral buckling alone, pneumatic retinopexy alone, or some combination of vitrectomy, gas, and buckling should be used is a very complex issue with few answers. In general, vitrectomy, gas, and laser should be used when vitreous opacities or traction make it unlikely that scleral buckling alone will succeed. Relative advantages of scleral buckling include less cataract progression, less cost, and proven high success rates in certain types of detachments. Advantages of vitrectomy include no impact on refraction, the extraocular muscles, or levator function. The highest success rate would be anticipated if vitrectomy and scleral buckles were used, but the cost and complexity are higher, and either the vitrectomy or buckling component may be unnecessary. Many surgeons, including the authors, use primary vitrectomy in most pseudophakic detachments. The authors are more inclined to use primary vitrectomy for superior detachments and buckling for inferior detachments. Evidence of traction on breaks, especially large horseshoe tears, suggests the need for vitrectomy. The presence of avulsed vessels also suggests the need for vitrectomy.

Surgical Sequence for Primary Vitrectomy

It is essential to remove as much peripheral vitreous as possible without damaging the lens or creating new retinal breaks. Scleral depression is very useful for this purpose. Although many surgeons use wide-angle visualization for peripheral vitrectomy, the authors find irrigating contact lenses to be faster and more efficient when combined with scleral depression.

All traction should be removed from each retinal break. It is crucial to remove traction on the anterior edge as well as from the more apparent flap. Amputation of the tip of the flap insures removal of this component of the traction.

If the breaks/tears can be seen easily after fluid/air exchange, they can be used for internal drainage of SRF. If access to the breaks is difficult, a posterior drainage retinotomy or perfluorocarbon liquids are required. Drainage retinotomy can be initiated by using the two-function manipulator or disposable bipolar endoilluminator to coagulate, weaken, and mark the site (Fig. 6.1). Outside the arcades, at the most posterior extent of the SRF is often a good location. Nasal is better than temporal for total detachments. A single tap on the vitreous cutter pedal can serve to make an ideal round retinotomy (Fig. 6.2). The soft-tip cannula is ideal for drainage of subretinal fluid (Fig. 6.3). Internal drainage of SRF should precede fluid/air exchange, especially with use of preexisting peripheral retinal

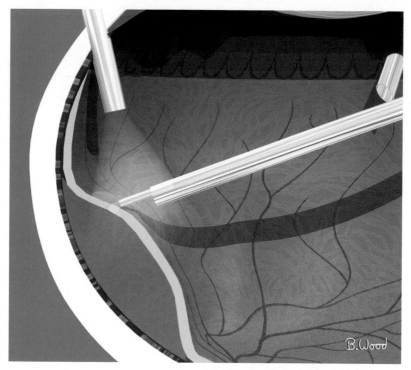

FIG. 6.1. The disposable bipolar endoilluminator is used to coagulate and mark the site prior to drainage retinotomy.

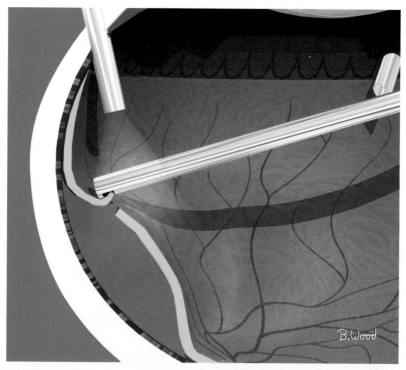

FIG. 6.2. A single tap on the vitreous cutter pedal makes a small, round retinotomy.

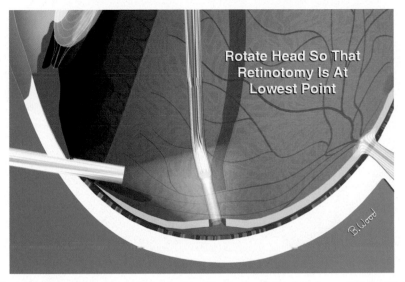

FIG. 6.3. The soft-tip cannula is the ideal instrument for draining subretinal fluid.

breaks for drainage. If IOL fogging occurs during fluid/air exchange, liquid perfluorocarbon can be used to displace the SRF anteriorly out the retinal breaks (Fig. 6.4). Endolaser retinopexy can be performed under perfluorocarbon liquids (PFCL). Fogging can be anticipated if a YAG capsulotomy has been performed and the anterior vitreous cortex has been disrupted. The Chang End-Aspirating laser probe is ideal for primary vitrectomy, PDR/TRD, and PVR cases because SRF can be removed continuously while treating the retinal breaks (Fig. 6.5).

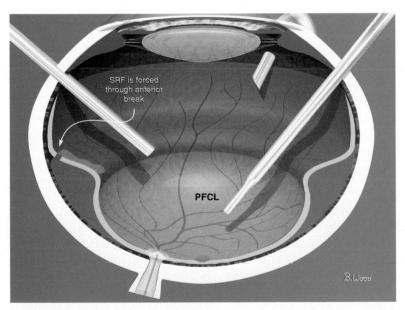

FIG. 6.4. If IOL fogging occurs during FAX, liquid perfluorocarbon can be used to force subretinal fluid anteriorly through retinal breaks.

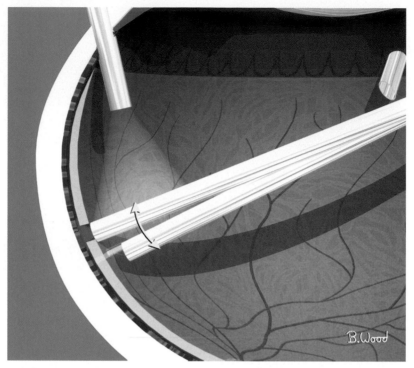

FIG. 6.5. The end-aspirating laser allows simultaneous retinopexy during aspiration of sub-retinal fluid.

Although many surgeons perform 360° laser treatment in primary vitrectomy and even macular hole cases, it is unknown whether this reduces postoperative retinal detachment. Some surgeons use laser indirect ophthalmoscopy (LIO) instead of endolaser. This approach theoretically increases nuclear sclerosis and corneal damage from laser energy absorption. It is likely that light scatter from the cornea and lens will increase macular damage as well. Iris damage often occurs with LIO during vitrectomy. It is unclear if there are any advantages to this approach.

It is unknown if scleral buckling is needed in primary vitrectomy for retinal detachment. The authors rarely use scleral buckling in vitrectomy cases in order to reduce induced refractive error, strabismus, pain, and ptosis.

SCLERAL BUCKLING

Sponges Versus Hard Silicone

The smooth surface and relative incompressibility of "hard" silicone make it superior to sponges for scleral buckling. Higher extrusion and infection rates make sponges less desirable (11,12). Sponges create a higher buckle immediately under the sutures and a lower buckle between the sutures. This may create a higher incidence of radial folds. The area of lesser buckling effect between sutures corresponds with regions of bulging under the conjunctiva, which creates a dellen-like effect, leading to exposure of the buckle (Fig. 6.6).

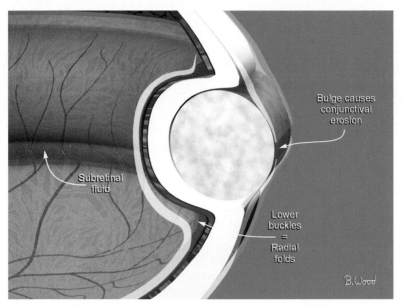

FIG. 6.6. The problems with sponges include conjunctival erosion and radial folds.

Implants Versus Explants

Although scleral dissection is an acceptable method of scleral buckling, its use is decreasing markedly because it is inflexible and time-consuming. The original justification for scleral dissection was the ability to avoid scleral damage from full-thickness diathermy. Although burying the buckle under a flap reduces extrusion, it increases intrusion, operating time, inflexibility, and the risk of scleral perforation.

Buckling with Vitreous Surgery

Scleral buckling is practiced with many variations for retinal reattachment (13,14). A rapid, simplified form of scleral buckling is advantageous when it must be combined with vitreous surgery and is preferred by the authors for all scleral buckling (Fig. 6.7). The elimination of vitreous traction coupled with complete intraoperative reattachment dictates a different approach to scleral buckling than is utilized without vitreous surgery. Like retinopexy, scleral buckling should be performed after completion of vitreous surgery and internal drainage of subretinal fluid, fluid/air exchange, and completion of SRF drainage. Only at this time can a realistic assessment of the extent of buckling required be made and iatrogenic breaks incorporated into the buckling location planning process.

The complete control over intraocular pressure (IOP) inherent to a sew-on infusion cannula permits extremely extensive and high scleral buckles without increased IOP. Vitreous surgery with any instrument has a baseline incidence of peripheral, aphakic-like, retinal detachments. This is analogous to the incidence of retinal detachment noted to accompany vitreous loss at cataract surgery. In addition, forces created by instrument introduction add to this baseline incidence. Peripheral vitreous is usually trapped on the inner portion of the sclerotomies at the time of wound closure, causing late retinal detachments from contraction of this vitreous.

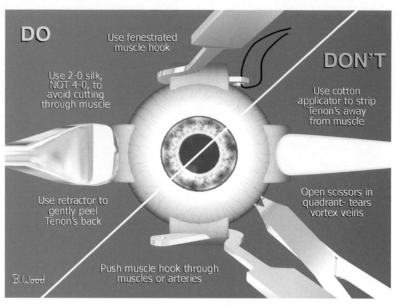

FIG. 6.7. A rapid, simplified form of scleral buckling is advantageous.

Encircling Bands

Prophylactic scleral buckling with an encircling band can then be thought of as making a new ora serrata to treat peripheral vitreoretinal traction preceding retinal detachment. Encircling bands for prophylactic buckling were used frequently in the early days of vitrectomy (15,16). This approach is rarely used today because of better cutters, techniques, fluidics, and dissection methods. Local anesthesia, outpatient surgery, and cost containment all contribute to the elimination of prophylactic buckling.

The method used for encircling bands will be described later for those occasions in which it will be required. Scleral belt loops are made after the retromuscle traction sutures are placed and before the infusion cannula sclerotomy is made. A hockey stick blade #57 (Grieshaber CS1 014) is used for the radial cuts, which are made 3 mm apart and 2 mm long at the equator. A disposable electrothermal cautery is used for hemostasis and tissue shrinkage. Forceps (0.3 Castroviejo) are used to lift the edge, and a bent, rounded end blade #69B (Grieshaber 681.28) is used to undermine the sclera between the radial cuts. Rows of retinopexy are no longer utilized to reduce inflammation and scarring. The band is pulled through the belt loops and under the rectus muscles with 0.3 Castroviejo forceps. The band is joined superonasally using a 3-0 Supramid suture with two individual passes and knots around the two bands. The band is not sutured to the sclera. Moderate imbrication effect is judged by external inspection, rather than arbitrarily using measurement of the band or IOP, both of which are unreliable and interdependent. By using scleral belt loops, the buckle is of equal height in each quadrant and the band will slip circumferentially with ease. The belt loops and the Supramid suture decrease the incidence of extrusion and infection, compared with other methods. The Watzke sleeve is more difficult to place, and tantalum clips have fallen out of popularity.

Circumferential Explants

Because of their narrow configuration, bands alone are usually not utilized to treat specific retinal breaks. If a circumferential explant can cover the posterior extent of a retinal break, it is utilized in preference to a radial explant. Circumferential explants require less exacting localization, do not distort the macula, and cover a broader extent of vitreous base pathology. Posterior breaks are managed with vitrectomy techniques. The principal author has not used radial buckles or sponges for more than 20 years in the buckling alone or vitrectomy setting.

Monofilament (5-0) nylon sutures are utilized with a single circumferential posterior scleral bite. In contrast to radial suture bites, the circumferential bite can be quite long without reducing the posterior extent of the buckle. The single circumferential posterior scleral bite reduces by one-half the chances of perforating the retina, as compared with paired bites. This posterior bite is always placed 3 mm and preferably 5 mm posterior to the most posterior aspect of the most posterior break. An excessively anterior positioning of the buckle causes many reoperations after scleral buckling procedures.

All anterior scleral bites are placed circumferentially in the scleral condensation, conforming to the rectus muscle insertions. This provides an area of thicker sclera for greater permanence. This muscle ring also conforms to the ora serrata; therefore a scleral suture bite placed here in a circumferential orientation cannot perforate the retina (Fig. 6.8). Extending all circumferential buckles to the ora serrata prevents the anterior leakage of SRF associated with narrow bands or buckles placed more posteriorly.

The explant is trimmed from a larger piece of silicone for a custom fit if a standard-width implant will not work. In every case, the explant width is made so that the outer surface of the explant conforms to the contour of the globe after tying up the sutures. Off-shelf explant with sutures placed 1 to 3 mm wider than the explant will not provide the

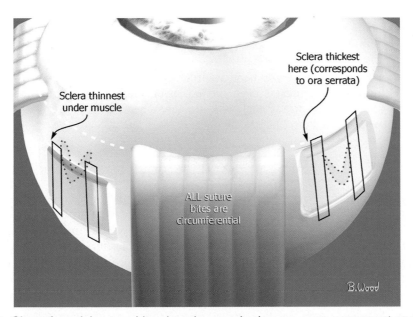

FIG. 6.8. Circumferential suture bites into the muscle ring are more permanent and cannot perforate the retina.

correct effect. If a large ratio of implant width to suture spread is utilized, the explant will be only partially imbricated into the sclera. This external protuberance wears a hole in the conjunctiva by creating a dellen-like effect, is similar to that observed with sponges, and provides a less substantial buckling effect. A slight chamfering of the cut edges of the silicone seems to provide a lesser chance of scleral or conjunctival erosion. Two or three mattress sutures per quadrant provide the most consistent buckling effect and reduce the chance of extrusion or sutures pulling through the sclera. Explants without grooves are preferred because they do not fold along the groove and bands are never combined with buckles using the author's technique.

The authors use the circumferential buckle method described earlier for all scleral buckling with or without vitreous surgery. All detached quadrants are buckled, direct needle drainage of subretinal fluid is used exclusively, and bands, sponges, and radial buckles are never used. An attempt is made to avoid the superior rectus as mentioned earlier, and only muscles absolutely necessary to exposure are engaged with traction sutures. Minimal retinopexy is used. Transscleral diode laser retinopexy is alternative to cryopexy; however, it cannot be used in highly pigmented patients and is more difficult to judge treatment intensity.

Scleral Buckling with a Broad Encircling Buckle

If proliferative vitreoretinopathy (PVR) is present, a 360°, moderate-height, broad buckle is utilized with the procedures described for circumferential buckles. Encircling sponges can result in anterior or posterior leakage. As PVR is a diffuse process, no attempt is made to customize the buckle contour; instead a uniformly high, broad, encircling buckle is utilized (see Fig. 7.13) (S. Charles, unpublished data, 1977).

The posterior circumferential bites are made as posteriorly as possible without compression of vortex veins, and the circumferential anterior bite is placed in the scleral condensation at the muscle ring. The usual suture spread is 10 to 12 mm, with the usual tire being 6 to 9 mm in width. Imbrication will then cause the buckle to be flush with the surface of the globe. The ends are joined with two interrupted 5-0 nylon sutures, with long bites through the implant material, and the knot is then buried. To provide a consistently smooth internal buckle contour, no band, encircling suture or overlapping is used. The direct needle-drainage technique is used for the intraoperative elimination of subretinal fluid before the encircling tire is anchored in place, when indicated, if this technique is used without vitrectomy (see Chapter 4).

Scleral Defects

Thin sclera can be covered in most cases with a circumferential scleral buckling or encircling tire, previously described. Preserved sclera and fascia lata add a degree of complexity, infection risk, and risk of dehiscence, and are rarely utilized. Full-thickness defects, unless extremely large, can usually be repaired by suturing good tissue edges together rather than by oversewing. This approach creates a scleral shortening effect that may be beneficial with PVR or wound-related cellular proliferation. A small leaking area can be handled with various tissue adhesives. Sponges appear to be more erosive to the sclera than hard silicone and are therefore not utilized.

REFERENCES

1. Foos RY. Posterior vitreous detachment. *Trans Am Acad Ophthalmol Otolaryngol* 1972;76:480.
2. Linder B. Acute posterior vitreous detachment and its retinal complications. *Acta Ophthalmol* 1966;87[Suppl]:1.

3. Foos RY. Anatomic and pathologic aspects of the vitreous body. *Trans Am Acad Ophthalmol Otolaryngol* 1973; 77:171.
4. Foos RY. Tears of the peripheral retina: pathogenesis, incidence, and classification in autopsy eyes. *Mod Probl Ophthalmol* 1975;15:68–81.
5. Byer NE. Clinical study of retinal breaks. *Trans Am Acad Ophthalmol Otolaryngol* 1967;71:461–473.
6. Byer NE. The natural history of asymptomatic retinal breaks. *Ophthalmology* 1982;89:1033–1039.
7. Byer NE. Long term natural history of lattice degeneration of the retina. *Ophthalmology* 1989;96:1369–1401.
8. Byer NE. Cystic retinal tufts and their relationship to retinal detachment. *Arch Ophthalmol* 1981;99:1788–1790.
9. Byer NE. Natural history of posterior vitreous detachment with early management as the premier line of defense against retinal detachment. *Ophthalmology* 1994;101:1503–1513.
10. McHugh DA, Schwartz S, Dowler JG, et al. Diode laser contact transscleral retinal photocoagulation: a clinical study. *Br J Ophthalmol* 1995;79:1083–1087.
11. Russo CE, Ruiz RS. Silicone sponge rejection: early and late complications in retinal detachment surgery. *Arch Ophthalmol* 1971;85:647.
12. Hahn YS, Lincoff A, Lincoff H, et al. Infection after sponge implantation for scleral buckling. *Am J Ophthalmol* 1979;87:180.
13. Devenyi RG, de Carvalho Nakamura H, et al. Combined scleral buckle and pare plana vitrectomy as a primary procedure for pseudophakic retinal detachments. *Ophthalm Surg Lasers* 1999;30:615–618.
14. Desai UR, Strassman IB. Combined pars plana vitrectomy and scleral buckling for pseudophakic and aphakic retinal detachments in which a break is not seen preoperatively. *Ophthalmic Surg Lasers* 1997;28:718–722.
15. Michels RG. Vitrectomy for the complications of diabetic retinopathy. *Arch Ophthalmol* 1978,96:237.
16. Hutton WL, Snyder WB, Vaiser A. Vitrectomy in the treatment of ocular perforating injuries. *Am J Ophthalmol* 1976;81:733.

7

Proliferative Vitreoretinopathy

Proliferative vitreoretinopathy (PVR) can be thought of as a reparative or scarring mechanism. Contact inhibition is lost because of mechanical disruption of a tissue such as the retinal pigment epithelium (RPE), and the response is migration, contraction, and moderate proliferation of cells. A defect in the internal limiting membrane (ILL, ILM) can be created by vitreous traction, a retinal break, or membrane dissection. Glial cells then migrate, proliferate to some extent, and contract the retinal surface as if to repair the retina/lLM defect. Retinal breaks "heal" as a result of this mechanism, as has been shown in macular hole surgery and retinotomies for submacular surgery. Similarly, if the retina is separated from the RPE, the RPE cells migrate to the retinal surface and the posterior surface of the posterior vitreous cortex (PVC). Monocytes can gain access to the retinal surface from the iris and ciliary body capillaries as a result of ocular inflammation. It is known that these cells can migrate, proliferate, and contract on the retinal surface (1–13).

Glial, RPE, and monocytic cells migrate along an existing substrate or to a new tissue surface. As cellular migration occurs, intracellular contraction of the cells occurs, creating tangential traction on the retina. All healing mechanisms studied have demonstrated a microtubule, smooth, musclelike contraction process occurring with many cells acting in concert. The myofibroblasts have coated pits, which have specific receptor sites for collagen, fibrin, and elastin. These pits contain fibronectin, which allow the cells to attach to collagen fibers (14,15). Growth factors (e.g., TGF Beta), metalloproteinases, fibronectin, and receptors for collagen, elastin, and fibrin are components of the migration and contraction phenomenon. Proliferation (mitotic activity) is thought by the authors to be of much lesser importance. The authors think of this as hypocellular periretinal scarring, which is analogous to hypocellular vitreous contraction. To emphasize the hypocellular nature of this process, the authors suggest that we take the *P* out of *PVR*. Tangential shortening of the cells occurs before collagen production, which may be thought of as a late stabilization phase. The generation of basement membrane and collagen can be thought of as a recreation of Bruch's membrane or the ILM, as if to duplicate the process that occurs in embryonic development.

Proliferative vitreoretinopathy can be localized and create isolated star folds, fixed folds, subretinal changes, or epimacular membranes (16–18). It can be more widespread, which gave rise to the no-longer-used term *massive periretinal proliferation*. If the proliferation of glial or RPE cells extended onto the contiguous posterior surface of the PVC, the older term *massive vitreous retraction* would have been used. At this time, there is no proof of the role of hyalocytes in the pathogenesis.

Scarring in the subretinal space can occur in many physical configurations, as discussed later (see the section entitled "Subretinal Proliferation"). A placoid configuration can create an inverted star fold configuration. Subretinal bands (strands) occur presumably as tubes of RPE cells proliferate along a fibrin strand. These then contract, causing an extended dendritic configuration. If the band is circumferential at the mid-retinal level, it can create an annular configuration with a resultant closed-cone retinal detachment.

CASE SELECTION

Vitrectomy Versus Scleral Buckling

Vitrectomy should be thought of as a mechanical approach to a mechanical problem not reparable by scleral buckling alone. It has no known prophylactic benefit in the prevention of PVR, nor is it an approach to be utilized only after several scleral buckles are tried (18). Simply stated, if it appears that vitrectomy will enhance the prognosis, it should be combined with the scleral buckling or used alone as the initial procedure.

Operability

Extensive star folds, even in a closed-cone (funnel) configuration, are usually operable (Fig. 7.1). If extensive membrane peeling has been performed, the recurrent proliferation may be more adherent to the retinal surface. Excessive retinopexy probably causes RPE and glial reproliferation, whereas retinal surface dissection probably causes glial proliferation. If extensive subretinal placoid proliferation is present, this is often inoperable. Redundant retina can simulate diffuse subretinal placoid proliferation, making clinical assessment difficult. The presence of large retinal breaks and extensive surface proliferation was thought of as inoperable before the advent of epi- and subretinal dissection, internal drainage of SRF, retinectomy, and silicone oil. In addition to the mechani-

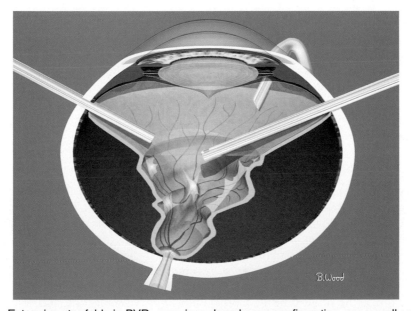

FIG. 7.1. Extensive star folds in PVR, even in a closed-cone configuration, are usually operable.

cally inoperable configurations, there are many patient-based and biologic decisions related to operability. If the patient has an apparently operable mechanical configuration but has had many recurrences after vitrectomy, surgery might be contraindicated because of biologic behavior, especially if the patient has another functional eye, has medical problems, or is very elderly. Iris neovascularization, glaucomatous cupping, and severe uveitis can influence the decision of operability as well.

Cases with extremely recent proliferative activity and an inflammatory component have a worse prognosis than inactive cases (19). In such cases, a period of observation and subconjunctival steroids should precede surgery (S Charles, unpublished data, 1979; RG Michels, personal communication). As described by SJ Ryan, a definite life cycle characterizes this reparative or scarring process. Recurrent proliferation is reduced if reoperation is delayed until the proliferation stabilizes and inflammation is minimal. Proliferative inactivity can be judged by the presence of minimal cells and flare, waning conjunctival hyperemia, increased comfort, and lack of further progression of epiretinal membranes.

SURGICAL SEQUENCE AND TECHNIQUES

Initial Steps

After the conjunctiva and Tenon's capsule are opened circumferentially 1 mm posterior to the limbus, a fenestrated muscle hook is used to place retromuscle traction sutures, if scleral buckling is to be performed. The operating microscope is used to facilitate the exposure of the old buckle as well as to place the new buckle. The infusion cannula is placed in the usual position 3 mm posterior to the limbus, verified to be in proper position through the microscope, and utilized to prevent hypotony if a previous buckle(s) is to be is removed. All the previous scleral buckling materials and sutures are removed unless a relatively wide encircling element has been utilized during a previous procedure. The exposure of the sclera is extended under each muscle to just behind the vortex veins (being careful to avoid these). If scleral dehiscences are present, it is probably better to close these with sutures placed in thicker sclera, resulting in a scleral resection effect, rather than to treat them with scleral patch grafts. Any open subretinal fluid (SRF) drainage site or sclerotomy closed with absorbable sutures should be sutured with an 8-0 monofilament nylon suture to prevent leakage and incarceration. The sclerotomies for the endoilluminator and active instruments should be made in the usual position 3 mm posterior to the limbus, avoiding previous sclerotomies.

Management of the Lens or Intraocular Lens

The crystalline lens should be removed in moderate to advanced PVR cases to permit careful peripheral vitreous dissection and decompartmentalization. Endocapsular lensectomy should be utilized unless extremely dense nuclear sclerosis demands combined extracapsular cataract extraction.

If a posterior chamber intraocular lens is present, it should be retained. Selected anterior chamber and iris plane lenses must be removed. Implant removal (see Chapter 3) can occasionally result in an intraoperative hemorrhage, cause corneal and iris damage, and compromise the surgical result. Corneal incisions, viscoelastics, and haptic cutting minimize the incidence of intraoperative hemorrhage. Cut haptics can be left if bleeding is anticipated because of fibrous scarring around the haptic. The hypotony that occurs during lens removal can theoretically cause choroidal hemorrhage. The patient's refraction is made myopic with a broad encircling buckle, rendering the IOL optically less advantageous. Simultaneous IOL implantation causes many PVR cases to fail and is frequently overutilized.

COMPARTMENTALIZATION

Serum components and inflammation play a role in the causation and acceleration of PVR. A source tissue produces growth factors, which then target substrate tissues. The target tissue (retina) is in the same compartment as the source in PVR, but on remote surfaces in proliferative diabetic retinopathy (VEGF, iris and trabecular meshwork). Viscoelastics, fibrin, inflammation, and blood can be thought of as culture media enhancing PVR. The lens or IOL creates a two-compartment eye, prolonging the cell culture–like environment, and provides a migration substrate. Removal of the lens in PVR cases increases the egress rate of cytokines, cells, and serum components such as fibronectin through the trabecular meshwork. Similarly, gases and silicone produce sequestration of cells and factors at the retinal-bubble interface enhancing PVR.

Vitrectomy

The anterior vitreous cortex (AVC) is removed first, along with all vitreous attachments to cataract and trauma wounds, and the iris. Very low suction force using the proportional suction control should be utilized to prevent retinal breaks from suction-induced vitreoretinal traction. The highest cutting rates should be used to increase fluidic stability. The PVC is frequently in contact with the AVC and removable in a single step. A posterior vitreous detachment (PVD) is almost always present in PVR cases. Hypocellular vitreous contraction causes the PVC and AVC to come together in a "frontal plane" (FP) configuration. *Core vitrectomy* is a misnomer; a core configuration does not exist in PVR eyes.

Anterior PVR

Anteroposterior vitreous fibers normally extend from the retina at the posterior edge of the vitreous base to the pars plana, ciliary body, and iris. Frequently, these fibers undergo hypocellular vitreous contraction and pull the equatorial retina anteriorly into a circumferential fold. The principal author first described this phenomenon as anterior loop contraction in 1975. A circumferential equatorial ring of epiretinal membrane or contracted equatorial vitreous is typically present in PVR. Hypocellular contraction of the AVC and PVC is also common in PVR cases. Collectively, these structures are known as anterior PVR. They are frequently incorrectly termed "*vitreous membranes* or the *vitreous base.* Anterior PVR must be relieved to allow retinal reattachment.

Scleral depression by the assistant facilitates anterior PVR dissection. The radial component of anterior PVR dissection can be done with the vitreous cutter if broad or delamination scissors if narrow (Fig. 7.2). The diamond-coated, end-opening forceps can be used to peel posterior ERMs in an anterior direction to the posterior edge of the vitreous base. Blunt dissection with the vitreous cutter and endoilluminator can be used to separate vitreous and ERM from peripheral retina (see Fig. 5.9). Delamination scissors can be used to delaminate or segment the circumferential component (Fig. 7.3).

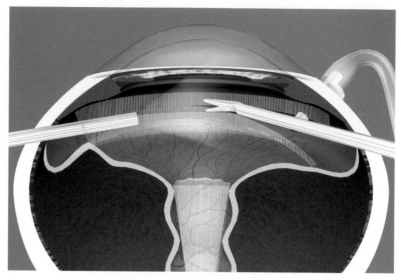

FIG. 7.2. The radial component of anterior loop traction is dissected with the right-angle scissors. ALT must be relieved to allow retinal reattachment.

Epiretinal Membranes

Membrane peeling can cause retinal breaks, hemorrhage, and defects in the ILM implicated in the recurrence of cellular migration, contraction, and proliferation. Often the epiretinal membranes peel easily with none of these problems and allow complete release of tangential traction (Fig. 7.4). End-opening, diamond-coated, 20-gauge forceps (Grieshaber 612.12) are the authors' choice for membrane peeling (Fig. 7.5). The principal author has not used pics since 1978. If the membranes are tightly adherent, they should be segmented and/or delaminated with 20-gauge horizontal delamination scissors. Forceps

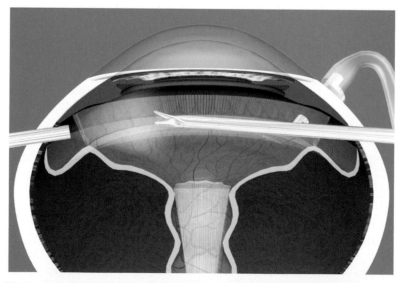

FIG. 7.3. Right-angle scissors are used to segment or delaminate the circumferential component of ALT.

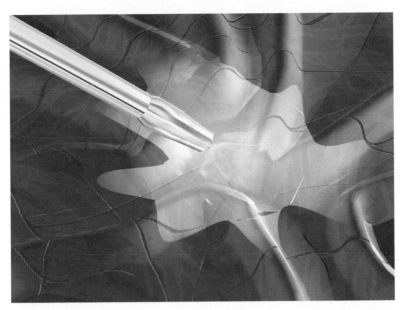

FIG. 7.4. Inside-out pinch-peeling of epiretinal membranes with the diamond-coated end-opening forceps often allows complete release of tangential traction without retinal breaks, hemorrhage, or ILM damage, and their subsequent complications.

membrane peeling or segmentation/delamination of the ERM causing a star fold, fixed fold, or area appearing to have retinal/retinal adherence must be completed, or retinectomy may be required. A specific attempt must be made to release the ERM, causing circumferential traction at the equator by using scissors segmentation or delamination. If this cannot be safely accomplished because of tight adherence to the retinal surface, this portion of ERM can be left intact and supported by the very broad and high buckle. Frequently, dense ERM can be delaminated from the retinal surface with delamination scissors with the blades parallel to the retinal surface. Segmentation of the denser portions of an ERM using the same scissors is very effective in releasing traction and tends to be underutilized (Fig. 7.6). When

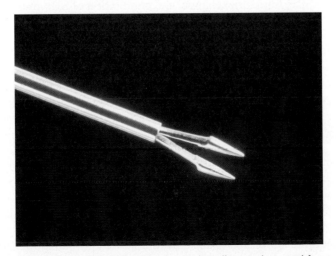

FIG. 7.5. Grieshaber 612.12 end-opening diamond-coated forceps.

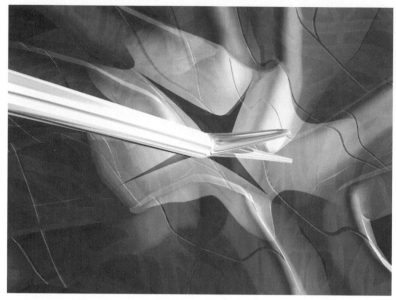

FIG. 7.6. Inside-out segmentation of denser portions of the ERM with right-angle scissors can be very effective and tends to be underutilized. When the entire surface of the retina can be visualized and the sharp angulations have been converted to rounded contours, dissection is complete.

the entire surface of the retina can be visualized and the sharp angulations have been converted to rounded contours, dissection is complete.

Subretinal Proliferation

Many anatomic forms of subretinal proliferation occur, just as there is variability in the configuration of ERMs. The term *strands* is a misnomer because of the frequent occurrence of placoid elements.

Placoid subretinal proliferation, if moderate in extent, is managed by attempting internal drainage of SRF, fluid/air exchange, and completion of SRF drainage. If the retina becomes attached, subretinal surgery and/or scleral buckling are not required. If there is extensive proliferation, subretinal forceps removal is required.

Dendritic proliferation can usually be managed by forceps removal (Fig. 7.7) or segmentation, internal drainage of SRF, fluid/air exchange, and completion of SRF drainage. The diamond-coated, end-opening forceps are pushed through the retina over the densest part of the subretinal proliferation (Fig. 7.8) and used to grasp and remove the tissue (Fig. 7.9). Care must be taken to avoid entrapping the retina in the forceps or damaging the RPE or choroid. Frequently the dendrite will break, releasing the traction.

Extension of dendritic proliferation in a rather posterior, circumferential configuration gives rise to an annular ring configuration. After completion of the vitrectomy and inside-out forceps membrane peeling, the scissors are placed in the subretinal space through an existing retinal break or a cut made in the retina over the subretinal annulus. Scissors allow the surgeon to transect the annulus at a considerable distance from the retinal defect used to gain entry to the subretinal space. The endoilluminator can be used to illuminate the subretinal space and to contact and palpate the retina to deter-

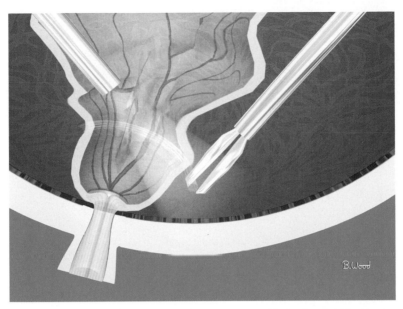

FIG. 7.7. Dendritic proliferation can usually be managed by subretinal forceps removal.

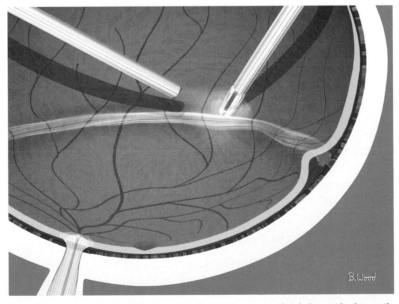

FIG. 7.8. The diamond-coated, end-opening forceps are pushed through the retina over the densest part of the subretinal proliferation and are used to grasp and remove the tissue through the retinotomy.

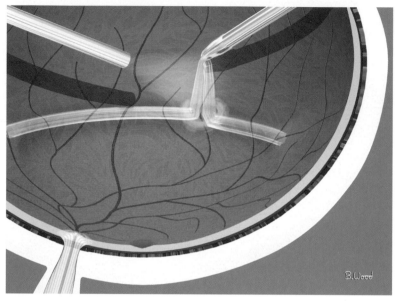

FIG. 7.9. Through sequential regrasping, the subretinal proliferation can be completely removed.

mine if the traction has been alleviated. At times, it is necessary to transect the annulus in several locations.

Following transection or removal of the annulus or dendritic membrane, internal drainage of SRF, then fluid/air exchange, and completion of SRF drainage, laser endophotocoagulation, and scleral buckling, when necessary, with a wide buckle are completed. If an appropriate encircling buckle is present, no additional buckling is required. Attachment and endophotocoagulation can be followed by air/gas exchange or air/silicone exchange. If extensive membrane is present in the subretinal space, a 90° or greater circumferential retinectomy can be performed to allow visualization and access to the subretinal space. Large retinectomies are almost never required to remove subretinal proliferation. Direct puncture retinotomies can allow access to very posterior subretinal proliferation. Internal drainage of SRF, fluid/air exchange, and completion of SRF drainage followed by endophotocoagulation, and air/silicone exchange are required in most of these severe PVR cases.

The Reattachment Experiment

The reattachment experiment is defined as the combination of internal drainage of SRF, fluid/air exchange, and completion of internal drainage of SRF to determine the need for further dissection. In contrast to the normally low transretinal pressure gradient, a somewhat higher gradient is created, forcing a moderately stiffened retina against the RPE. The air pump connected to the infusion cannula and the soft-tip cannula should be utilized for this step. This should be followed by air/gas exchange or air/silicone exchange at the end of the procedure. On occasion, this step will uncover areas of ERM not seen before the retinal cone was opened up. Forceps membrane peeling, delamination, or segmentation of these now visible membranes can be performed under air, further releasing tangential traction.

\ Moderate to small amounts of subretinal air appearing during the reattachment experiment indicate that the traction has not been completely eliminated, which can be rectified by scleral buckling if not already in place. The subretinal air will frequently reenter the intraocular cavity as scleral buckling pushes the pigment epithelium in contact with the retina. Until the remaining traction on the retina is relieved, it is impossible to remove subretinal air unless the eye is refilled with infusion fluid. It is better to leave the subretinal air in place and proceed with further peeling, segmentation delamination, subretinal surgery, retinectomy, and/or scleral buckling. Very anterior, direct needle drainage of subretinal air after tying up the buckle sutures will allow its complete removal.

At times, retinal defects will enlarge greatly or spontaneous defects will occur as the reattachment experiment is performed. This will allow the release of tangential traction on foreshortened retinas and permit retinal conformation with the pigment epithelium. These defects occasionally are extensive, leading to inoperability, but in many cases are helpful in allowing retinal reattachment.

The basic mechanical problem in PVR retina is retinal foreshortening combined with the requirement of the retina to conform to the inner surface of the rigid eye wall. The tensile strength and contraction forces of periretinal membranes exceed the strength of the retina and the normal transretinal pressure gradient by a factor of approximately 100.

High scleral buckles coupled with marked retinal foreshortening may push the posterior retina away from the RPE. Scleral resection is technically difficult, has a limited effect, and works only for uniform foreshortening in several quadrants.

RETINECTOMY

Steep folds can result from retinal incarceration in the sclera at the prior sclerotomies, trauma sites, or previous drainage sites. If a single fold occurs, a retinal cut made perpendicular to the long axis of the fold will release the traction, analogous to a plastic surgeon releasing a scar. Multiple steep folds radiating from an epicenter of periretinal membrane may require retinectomy, including or surrounding the epicenter. In general, radial folds require circumferential cuts, just as the typical equatorial, circumferential fold requires a radial cut.

Diffuse retinal foreshortening that cannot be managed by membrane peeling/segmentation/delamination requires large circumferential retinectomies (Fig. 7.10). Other surgeons use the term *relaxing retinotomies,* indicating that no retina is removed with their approach. The retinectomy approach was developed by the author to remove all tissue anterior to the circumferential "relaxing" retinotomy. The advantage of complete removal is less hypotony from epiciliary tissue, less iris neovascularization from ischemic tissue, and less anterior movement of a silicone oil bubble due to contraction of the circumferential ring of pars plana tissue. Cases requiring large circumferential retinectomies are managed similar to giant breaks with PVR using silicone oil but usually not scleral buckling.

The need for large retinectomies frequently cannot be anticipated in the office. Excessive retinectomies can result from underestimation of the effectiveness of periretinal dissection methods. Large retinectomies are needed only after failure of the reattachment experiment. In all cases, the retinal reattachment experiment should be attempted after completion of periretinal membrane dissection and stopped immediately if subretinal air appears. Incremental retinectomy with endodiathermy applied to retinal vessels to be transected should be alternated with incremental additional drainage of SRF. This process

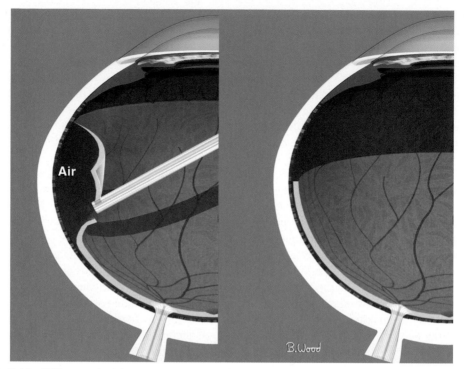

FIG. 7.10. Diffuse retinal foreshortening that cannot be managed by membrane peeling/segmentation/delamination requires large circumferential retinectomies.

should cease only when the retina is so rigid it cannot be mechanically unfolded or it becomes completely reattached (20).

The contributing factors in achieving intraoperative reattachment include surface tension of the fluid/air interface, size of the retinal breaks, retinal stiffness, and the contour of the eye wall (see Chapter 4). When periretinal membrane dissection is completed and the reattachment experiment is applied, further mechanical forces on the retina may become apparent. Mechanically holding the retina in position as reattachment is attempted can be useful at times (21). This can be accomplished with the endoilluminator, the vitreous cutter, or a soft-tip cannula.

VISCOELASTICS AS VITREOUS SUBSTITUTES

Viscoelastics are non-Newtonian fluids and have exceedingly low surface tension (tamponade) effects. They are pseudoplastic and will slowly deform and pass through a small retinal break very easily. In addition, viscoelastics acts as a sustained-release medium for cells and cytokines. For these reasons viscoelastics have no place in the authors' PVR armamentarium.

SILICONE

Silicone oil was first utilized without vitreous surgery techniques as a surface tension and dissection device, producing ERM peeling by forcing the retina back with concurrent drainage of SRF (22–27). This method will not work with more extensive ERM or subretinal proliferation. Recent studies with improved silicone oil (28–37) have not shown the retinal toxicity noted in previous years. Inferior peripheral iridectomy as developed by Ando (38) allows aqueous humor to pass from the ciliary processes into the anterior chamber to supply metabolites to the corneal endothelium.

Aqueous access to the cornea reduces silicone keratopathy. Keratopathy occurs in less than 10% of cases with long-term oil (S. Charles, data presented at the Vitreous Society, 1996, using Adatomed 5000cs). Reduction of lower-molecular-weight components, by using higher average molecular weight and therefore higher viscosity, and purification to remove metal ions dramatically reduces silicone emulsification, corneal changes, and glaucoma.

The physical effects of silicone are based on its interfacial (surface) tension resulting from its immiscibility with water (aqueous). The ability to restore a transretinal pressure gradient is a function of the size and shape of the retinal break and the tangential forces (stiffness) on the retina (Fig. 7.11). Viscosity is not a factor in the transretinal pressure gradient, and the silicone/aqueous interfacial tension is 25 dyne/cm, which is much less than that of an air/gas/fluid interface at 70.

Long-term rhegmatogenous confinement (tamponade) may obviate the need for retinopexy, therefore reducing reproliferation in response to tissue destruction (39). Long-term tamponade limits the rhegmatogenous component from contraction-created breaks and those missed at the time of surgery. Silicone may act to prevent the wetting of the reti-

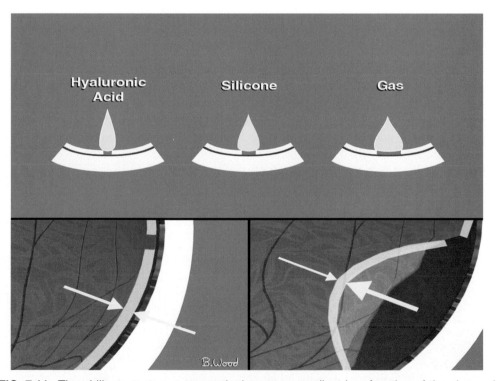

FIG. 7.11. The ability to restore a transretinal pressure gradient is a function of the size and shape of the retinal break and the tangential forces (stiffness) on the retina. Viscosity is not a factor in the transretinal pressure gradient, as the silicone/aqueous interfacial tension is 25 dyne/cm, which is much less than that of an air/gas/fluid interface at 70 dyne/cm.

nal surface by cytokines implicated in reproliferation (J. Lean, personal communication). Silicone can reduce reproliferation by retinopexy avoidance but appears to have no direct role in suppressing or stimulating reproliferation. Silicone may also increase reproliferation because of sequestration of cells and cytokines at the silicone/retinal interface and prevention of access of pharmacologic agents to the retina surface (see Fig. 5.15).

Retinectomy and multiple previous procedures using gas are relative indications for using silicone in PVR. The patient must be informed about possible corneal problems, glaucoma, and the possibility of silicone removal.

RETINAL SUTURES, TACKS, AND INTENTIONAL INCARCERATION

Permanent fixation of the retina to the sclera has been utilized to prevent inward curling or posterior sliding of large retinal flaps or the edges of retinectomies. These methods have the risk of retinal/choroidal hemorrhage, tissue damage, and the creation of retinal breaks. Retinal tacks are more safely and easily utilized than sutures or intentional retinal incarceration. They can be repositioned as well as removed later. Different materials have been used for the construction of retinal tacks: polyacetal (42), steel (43), titanium (44,45), and certain alloys (H. Grieshaber). Sutures and incarceration are time-consuming and frequently place additional traction on the retina. No permanent fixation method can prevent surface contraction and detachment. Tacks cause bleeding, reproliferation, distortion, and secondary breaks, and have not been utilized by the principal author for many years.

RETINOPEXY

After the reattachment experiment has been successfully completed, endophotocoagulation can be applied to retinal breaks. Post reattachment retinopexy (S. Charles) permits treatment of both the retina and the RPE for stronger adherence. It may limit migration of RPE cells implicated in PVR. Because retinopexy is implicated in PVR formation (40,41) and inflammation can cause retinal/retinal adherence, retinopexy should be limited to the retinal breaks or suspected break areas. Panretinal photocoagulation has never been used by the authors for PVR because it can cause reproliferation and fibrin syndrome. Similarly, the authors never use many rows of treatment but rather surrounds retinal defects with a moderately wide row of confluent laser (Fig. 7.12) unless silicone is used for retinopexy avoidance in highly active or inflamed cases. The authors do not use cryopexy because it has been implicated in PVR (40,41).

Retinoplasty

Retinoplasty using a synthetic adhesive such as cyanoacrylate (46,47) could theoretically replace all vitreous substitutes and retinopexy. An ideal polymer retinal patch should be very flexible, more elastic than the retina, and less permeable than the retina, and should not adhere to the RPE. Aqueous humor (the ideal vitreous substitute) could be used in place of gas or silicone if a retinal patch were available.

Scleral Buckling

Since PVR is a diffuse problem, no attempt is made to localize buckles to certain areas in most cases. A broad encircling tire is utilized in almost all scleral buckling cases, with extremely broad radial separation of the sutures (Fig. 7.13). The authors' preferred suture is 5-0 monofilament nylon because it does not slip, does not require an assistant

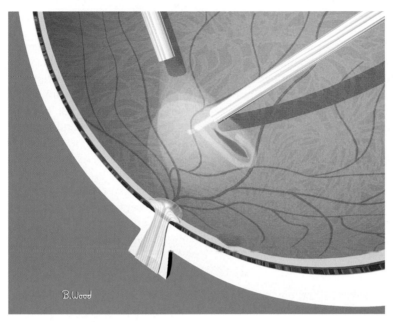

FIG. 7.12. After the reattachment experiment has been successfully completed, endopho-tocoagulation can be applied to retinal breaks in a moderately wide row of confluent laser treatment.

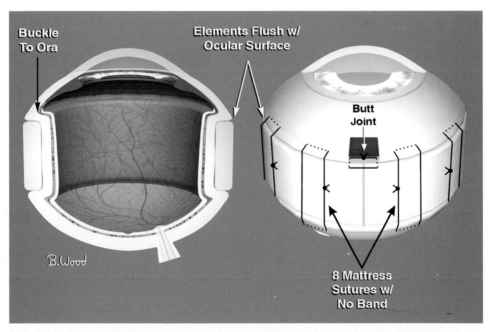

FIG. 7.13. 5-0 monofilament nylon sutures are used for the broad encircling tire, with bites placed circumferentially in the muscle ring, and a single circumferential posterior bite at or just behind the vortex veins. The ends of the tire are butt-joined (end-to-end) using two 5-0 nylon sutures.

to hold the knot during tying, and does not have interstices, which might harbor bacteria. All anterior bites are placed circumferentially in the muscle ring with a single circumferential posterior bite at or just behind the vortex veins. Two sutures are used in each quadrant so that the buckling effect is the result of imbrication of the buckle into the globe from these sutures. Sponges are not utilized because of the uneven buckle surface they cause and the risk of extrusion. By extending the buckle to the ora, anterior leakage of SRF is avoided and any residual circumferential, anterior PVR, or sclerotomy-related traction is supported. The ends of the tire are butt-joined (end-to-end) using two 5-0 nylon sutures. Most of the buckling effect comes from the disparity between suture bite separation and buckle width. The goal is to cause the outer surface of the explant to conform to the curvature of the nonbuckled portion of the globe. The buckle should extend posteriorly up to the vortex veins. Localized buckles distort the contour of the eye wall and push stiff retina inward. If SRF or subretinal air is present before the buckle is tightened up, it should be allowed to remain until the buckle is complete. Direct, needle drainage of SRF can then be accomplished without having to reenter the eye.

REOPERATION

If PVR is severe but no buckle is present, the initial approach is lens removal (if phakic), inside-out forceps membrane peeling, internal drain of SRF, air/gas exchange with 16% C_3F_8, endophotocoagulation, and a broad, high, 360° hard silicone scleral buckle. If this fails, the usual approach is further peeling, possible retinectomy or subretinal surgery as indicated, laser endophotocoagulation to surround the retinal breaks, and air/silicone exchange. If breaks or retinectomies are extensive, air/silicone exchange should be utilized at reoperation. The authors tend to use silicone oil on first-time reoperations in recent years because of the availability of higher-quality oil.

RESULTS

Results are highly dependent on case selection, surgical methods, and surgical experience. Using conventional techniques of vitreous surgery, about 50% to 85% of cases achieved long-term retinal reattachment (48–50). With the previously described methods and case selection criteria, 90% of cases can be repaired surgically, with more than 74% remaining attached over the long term (51,52). About 50% of the cases sustain improved vision of better than 5/200, but many cases require more than one procedure (53).

COMPLICATIONS

Proliferative Vitreoretinopathy Recurrence

A recurrence of PVR with secondary retinal separation is the most frequent complication. In approximately one-half of the recurring cases, further scissors segmentation/delamination, air/silicone exchange and endolaser photocoagulation can cause successful reattachment.

Although the use of intraocular steroids and 5-fluorouracil and its derivatives (54–61) for PVR cases has been described, therapeutic efficacy has not been proven. It appears that the migration phase of the RPE cells is more important than the proliferation phase in the development of PVR. As these drugs have a short half-life, better delivery systems are required than those presently available. Cytotoxic agents have low therapeutic ratios, which is a significant problem, especially when coupled with the highly variable drug elution rate of sustained-release delivery systems.

Inflammation

Because retinal breaks are exclusively treated with laser endocoagulation, the usual exudative detachment and fibrin syndrome associated with two or three rows of cryopexy are eliminated. A very rare patient will experience severe inflammation and transient iris neovascularization, and go on to (develop) phthisis bulbi. This rare complication could be from anterior segment necrosis syndrome, sympathetic uveitis, or some yet unexplained etiology but is usually due to excessive retinopexy or operating on inflamed eyes. Subconjunctival repository steroids without systemic steroids are used in every PVR case unless the patient is a steroid responder.

REFERENCES

1. Machemer R, Van Horn D, Aaberg TM. Pigment epithelial proliferation. *Am J Ophthalmol* 1978;85:181.
2. Van Horn DL, Aaberg TM, Modene R, et al. Glial cell proliferation in human retinal detachment with massive periretinal proliferation. *Am J Ophthalmol* 1977;84:383.
3. Machemer R. Role of the pigment epithelium in vitreous pathology. *Trans Ophthalmol Soc UK* 1975;95:402.
4. Machemer R, Laqua H. Pigment epithelium proliferation in retinal detachment (massive periretinal proliferation). *Am J Ophthalmol* 1975;80:1.
5. Machemer R. Massive periretinal proliferation (MPP) 1. Pigment epithelial proliferation. *Mod Probl Ophthalmol* 1975;15:227.
6. Mandelhorn M, Machemer R, Fineberg E, et al. Proliferation and metaplasia of intravitreal retinal pigment epithelium cell autotransplants. *Am J Ophthalmol* 1975;80:227.
7. Laqua H, Machemer R. Clinical-pathological correlation in massive periretinal proliferation. *Am J Ophthalmol* 1975;80:913–929.
8. Laqua H, Machemer R. Glial cell proliferation in retinal detachment (massive penretinal proliferation). *Am J Ophthalmol* 1975;80:602.
9. Campochiaro PA, Jerdan JA, Cardin A, et al. Vitreous aspirates from patients with proliferative vitreoretinopathy stimulate retinal pigment epithelial cell migration. *Arch Ophthalmol* 1985;103:1403-1405.
10. Campochiaro PA, Jerdan JA, Glaser BM. Serum contains chemoattractants for human retinal pigment epithelial cells. *Arch Ophthalmol* 1984;102:1830.
11. Campochiaro PA, Glaser BM. Platelet-derived growth factor is chemotactic for human retinal pigment epithelial cells. *Arch Ophthalmol* 1985;103:576.
12. Pastor JC. Proliferative vitreretinopathy: an overview. *Surv Ophthalmol* 1998;43:3–18.
13. Campochiaro PA. Pathogenesis mechanisms in proliferative vitreoretinopathy. *Arch Ophthalmol* 1997;115:237–241.
14. Kohno T, Sorgente N, Ryan SJ. Fibronectin distribution at the vitreoretinal interface. *Invest Ophthalmol Vis Sci* 1983;24[Suppl]:240.
15. Kohno T, Sorgente N, Patterson R, et al. Fibronectin and Laminin distribution in bovine eye. *Jpn J Ophthalmol* 1983;27:496.
16. Anderson DH, Stern WH, Fisher SK, et al. The onset of pigment epithelial proliferation following retinal detachment. *Invest Ophthalmol* 1981;21:10.
17. Machemer R. Pathogenesis and classification of massive penretinal proliferation. *Br J Ophthalmol* 1978;62:737.
18. Machemer R, Aaberg TM, Freeman HM, et al. An updated classification of retinal detachment with proliferative vitreoretinopathy. *Am J Ophthalmol* 1991;112:159–165.
19. Charles S. Presentation at 11th Annual Estelle Doheny Eye Foundation Conference. Los Angeles, CA, September 1979.
20. Han DP. Relaxing rentinotomies and retinectomies: surgical results and predictors of visual outcome. *Arch Ophthalmol* 1990;108:694–697.
21. Glaser BM. A new method of treating giant tears without patient rotation with the use of intraocular gas and silicone oil. Presentation at Annual Meeting of American Academy of Ophthalmology. Atlanta, GA, October 2, 1985.
22. Cibis PA, Becker B, Okun E, et al. The use of liquid silicone in retinal detachment surgery. *Arch Ophthalmol* 1962;68:590.
23. Cibis PA. Vitreous transfer and silicone injections. *Trans Am Acad Ophthalmol Otolaryngol* 1964;68:983.
24. Okun E. Intravitreal surgery utilizing liquid silicone: a long-term followup. *Trans Pac Coast Otolaryngol Ophthalmol Soc* 1968;49:141.
25. Okun E, Arribas NP. Therapy of retinal detachment complicated by massive preretinal fibroplasia (long-term followup of patients treated with intravitreal liquid silicone). In: *New Orleans Academy of Ophthalmology Symposium on Retina and Retinal Surgery*. St. Louis: CV Mosby, 1969:278–293.
26. Scott JD. The treatment of massive vitreous retraction by the separation of preretinal membranes using liquid silicone. *Mod Probl Ophthalmol* 1975;15:285.

27. Scott JD. A rationale for the use of liquid silicone. *Trans Ophthalmol Soc UK* 1977;97:235.
28. Labelle P, Okun E. Ocular tolerance to liquid silicone: an experimental study. *Can J Ophthalmol* 1972;7:199.
29. Ober RR, Blanks JC, Ogden TE. Experimental retinal tolerance to liquid silicone. *Retina* 1983;33:77.
30. Ober RR, Ryan SJ, Minckler DS, et al. Ocular tolerance to liquid silicone: an experimental study. *Invest Ophthalmol Vis Sci* 1980;19[Suppl]:47.
31. Meredith TA, Lindsey DT, Edelhauser HF, et al. Electroretinographic studies following vitrectomy and intraocular oil injection. *Br J Ophthalmol* 1985;69:254.
32. Momirov D, Van Lith GHM, Zivojnovic R. Electroretinogram and electro-oculograms of eyes with intravitreously injected silicone oil. *Ophthalmologica* 1983;186:183.
33. Freeman KD, Gregor ZJ. Electrophysiological responses after vitrectomy and intraocular tamponade. *Trans Ophthalmol Soc UK* 1985;104:129.
34. Foerster M, Esser J, Laqua H. Silicone oil and its influence on electrophysiologic findings. *Am J Ophthalmol* 1985;99:201.
35. Abrams GW, Azen SP, McCuen BW 2nd, et al. Vitrectomy with silicone oil or long acting gas in eyes with severe PVR: results of additional and long-term follow-up. Silicone Study Report 11. *Arch Ophthalmol* 1997;115: 335–344.
36. Diddie KR, Azen SP, Freeman HM, et al. Anterior proliferative vitreretinopathy in the silicone study. Silicone Study Report Number 10. *Ophthalmology* 1996;103:1092–1099.
37. Vitrectomy with silicone oil or pleurofluorocarbon gas in eyes with severe PVR: results of a randomized clinical trial. Silicone Report 2. *Arch Ophthalmol* 1992;110:780–792.
38. Ando F. Intraocular hypertension resulting from pupillary block by silicone oil. *Am J Ophthalmol* 1985;99:87.
39. Charles S. Vitrectomy for retinal detachment. *Trans Ophthalmol Soc UK* 1980;100:542.
40. Campochiaro PA, Kaden IH, Vidaurri-Leal JS, et al. Cryotherapy enhances intravitreal dispersion of viable retinal pigment epithelial cells. *Arch Ophthalmol* 1985;103:434.
41. Glaser BM, Vidaurri-Leal J, Michels RG, et al. Cryotherapy during surgery for giant retinal tears enhances dispersion of viable retinal pigment epithelial cells. *Ophthalmology* 1993;100:466–470.
42. Ando F, Kondo J. A plastic tack for the treatment of retinal detachment with giant tear (letter). *Am J Ophthalmol* 1983;95:260.
43. De Juan E, Hickingbotham D, Machemer R. Retinal tacks. *Am J Ophthalmol* 1985;99:272.
44. Aaberg TM. Presentation at Duke advanced vitrectomy course. Durham, NC, April 1985.
45. Aaberg TM. Presentation at American Retina Society meeting. Cleveland, OH, November 1985.
46. McCuen BW, 2nd, Hida T, Sheta SM, et al. Experimental transvitreal cyanoacrylate retinopexy in a primate model. *Am J Ophthalmology* 1987;94:337–340.
47. McCuen BW, 2nd, Hida T, Sheta SM. Transvitreal cyanoacrylate retinopexy in management of complicated retinal detachment. *Am J Ophthalmology* 1987;103:782–789.
48. Machemer R, Laqua H. A logical approach to the treatment of massive periretinal proliferation. *Ophthalmology* 1978;85:584.
49. Machemer R. Massive periretinal proliferation: a logical approach to therapy. *Trans Am Ophthalmol Soc* 1977; 75:556.
50. Sternberg P, Machemer R. Results of conventional vitreous surgery for proliferative vitreoretinopathy. *Am J Ophthalmol* 1985;100:141.
51. Charles S. Methodology and research on proliferative vitreoretinopathy. Presented at Retina Society Meeting. Cleveland, OH, November 1985.
52. Charles S. Vitreous surgery for proliferative vitreoretinopathy. Presented at Vitreous Society Meeting. Orlando, FL, October 1985.
53. Lewis H, Aaberg TM. Causes of failure after repeat vitrectomy for recurrent proliferative vitreoretinopathy. *Am J Ophthalmol* 1991;15;111:15–19.
54. Machemer R, Sugita G, Tano Y. Treatment of intraocular proliferations with intravitreal steroids. *Trans Am Ophthalmol Soc* 1979;77:171.
55. Tano Y, Chandler D, Machemer R. Treatment of intraocular proliferation with intravitreal injection of triamcinolone acetonide. *Am J Ophthalmol* 1980;90:810.
56. Chandler DB, Rozakis G, De Juan E, et al. The effect of triamcinolone acetonide on a refined experimental model of proliferative vitreoretinopathy. *Am J Ophthalmol* 1985;99:686.
57. Stern WH, Lewis GP, Erickson PA, et al. Fluorouracil therapy of proliferative vitreoretinopathy after vitrectomy. *Am J Ophthalmol* 1983;96:32.
58. Blumenkranz MS, Ophir A, Claflin Al, et al. Fluorouracil for the treatment of massive periretinal proliferation. *Am J Ophthalmol* 1982;94:458.
59. Santana M, Wiedemann P, Kirmani M, et al. Daunomycin in the treatment of experimental proliferative vitreoretinopathy-retinal toxicity of intravitreal daunomycin in the rabbit. *Graefes Arch Clin Exp Ophthalmol* 1984; 221:210.
60. Wiedemann P, Sorgente N, Bekhor C, et al. Daunomycin in the treatment of experimental proliferative vitreoretinopathy–effective doses *in vitro* and *in vivo*. *Invest Ophthalmol Vis Sci* 1985;26:719.
61. Wiedemann P, Sorgente N, Kirmani M, et al. Daunorubicin in the treatment of experimental MPP-effective doses *in vitro* and *in vivo*. *Invest Ophthalmol Vis Sci* 1983;24[Suppl]:241.

8

Giant Breaks

Giant retinal breaks are traditionally defined as breaks extending for greater than 90°. Because of the propensity of the retina to fold over, surgical management of these detachments was very difficult until the advent of vitrectomy and intraocular gas. The next major advance occurred when Chang initiated the application of perfluorocarbon liquids to giant break surgery (1). It is now relatively straightforward to achieve surgical success in most cases. The long-term success rate is determined by the incidence of proliferative vitreoretinopathy (PVR). Although vitreous dynamics, trauma, and hereditary peripheral retinal changes play a role, the exact pathogenesis of giant breaks remains unclear. The high incidence of associated PVR presumably relates to the exposure of vast areas of retinal pigment epithelium (RPE) and retinal glial cells to the vitreous matrix. RPE cells migrate along the vitreous and retinal surfaces. The exposed edge of retina presumably enables glial cells to migrate to the retinal surface as well. Vitreous is virtually never observed on the photoreceptor side of the retina in these cases.

The differentiation between inward folding of the internal limiting membrane (ILM), and PVR; although one can often distinguish between giant breaks and giant disinsertions, does not seem to play a role in management strategies or prognosis.

CASE SELECTION

Quadrantic giant breaks can be managed effectively with scleral buckling alone if there is minimal folding of the retina. Moderate degrees of folding can be managed by adding expanding C_3F_8 gas to the scleral buckling modality. More extensive breaks with retinal folding are best managed with vitrectomy and perfluorocarbon liquids. Giant breaks combined with PVR; vitreous to a wound, dislocated lenses, or vitreous hemorrhage are absolute indications for vitrectomy, regardless of the size of the break.

SURGICAL SEQUENCE AND TECHNIQUES

Patient Education

The patients should be psychologically prepared for 3 weeks in the facedown position after surgery with gas, unless perfluorocarbon liquids (1 week) are used instead of gas.

Incisions

Typical conjunctival incisions for vitrectomy should be made. The sclerotomies are made in the usual fashion, 3 mm posterior to the limbus; after checking full-thickness insertion, the infusion cannula is turned on. Muscle traction sutures are not required because scleral buckling is not efficacious.

Management of the Lens

The crystalline lens should probably be removed in almost all folded-over breaks, in 180° or greater giant breaks, and in many breaks of lesser extent. Lensectomy permits removal of the anterior vitreous cortex (AVC) and, more specifically, the anterior loop traction (anterior PVR).

Endocapsular lensectomy with the Alcon or equivalent 20-gauge fragmenter should be utilized if the lens is to be removed. The mobility of the retina and vitreous in these cases dictates caution during lensectomy. The fragmenter should not be permitted to pull on the vitreous in any instance. An anterior vitrectomy should precede lensectomy to prevent vitreous traction by the fragmenter. A lensectomy can be performed with the vitrectomy cutter, if the patient has a soft lens.

Special care should be taken to avoid contacting the iris because iris bleeding and mechanically induced miosis can compromise the surgical procedure. The diamond-coated, end-opening forceps should be used to remove the lens capsule. Excellent mydriasis should be maintained pharmacologically, by prevention of hypotony, and by avoidance of contact with the iris.

Vitrectomy

Vitreous removal should be performed using very low suction force with proportional suction control and high cutting rates because of marked retinal mobility. The vitreous is rarely attached to the posterior edge of the giant break.

The vitreous must be trimmed to the anterior retinal surface to prevent vitreous entrapment in the SRF drainage cannula and to prevent late vitreous traction from causing redetachment (Fig. 8.1). It is normal to remove portions of detached nonpigmented pars plana epithelium anterior to the break during the trimming of the peripheral vitreous.

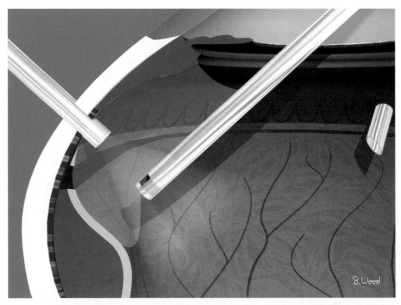

FIG. 8.1. The peripheral vitreous must be trimmed to the surface of anterior retina to prevent imbrication into the suction cannula.

Fluid/Air/Gas Exchange

Internal drainage of subretinal fluid and fluid/air exchange can be performed without perfluorocarbon liquids in certain cases. Internal drainage of subretinal fluid must precede fluid/air exchange and continue during exchange. A soft-tip extrusion cannula should be positioned just anterior to the edge of the giant break (Fig. 8.2). The retina will be gently pulled into position as the SRF is drained. Rotating the eye toward the giant break enables drainage of the vitreous fluid simultaneous with the subretinal fluid and facilitates complete drainage of SRF and better repositioning of the retina.

Air can be used for intraoperative surface tension management in 90° to 180° giant breaks but should not be used for larger or folded-over breaks. If air is used in these cases, the retina will be forced posteriorly and can become a folded mass over the optic nerve. In contrast, perfluorocarbon liquids permit removal of all subretinal fluid (SRF) and position the retina in a nonfolded state near its original position, permitting laser retinopexy to both RPE and the retina.

Perfluorocarbon Liquids

Perfluorocarbon liquids are surface tension management agents similar to silicone oil, air, and gas. Silicone and gas float because their density is less than that of infusion fluid. Perfluorocarbon liquids are denser than infusion fluid and retina, and migrate to the lowest part of the eye. Retina is less dense than PFC liquids and therefore floats, limited only by vitreoretinal traction and its inherent stiffness. Similarly, SRF is less dense than PFC liquids and floats up through the giant break and into the anterior vitreous cavity.

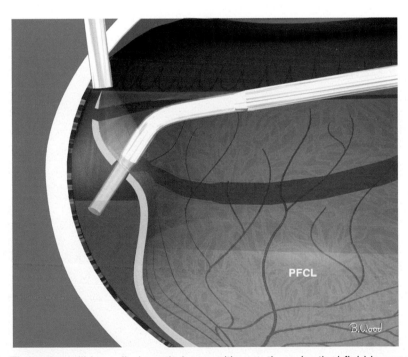

FIG. 8.2. The retina will be pulled gently into position as the subretinal fluid is removed with the suction cannula.

Perfluorocarbon liquid should be injected on the anterior side of the retina, near the optic nerve with a 23–27-gauge, blunt cannula. Because the endoilluminator is plugging one sclerotomy and both PFC liquid and BSS are incompressible, BSS Plus must be allowed to leak around the cannula to allow normalization of the IOP. The PFC liquid should be injected until the retina is unfolded and all subretinal fluid is gone. PFC liquids must reach the pars plana when injection is complete. The BSS-PFC interface is very difficult to see, especially with Vitreon, making estimation of the PFC level difficult. The endoilluminator should be repositioned until a light reflex from the interface is visible.

If PFC liquids are used when giant breaks and PVR coexist, care must be taken to avoid PFC liquids from entering the subretinal space. PFC liquids will enter the subretinal space when the difference between forces due to specific gravity and intrafacial tension effects is less than the combined stiffness of the retina and PVR membranes (2–4).

Retinopexy

Confluent laser retinopexy should be used at the posterior margin of the retinal break (Fig. 8.3). Multiple spots with interspersed untreated spaces necessitate a larger treatment area and create the problem of leakage of SRF between the spots. Care should be taken to extend the laser (treatment) around the ends of the break to the pars plana to avoid SRF migration (5–7). Treatment intensity is more difficult to judge with red or near-IR laser energy. Cryo is thought to cause increased PVR (8–13) and retinal slippage compared with laser. Transscleral diathermy can damage the sclera but can be very effective in an air-filled eye. Transscleral laser is less predictable and, like cryo and diathermy, requires exposure of the scleral surface (14).

Postoperative Surface Tension Management

The options for postoperative surface tension management include perfluorocarbon liquids, silicone, and gas. The advantage of PFC liquids is that the slippage that occurs at

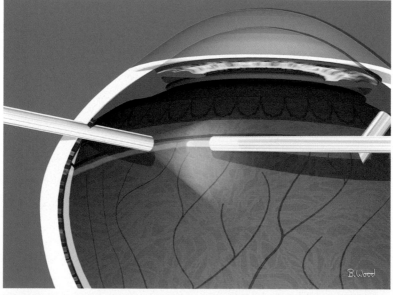

FIG. 8.3. Confluent laser retinopexy should be applied to the posterior margin of the giant break and should be extended around the ends of the break to the pars plana.

the time of PFC/gas or PFC/silicone exchange is avoided. The disadvantage is that a surgical procedure is required to remove the PFC liquids. Vitreon is approved for short-term postoperative use, but perfluon is preferred by the authors. Gas will absorb eliminating the need for removal. Gas expands with air travel, bubble size decreases with time, and the view is problematic for the patient and physician. Silicone is the best option for PVR combined with giant breaks. The exchange from PFC liquids to gas or silicone causes posterior slippage in many cases.

Laser retinopexy must be applied before this slippage occurs in order to position the laser correctly. The patient must be positioned prone immediately after surgery if gas or silicone is used and continuously in order for the retina to move back to a nonredundant position. On some occasions, permanent folds will occur. Retinal folds do not represent a serious problem unless the macula is involved or very large areas of RPE are exposed. Damage to the retina and/or RPE occurring in a prolonged attempt to eliminate folds may unnecessarily stimulate PVR.

It is tempting to allow the patient to position part-time or position other than prone, or to shorten the prone period. These compromises reduce success rates. Short-term PFC patients must be supine for 7–10 days before the PFC is removed.

RESULTS

With the previously described methodology, about 95% of cases can be successfully reattached in the operating room and remain reattached for the first 3 weeks. However, the long-term results range from 50% to 90%, depending on PVR, surgical techniques, and case selection (15,16). PVR can be managed by reoperation with the approach described earlier (Fig. 8.4). Epimacular membranes (macular pucker) occur in a significant number of cases and can be managed effectively with substantial visual recovery after vitrectomy revision and diamond-coated, end-opening, inside-out, forceps membrane peeling.

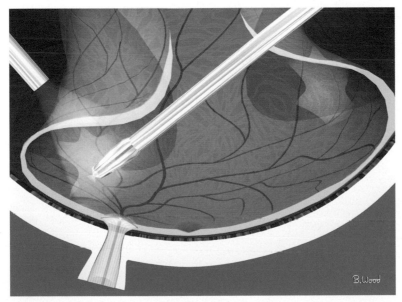

FIG. 8.4. Epiretinal and epimacular membranes can be managed with inside-out membrane peeling using end-opening, diamond-coated forceps.

MANAGEMENT OF THE FELLOW EYE

The high incidence of bilaterality in the nontraumatic, genetically determined cases of giant breaks is of great concern (17). The potential for giant breaks in the other eye raises the question of prophylaxis to the other eye. It is known that retinal breaks and even giant breaks frequently occur at the posterior margin of previous retinopexy marks. It is well known that hypocellular vitreous contraction can pull the retina away from a high, broad scleral buckle. The authors currently laser retinal breaks in the other eye, but do not perform 360° retinopexy or scleral buckling.

REFERENCES

1. Chang S, Lincoff H, Zimmerman NJ, et al. Giant retinal tears: surgical techniques and results using perfluorocarbon liquids. *Arch Ophthalmol* 1989;107:761.
2. Glaser BM, Carter JB, Kupperman BD, et al. Perfluo-octane in the treatment of giant retinal tears with PVR. *Ophthalmology* 1991;98:1613.
3. Darmakusma IE, Glaser BM, Sjaarda RN, et al. The use of perfluoro-octane in the management of giant retinal tears without PVR. *Retina* 1994;14:323.
4. Verstraeten T, Williams GA, Chang S, et al. Lens-sparing vitrectomy with perfluorocarbon liquid for the primary treatment of giant retinal tears. *Ophthalmology* 1995;102:17.
5. Charles S. Endophotocoagulation. *Retina* 1981;1:117.
6. Yoon YH, Marmour MF. Rapid enhancement of retinal adhesion by laser photocoagulation. *Ophthalmology* 1988;95:1385.
7. Powell JO, Bresnick GH, Yanoff M, et al. Ocular effects of argon laser radiation. II. Histopathology of chorioretinal lesions. *Am J Ophthalmol* 1971;71:1267.
8. Campochiaro PA, Kaden IH, Vidaurri-Leal JS, et al. Cryotherapy enhances viable intravitreal dispersion of retinal pigment epithelial cells. *Arch Ophthalmol* 1984;103:434.
9. Kreissig I, Lincoff H. Mechanism of retinal attachment after cryosurgery. *Trans Ophthalmol Soc UK* 1975;95:148.
10. Johnson RN, Irvine AR, Wood IS. Endolaser, cryopexy, and retinal reattachment in the air-filled eye: a clinicopathologic correlation. *Arch Ophthalmol* 1987;105:231.
11. Jaccoma EH, Conway BP, Campochiaro PA. Cryotherapy causes extensive breakdown of the blood retina barrier: a comparison with argon laser photocoagulation. *Arch Ophthalmol* 1985;103:1728.
12. Campochiaro PA, Kaden IH, Vidaurri-Leal J, et al. Cryotherapy enhances intravitreal dispersion of viable retinal pigment epithelial cells. *Arch Ophthalmol* 1985;103:434.
13. Glaser BM, Vidaurri-Leal J, Michels RG, et al. Cryotherapy during surgery for giant retinal tears and intravitreal dispersion of viable pigment epithelial cells. *Ophthalmology* 1993;100:466.
14. Haller JA, Lim J, Goldberg MF. Pilot trial of transscleral diode laser retinopexy in retinal detachment surgery. *Arch Ophthalmol* 1993;111:952.
15. Freeman HM, Schepens CL, Couvillion GC. Current management of giant retinal breaks 11. *Trans Am Acad Ophthalmol Otolaryngol* 1970;74:59.
16. Machemer R, Allen AW. Retinal tears 180 degrees and greater: management with vitrectomy and vitreoretinal gas. *Arch Ophthalmol* 1976;94:1340.
17. Freeman HM. Fellow eyes of giant retinal breaks. *Mod Probl Ophthalmol* 1979;20:267.

9

Pneumatic Retinopexy and Office Fluid Air and Gas Exchange

Air was used by Ohm and Rosengren over a half century ago for the repair of retinal detachments. Dominguez (1), and subsequently Hilton and Grizzard (2), reported the use of in-office injection of expanding gas for the repair of primary, rhegmatogenous retinal detachment. Initially, cryoretinopexy was applied before gas injection, while others used laser retinopexy after reattachment, analogous to the post reattachment retinopexy concept developed by the principal author for vitreous surgery (3,5,7,9–12).

Retinal reattachment surgery outcome data are very difficult to interpret because of the large number of variables, vast array of surgical options and combinations of techniques, as well as the relatively low number of cases per surgeon. Some surgeons state that pneumatic retinopexy causes PVR, and in spite of this, they inject gas after scleral buckling. Although it is clear that pneumatic retinopexy should not be used for cases with PVR or marked vitreous traction, it is unknown with statistical accuracy what the indications should be. It is clear that single, superior retinal breaks are the ideal cases for pneumatic, but these cases can also be repaired with very high success rates by scleral buckling. Yarian and associates were major advocates of pneumatic retinopexy and participated in the pneumatic retinopexy multicenter, randomized trial but have advocated use of the Lincoff balloon. Pneumatic retinopexy costs less than scleral buckling or primary vitrectomy. Tornambe practices in a region with many capitated managed-care plans, is a cost savings advocate, and remains a staunch advocate of pneumatic retinopexy. Tornambe currently advocates use of 360° laser retinopexy in these cases, which raise the issue of potential stimulation of PVR (4,6,8). The principal author utilized pneumatic retinopexy in a wide variety of cases since 1988 but uses the technique less frequently in recent years because of failures due to progressive contraction of the vitreous, new retinal breaks, unpredictability, and PVR. Patients with medical problems combined with simple, superior retinal detachments are the best candidates for pneumatic retinopexy.

SURGICAL SEQUENCE

The authors use topical viscous lidocaine anesthesia applied first as a drop and then with a sterile applicator at the intended pars plana injection site. Retrobulbar or peribulbar anesthesia is required in some cases.

The patient should be prepped with Betadine 5% after anesthesia is achieved. A sterile speculum is required to prevent the needle from contacting the nonsterile lid margins and lashes. The surgeon should use sterile gloves, sterile technique, and a filter when drawing up the gas and performing the procedure.

The authors routinely use C_3F_8 gas rather than SF_6 because it expands three to four times its original size, compared with two times for SF_6 (13–19). Greater expansion means that less gas can be injected and therefore less paracentesis will be required.

Injection of gas is best performed with the patient lying on his or her side or back (Fig. 9.1), *not* supine, seated, leaning over the examining table or at the slit lamp. Multiple bubbles (fish eggs) are completely preventable if the injection is performed at the highest point of the eye with the needle advanced just past the pars plana epithelium. By using this method, all gas is injected into the original bubble, preventing multiple bubbles (Fig. 9.2). A 30-gauge needle should be used to reduce leakage of gas after the injection. A tuberculin or 3-mL syringe is used for the gas injection. Repetitive in-and-out movement of the needle into the eye is avoided if the patient is on his or her side, decreasing the risk of endophthalmitis. By placing the needle only 3 mm into the eye, inadvertent contact with the lens and retina is reduced. It is difficult for a patient on his side to raise his head and bring the needle into contact with the retina. Approximately 0.3 to 0.6 mL of gas is injected, although the most appropriate volume is controversial. It is the authors' opinion that higher volumes give higher success rates but demand paracentesis. The authors use paracentesis in all cases and have recently switched to paracentesis before gas injection. Immediately after the injection, the reclining patient chair is tilted up to the seated position at the slit lamp, with the speculum remaining in place. Sitting the patient up has the added advantage of rolling the bubble away from the injection site, eliminating the need for an applicator stick to prevent leakage. A 30-gauge needle is advanced parallel and adjacent to the limbus through inferior clear cornea into the anterior chamber. Oblique entry ensures a self-sealing wound. Needle placement over the iris instead of the pupil reduces the risk of lens damage. The patient usually reports no light perception immediately after the injection, but light perception returns as soon as the paracentesis reduces the intraocular pressure.

Laser retinopexy is usually performed 1 or 2 days after the gas injection when the subretinal fluid has pumped out. The laser indirect ophthalmoscope is preferred to the three-mirror contact for post reattachment retinopexy (Fig. 9.3). If there are concerns about the

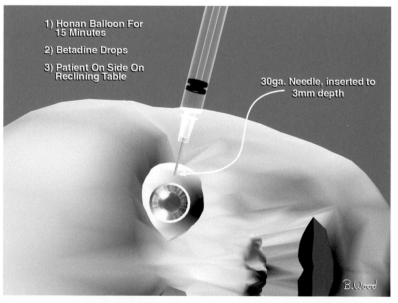

FIG. 9.1. Gas injection is performed with the patient lying on his or her side and the needle inserted into the highest point of the eye.

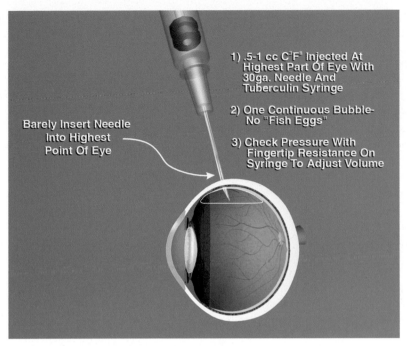

FIG. 9.2. With the patient lying on his or her side and the needle inserted only 3 mm, inadvertent contact with the lens or retina is reduced.

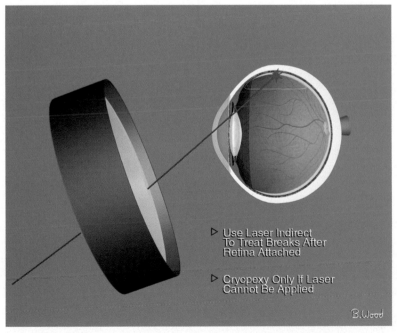

FIG. 9.3. Retinopexy is performed with the laser indirect ophthalmoscope, 1 or 2 days after gas injection.

ability to visualize the breaks after reattachment, preattachment retinopexy with transscleral cryopexy can be utilized.

IN-OFFICE FLUID/GAS EXCHANGE

Postvitrectomy retinal detachment without traction or PVR; or patients with hemorrhaging can be managed by in-office fluid/gas exchange using isoexpansive concentrations of C_3F_8 (16%) or SF_6 (25%) (Fig. 9.4). The injection needle is positioned 4 mm posterior to the limbus at the highest part of the eye, as in pneumatic retinopexy. The needle is advanced only 3 mm into the eye to avoid multiple bubbles. This 30-gauge needle is connected via a short piece of tubing to a 30- to 60-mL air/gas–filled syringe operated by the assistant. A second 25- to 30-gauge needle, depending on the viscosity of the intraocular fluid, is positioned 4 mm posterior to the limbus, at the lowest portion of the eye. This needle is connected to a tuberculin syringe, with the plunger removed, to act as a handle. The open end of this needle is positioned over a waste can to collect the fluid. The exchange is continued until gas appears in the egress needle. The egress needle is withdrawn and the intraocular pressure is adjusted using the gas syringe and tactile assessment of the IOP with a sterile applicator stick.

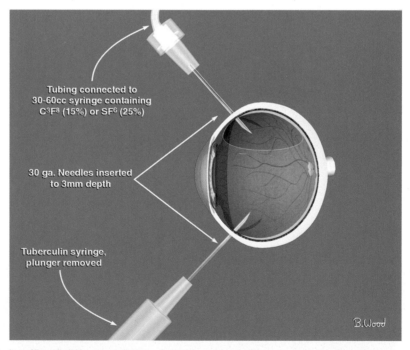

Tubing connected to
30-60cc syringe containing
C^3F^8 (15%) or SF^6 (25%)

30 ga. Needles inserted
to 3mm depth

Tuberculin syringe,
plunger removed

B.Wood

FIG. 9.4. In-office fluid/gas exchange is performed similarly to pneumatic retinopexy, with the addition of a second 30-gauge needle for fluid drainage. This second needle is attached to a tuberculin syringe with the plunger removed.

REFERENCES

1. Dominguez A. Cirugia precoz y ambulatoria del desprendimento de retina. *Arch Soc Esp Oftamol* 1985;48: 47–54.
2. Hilton GF, Grizzard WS. Pneumatic retinopexy: a two-step outpatient operation without conjunctival incision. *Ophthalmology* 1986;93:626.
3. McDonald HR, Abrams GW, Irvine AR, et al. Management of subretinal gas following attempted pneumatic retinal reattachment. *Ophthalmology* 1987;94:319–326,
4. Hilton GF, Tornambe PE. pneumatic retinopexy: an analysis of intraoperative and postoperative complications. *Retina* 1991;11:285–294.
5. Hilton GF, Kelly NE, Salzano TC, et al. Pneumatic retinopexy: a collaborative report of the first 100 cases. *Ophthalmology* 1987;94:307-314.
6. Ryan SJ. *Retina,* vol 3, 2nd ed. St. Louis: CU Mosby: 1994:2093–2112.
7. Roy FH. *Master techniques in ophthalmic surgery.* Baltimore: Williams & Wilkins, 1995:1118–1119.
8. Wilkinson CP, Rice TA. *Michels retinal detachment.* St Louis: CV Mosby, 1997:596–612.
9. Tornambe PE, Hilton GF, Brinton DA, et al. Pneumatic retinopexy. A two-year follow-up study of the multicenter clinical trial comparing pneumatic retinopexy with scleral buckling. *Ophthalmology* 1991;98:1115-1123.
10. Vygantas CM, Peyman GA, Daily MJ, et al. Octafluorocyclobutane and other gases for vitreous replacement. *Arch Ophthalmol* 1973;90:235.
11. Norton EWD. Intraocular gas in the management of selected retinal detachments. *Trans Acad Ophthalmol Otolaryngol* 1973;77:OP-85.
12. Lincoff H, Mardirossian J, Lincoff A, et al. Intravitreal longevity of three perfluorocarbon gases. *Arch Ophthalmol* 1980;98:1610.
13. Constable IJ, Swann DA. Vitreous substitution with gases. *Arch Ophthalmol* 1975;93:416.
14. DeJuan E Jr, McCuen B, Tiedeman J. Intraocular tamponade and surface tension. *Surv Ophthalmol* 1985;30:47.
15. Stinson TW III, Donion JV Jr. Interaction of intraocular air and SF6 with nitrous oxide: a computer simulation. *Anesthesiology* 1982;56:385.
16. Lincoff H, Coleman J, Kreissig I, et al. The perfluorocarbon gases in the treatment of retinal detachment. *Ophthalmology* 1983;90:546.
17. Fineberg E, Machemer R, Sullivan P. SF_6 for retinal detachment surgery: a preliminary report. *Mod Probl Ophthalmol* 1974;12:173.
18. Lincoff H, Maisel JM, Lincoff A. Intravitreal disappearance rates of four perfluorocarbon gases. *Arch Ophthalmol* 1984;102:928.
19. Lowe MA, McDonald HR, Campo RV, et al. Pneumatic retinopexy: surgical results. *Arch Ophthalmol* 1988;106: 1672.

10

Epimacular Membranes

Membranes on the macular surface can result from several pathogenic mechanisms with the common theme of tissue damage and subsequent repair (1–5). Epimacular membranes are hypocellular, largely collagen structures. Epimacular membranes are also called *macular puckers, cellophane maculopathy, surface-wrinkling retinopathy,* and *premacular fibrosis.* Each of these names has certain deficiencies; hence the currently most widely accepted name, *epimacular membranes.*

PATHOGENESIS

The so-called idiopathic type of epimacular membrane is caused by glial migration and proliferation from a defect in the internal limiting membrane created by a posterior vitreous separation (6). Retinal breaks, retinopexy, photocoagulation, inflammation, and vascular disease (7) can lead to glial proliferation (8–12) on the retinal surface. Retinal pigment epithelial cells (13,14) can migrate through a retinal break and proliferate on the retinal surface just as they do in proliferative vitreoretinopathy (PVR). Epimacular membranes can be thought of as localized glial or RPE-induced proliferative vitreoretinopathy.

ETIOLOGY OF VISUAL LOSS

Hypocellular contraction of the epimacular membrane causes nonrhegmatogenous elevation of the macula thought by the authors to be responsible for a major fraction of the associated visual loss. Reversible macular edema secondary to macular separation from the fluid-pumping mechanism of the retinal pigment epithelium contributes to visual loss as well. Although it is widely stated that traction on the ILM can produce macular edema, it is unclear what the mechanism would be and the concept remains unproven. Although the terms *macular pucker* and *surface wrinkling retinopathy* emphasize retinal distortion, some patients have marked improvement in postoperative vision in spite of persistent retinal distortion and metamorphopsia.

HISTORY

The typical epimacular membrane patient experiences a relatively rapid loss of vision accompanied by metamorphopsia over a period of several weeks, followed by relative stabilization of visual function. In spite of this typical history, it is common practice for doctors to advise a patient with a recent history of visual loss to, for example, the 20/50 level, that they should wait until the vision is reduced to 20/80 or worse before considering surgery.

In fact, the vision will usually stabilize at a visual level at or near that noted on initial presentation. Because visual results are better with better preoperative vision and shorter duration, it is better practice to make a decision on surgical intervention on the first visit.

CASE SELECTION

As with all surgical procedures, the decision to operate is a multifactorial process based on symptoms, extent of visual loss, visual needs, status of the other eye, age, duration, medical status, and presence of other ocular diseases. There is no substitute for ethical, sound clinical judgment in making the decision to operate.

The principal author's visual acuity threshold for surgery has moved from 20/200 to 20/40 in selected cases, as the methodology has improved. The principal author operates on patients with preoperative vision of 20/40, if the patient is significantly symptomatic, in good health, relatively young, and aware of the issues. Duration is a relative rather than an absolute criterion because cases of 10 years' duration have had significant visual improvement following surgery. This remarkable visual improvement is presumably because the minimal amount of subretinal fluid present in these cases leads to minimal irreversible photoreceptor degeneration, just as is the case in central serous retinopathy. Macular edema, except in the vascular disease subgroup, is probably secondary to macular elevation, typically reversible and not a contraindication to vitreoretinal surgery. Knowledge that the patient had poor vision before the membrane occurred is an absolute contraindication to surgery. The slow recovery of vision after retinal reattachment surgery coupled with the typical 1-month onset of epimacular membrane (EMM) makes it difficult to make a surgical decision in this situation. Patients with severe hereditary photoreceptor degeneration or a previous central retinal artery occlusion frequently have wrinkling of the retinal surface without an epiretinal membrane because of marked decrease in retinal thickness. Surgery is contraindicated in these situations (15–27).

SURGICAL SEQUENCE AND TECHNIQUES

Vitreomacular Traction Syndrome

The posterior vitreous cortex is rarely adherent to typical epimacular membranes. Some patients have macular elevation secondary to hypocellular contraction of the posterior vitreous cortex combined with marked adherence of the vitreous to the macula (28–30). This entity is known as vitreomacular traction syndrome. When operating on these cases, care must be taken to avoid tearing the fovea by imbrication of the vitreous into the port of the vitreous cutter. Horizontal scissors can be used to delaminate the posterior vitreous cortex from the fovea before any removal of the vitreous (Fig. 10.1).

Nonrhegmatogenous Proliferative Vitreoretinopathy

Some patients have multiple star folds from PVR in addition to an epimacular component. Removing these additional epiretinal membranes is a stimulus for recurrent PVR and is unnecessary unless they are causing macular elevation or distortion.

Need for Vitrectomy at the Time of Membrane Peeling

The need to remove the vitreous at the time of epiretinal membrane surgery has not been established. The principal author initially suggested the concept of membrane

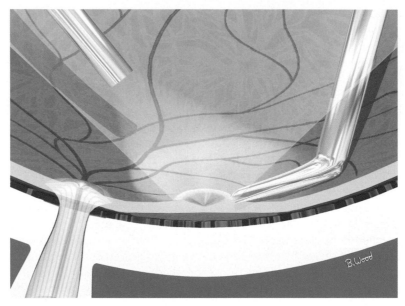

FIG. 10.1. When vitreomacular traction is present, the horizontal scissors are used to delaminate the posterior vitreous cortex from the fovea before any vitreous removal.

without vitreous removal but stopped advocating this approach after several hundred cases because of the following reasons: If vitrectomy is performed, it will prevent late complications from hypocellular vitreous contraction and patients will not complain of floaters. Vitrectomy can lead to postoperative rhegmatogenous retinal detachment because of intraoperative suction forces, cutter movement–induced traction, and vitreous incarceration in the sclerotomies. If the vitreous has been removed, a postoperative retinal detachment can be managed by in-office, two-needle, fluid/gas exchange and laser retinopexy. Anterior vitreous cortex removal is probably correlated with an increased incidence of posterior subcapsular cataract probably related to fluid turbulence. Avoiding the anterior vitreous cortex may reduce postoperative posterior subcapsular cataract and rhegmatogenous retinal detachment.

Epiretinal Membrane Removal

Machemer developed the concept of membrane peeling in 1972 soon after his introduction of vitrectomy. Originally, peeling was performed with a bent needle. O'Malley subsequently developed the concept of using a rounded, angulated instrument he called a pic to perform the peeling. The principal author and the late Ron Michels popularized the pic method. Bent needles and pics require the presence of a visible outer margin of the EMM frequently called an "edge." Alternatively, searching for an edge must be done with the accompanied risk of making a retinal break. The principal author subsequently developed the concept of inside-out forceps membrane peeling initially because of the difficulty of finding an "edge" in certain cases. In contrast to Machemer's outside-in membrane-peeling method, inside-out peeling is initiated by surface grasping the epimacular membrane with end-opening forceps (Fig. 10.2) or in some cases by making a slit in the apparent center of the epimacular membrane using the microvitreoretinal (MVR) blade (Fig. 10.3). The MVR blade is the same one used to make the

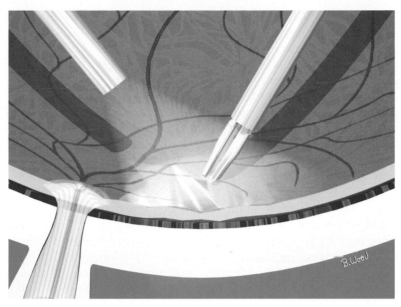

FIG. 10.2. Inside-out membrane peeling is initiated by grasping the denser epicenter of the EMM with the conformal forceps.

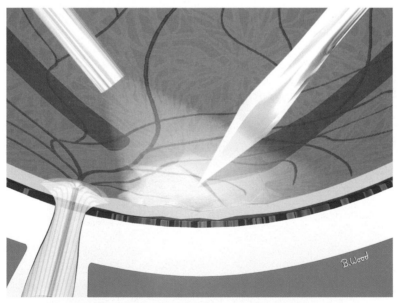

FIG. 10.3. If adequate purchase on the membrane cannot be obtained by pinch-peeling, a slit is made with the MVR blade to develop an edge for grasping.

sclerotomies. The MVR blade should not be bent, as there is no intent to place it between the membrane and the retina. The center of the membrane can be identified by noting the orientation of radial striae, the most elevated retinal region, the most opaque region of the membrane, and relative movement of the membrane with respect to the retina induced by lateral movement of the forceps or MVR blade tip. End-opening forceps with diamond coating were developed by one of the authors (SC) and Hans Grieshaber for surface grasping and must have precise alignment of the of the blade tips (Fig. 10.4). Others have developed effective end-opening forceps without diamonds (Fig. 10.5). The peeling should be accomplished by moving the forceps tangentially along the surface of the retina. This motion should be continued in a circular fashion similar to capsulorhexis (Fig. 10.6). If the membrane tears, it can be regrasped without removing any membrane from the forceps because the diamonds and microteeth will penetrate several layers of membrane and facilitate removal of the membrane through the pars plana as well. The surgeon should always observe the fovea during the peeling process rather than focusing on the forceps in order to prevent tearing the fovea. Areas of stronger adherence to the ILM can be detected by noting fine fibers being lifted from the retinal surface during the peeling process. Scissors delamination rather than peeling is utilized if strong adherence to the fovea, vessels, or any region of the retina is noted during the peeling process. Right-angle 20-gauge delamination scissors (Charles modification of the Grieshaber Sutherland scissors) with the blades roughly parallel to the retinal surface can be used to delaminate the glial attachment points (Fig. 10.7) without inducing trauma to the ILM. If there are marked folds, the blunt, polished end of the vitrectomy instrument can be used to gently push the retinal folds into better position; a method called *burnishing*. Moderate-sized peeled or delaminated membrane pieces should be removed through the pars plana with the forceps. If the membrane is very large or dense it should be removed with the vitrectomy probe.

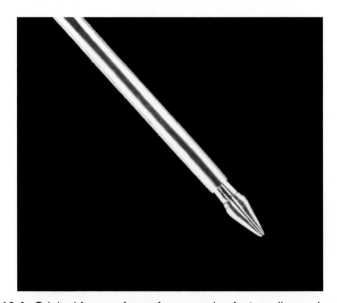

FIG. 10.4. Original forceps for surface grasping feature diamond coating.

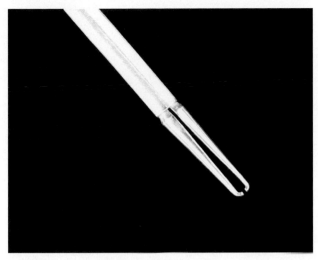

FIG. 10.5. The conformal forceps designed by Charles has no diamond coating and is now the preferred forceps.

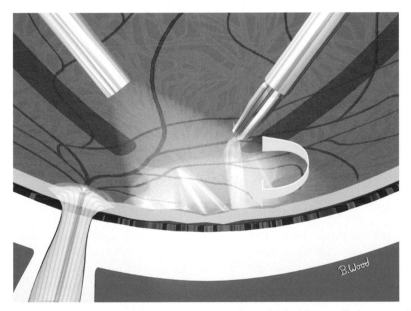

FIG. 10.6. Membrane peeling is affected in a circumferential fashion, pulling tangentially from the edge, as in capsulorhexis.

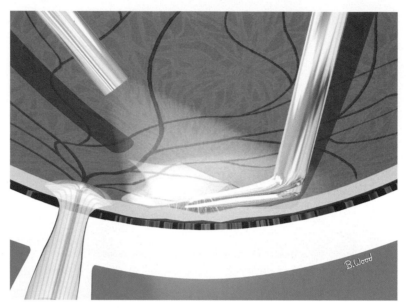

FIG. 10.7. If the membrane appears strongly adherent during the peeling process, right-angle scissors are used to delaminate the glial attachment points, without trauma to the ILM.

Management of Retinal Breaks

No posterior retinal breaks occurred in the principal author's prospective, consecutive, single-surgeon series of more than 1,200 consecutive cases; all other series report a 5% to 6% incidence of retinal breaks. The peripheral retina should be inspected at the end of the case and all retinal breaks with elevated edges should be managed with fluid/air exchange, air/gas exchange with 25% SF_6, and laser endophotocoagulation around the break(s). Laser alone can be used if the edges are not elevated and it is a posterior break. Scleral buckling is not required in these cases.

Management of Coexistent Cataract

The authors recommend that cataract surgery be performed before vitreous surgery if a visually significant cataract is present. This approach increases cost and subjects the patient to increased anesthesia and operative risk but enables a superior view at vitrectomy and optimal refractive status. Epimacular membrane surgery requires excellent visualization and should not be attempted if greater than 2+ nuclear sclerosis or a significant posterior subcapsular cataract is present. The fact that vitreous surgery causes progression of preexisting nuclear sclerotic cataract in a significant number of cases should be taken into account when considering when to remove the lens.

Cataract surgery can be combined with vitreous surgery using many different approaches. Some recommend that the cataract surgeon or the vitreoretinal surgeon perform phakoemulsification and intraocular lens insertion before initiating vitreous surgery. This is not an ideal approach because pigment release from the iris, viscoelastics, miosis, and corneal changes frequently adversely affects the view for membrane peeling. The author recommend prior cataract surgery or use of endocapsular lensectomy before the vitreous surgery. The authors also recommend preservation of the anterior lens capsule as first reported by Blankenship and Kokame. A posterior chamber intraocular lens is inserted in the ciliary sulcus through a clear corneal or scleral tunnel incision after the vitrectomy and membrane peeling. The principal author has modified Blankenship's technique by performing a circular posterior capsulorhexis rather than entering the lens through the equatorial capsule. Posterior cortical clearing hydrodissection is then performed. A 20-gauge four-crystal fragmenter (Alcon) is then used to remove the nucleus and epinucleus while carefully avoiding the anterior lens capsule. Aspiration is used to clean all cortex off the lens capsule. Any lens material that falls posteriorly can be removed with the fragmenter after vitreous removal is accomplished. The lens fragments should be picked up with suction mode before engaging fragmentation with the footpedal. The vitreous cutter in aspiration-only mode can be used to remove cortex from the lens capsule. After the cortical pieces are removed from the capsular bag, the cutter can be activated to facilitate removal. Careful cortical removal/capsule polishing probably obviates the need for primary anterior capsulotomy. The authors currently use acrylic (Acrysof by Alcon), foldable lenses inserted through a 3.2-mm keratome incision.

VISUAL RESULTS

About 40% of the patients in the author's (SC) series had improved vision to 20/40 or better. Approximately 56% improved to 20/80 or better. More than 85% of the patients improved two lines or greater in visual acuity. Those with greater visual loss (1/200 to 5/200) preoperatively improve to approximately the 20/200 level postoperatively. Those in the 20/200 region preoperatively typically return to the 20/50 to 20/60 level postoperatively. Those with 20/50 vision preoperatively usually return to the 20/20 to 20/25 level.

COMPLICATIONS

Retinal Breaks

No posterior retinal breaks were caused in the principal author's series of more than 1,200 consecutive vitrectomies for EMM. All other authors have reported an incidence of 5% to 7%. Although the author's series was not randomized to outside-in versus inside-out peeling, this marked difference probably indicates that inside-out, forceps membrane peeling is a safer method than using pics and outside-in peeling.

Rhegmatogenous Retinal Detachment

The author's series had a similar incidence of postoperative retinal detachment to that reported by other authors (<5%). This complication is related to inadvertent force on the vitreous base during vitreous removal, instrument introduction forces, and incarceration of vitreous in the sclerotomies. This complication can be decreased by using high-quality cutters (InnoVit), low suction force (<80 mm Hg), and highest possible cutting rates, and by avoiding pulling the cutter away when cutting is activated. The retinal periphery should be inspected with the indirect ophthalmoscope at the end of the case and any retinal breaks treated with endolaser, laser indirect ophthalmoscope (LIO), or cryopexy and fluid/gas exchange with 25% SF_6.

Proliferative Vitreoretinopathy Recurrence

If PVR was successfully repaired before the development of a membrane, it can be stimulated to recur by epimacular membrane surgery. Usually, the PVR-induced redetachment can be successfully repaired with repeat vitrectomy and silicone oil, but little improvement in pre-EMM surgery vision is then obtained.

Cystoid Macular Edema

The author's series noted a preoperative cystoid macular edema (CME) incidence of 3.2%. This incidence was based on clinical observation, as routine fluoroscein angiography was not performed. The McDonald et al. series reports a 3% incidence of CME.

Endophthalmitis

The author's series of more than 1,200 cases had no cases of postoperative endophthalmitis, whereas the literature reports an average incidence of 0.7%. The principal author uses a one-piece surgical drape that is folded over the lid margins and a microscope drape in all cases. Subconjunctival Tobramyan and Ancef are injected with a cannula at the end of the case. High-quality infusion fluid (Alcon BSS Plus) is used in all cases. Absorbable sclerotomy sutures are not used.

Recurrence of Epimacular Proliferation

Approximately 1.6% of treated EMM cases resulted in clinically significant recurrent epimacular membranes (17,31–34) in the author's series of more than 1,200 cases. Successful reoperation can usually be performed with sustained visual improvement. The recurrence rate emphasizes the reparative nature of the process and the damage to the retinal surface associated with membrane peeling. All patients probably have some repair of the retinal surface after membrane peeling. The criterion for defining a recurrence has not been established in the literature. In some patients, the folds disappear completely and a recurrence can easily be determined if folds recur. In other patients, the recurrent membrane causes macular elevation with minimal striae and the membrane is more difficult to visualize. Decreased visual function is usually the best indicator of clinically significant recurrences if the patient had initially experienced gradual visual improvement. Visually significant cataract must be ruled out before the visual loss can be attributed to the macula.

Retinal Whitening

Immediate postoperative retinal whitening occurs at the removal site in a significant percentage of cases. This disappears spontaneously in several days and does not seem to affect the visual outcome. It is probable that this phenomenon represents ganglion cell axoplasmic flow stasis. Michels noted that retinal whitening is present preoperatively in a significant number of cases.

Cataract

Posterior subcapsular cataracts after vitrectomy are largely avoidable. Posterior subcapsular cataracts can be caused by using low-quality infusion fluids such as lactated Ringers solution rather than glutathione bicarbonate Ringers (Alcon BSS Plus).

The observed increase in the incidence of nuclear sclerosis associated with EMM surgery is thought by the authors to result from ultraviolet irradiance and heating from infrared light exposure from the microscope light source and/or the endoilluminator. The principal author's series of more than 1,200 cases resulted in 7% of the patients requiring cataract surgery from progression of nuclear sclerosis after vitrectomy. The incidence of progression of nuclear sclerosis has been reported to range from 7% to well over 50%. This wide variation could be accounted for by many factors, including follow-up period, definition of clinical significance, postoperative refraction, operating time, intraoperative cataract surgery, light source ultraviolet and infrared (IR) content, and unknown factors. The principal author has used cooling of the infusion fluid for the past 10 years in an attempt to reduce heating of the nucleus secondary to infrared irradiation. Cooling lessens the effect of the ultraviolet light as well. Heating and ultraviolet exposure are thought by many cataract researchers to be factors in the development of nuclear sclerosis.

REFERENCES

1. Kampik A, Kenyon KR, Michels RG, et al. Epiretinal and vitreous membranes: comparative study of 56 cases. *Arch Ophthalmol* 1981;99:1445–1454.
2. Pearlstone AD. The incidence of idiopathic preretinal macular gliosis. *Ann Ophthalmol* 1985;17:378.
3. Scudder MJ, Eifrig DE. Spontaneous surface wrinkling retinopathy. *Ann Ophthalmol* 1982;94:44.
4. Sidd RJ, Fine SL, Owens SL, et al. Idiopathic preretinal gliosis. *Am J Ophthalmol* 1982;94:44.
5. Wise GN. Clinical features of idiopathic preretinal macular fibrosis. *Am J Ophthalmol* 1975;79:349.
6. Roth AM, Foos RY. Surface wrinkling retinopathy in eyes enucleated at autopsy. *Trans Am Acad Ophthalmol Otolaryngol* 1971;75:1047.
7. Wise GN. Clinical features of idiopathic preretinal macular fibrosis. *Am J Opthalmol* 1975;79:349.
8. Kenyon KR, Michels RG. Ultrastructure of epiretinal membrane removed by pars plana vitreoretinal surgery. *Am J Opthalmol* 1977;83:815.
9. Clarkson SG, Green WR, Massof D. A histopathologic review of 168 cases of preretinal membrane. *Am J Opthalmol* 1977;84:1.
10. Green WR, Kenyon KR, Michels RG, et al. Ultrastructure of epiretinal membranes causing macular pucker following retinal reattachment. *Trans Ophthalmol Soc UK* 1979;99:63.
11. Kampik A, Green WR, Michels RG, et al. Ultrastructural features of idiopathic progressive epiretinal membrane removed by vitreous surgery. *Am J Opthalmol* 1981;90:797.
12. Michels RG. A clinical and histopathological study of epiretinal membranes affecting the macula and removed by vitreous surgery. *Trans Am Ophthalmol Soc* 1982;80:580.
13. Laqua H. Pigmented macular pucker. *Am J Opthalmol* 1978;86:56.
14. Lindsey PS, Michels RG, Luckenbach M, et al. Ultrastructure of epiretinal membrane causing retinal starfold. *Ophthalmology* 1983;90:578.
15. Michels RG. Surgical treatment of macular pucker. In: Stirpe M, Convers M., Blankenship G., et al., eds. *Advances in vitreoretinal surgery.* Rome: Filia, 1987.
16. Shea M. The surgical management of macular pucker. *Can J Ophthalmol* 1979;2:110.
17. Wilkinson CP. Recurrent macular pucker. *Am J Opthalmol* 1979;88:1029.
18. Machemer R. A new concept for vitreous surgery: two instrument techniques in pars plana vitrectomy. *Arch Ophthalmol* 1974;92:407–441.
19. Trese MT, Chandler DB, Machemer R. Macular pucker: prognostic criteria. *Graefes Arch Clin Exp Ophthalmol* 1983;221:12–15.
20. Margherio RR, Cox MS, Trese MT, et al. Removal of epimacular membranes. *Ophthalmology* 1985;92:1075–1083.
21. McDonald HR, Verre WP, Aaberg TM. Surgical management of idiopathic epiretinal membranes. *Ophthalmology* 1986;93:978–983.
22. De Bustros S, Thompson JT, Michels G, et al. Vitrectomy for idiopathic epiretinal membranes causing macular pucker. *Br J Ophthalmol* 1988;72:692–695.
23. Rice TA, de Bustros S, Michels RG, et al. Prognostic factors in vitrectomy for epiretinal membranes of the macula. *Ophthalmology* 1986;93:602–610.
24. Charles S. General posterior segment techniques. In: Charles S, ed. *Vitreous microsurgery.* Baltimore: Williams & Wilkins, 1987:98.
25. Margherio RR. Discussion of Michels RG. Vitrectomy for macular pucker. *Ophthalmology* 1984;91:1387–1388.
26. Gass JDM. *Stereoscopic atlas of macular diseases, 4th ed.* St. Louis: CV Mosby, 1997:288–299, 938, 940, 944.
27. Barr CC, Michels RG. Idiopathic nonvascularized epiretinal membranes in young patients: report of six cases. *Ann Ophthalmol* 1982;14:335–341.
28. Smiddy WE, Michels RG, Glaser BM, et al. Vitrectomy for macular traction caused by incomplete vitreous separation. *Arch Ophthalmol* 1988;106:624–628.
29. Melberg NS, Williams DF, Balles MW, et al. Vitrectomy for vitreomacular traction syndrome with macular detachment. *Retina* 1995;15:192–197.
30. Bellhorn MB, Friedman AH, Wise GN, et al. Ultrastructural and clinicopathologic correlation of idiopathic preretinal macular fibrosis. *Am J Ophthalmol* 1975;79:366–373.
31. Michels RG. Vitreous surgery for macular pucker. *Am J Opthalmol* 1981;92:628.
32. Michels RG. Surgery of macular pucker. In: Fine SL, Owens SL, eds. *Management of retinal vascular and macular disorders.* Baltimore: Williams & Wilkins, 1983:120–130.
33. Michels RG. Vitrectomy for macular pucker. *Ophthalmology* 1984;91;1384.
34. Michels RG. Macular pucker. In: Fraunfelder FT, Roy FH. *Current ocular therapy, 2nd ed.* Philadelphia: WB Saunders, 1984:440–442.

11

Macular Holes

Until 1991 it was thought that macular holes were untreatable, unpreventable, and of unknown pathogenesis. In that year Kelly and Wendel developed the concept of using vitrectomy and fluid/gas exchange to treat these patients (1). Initially there was great skepticism about the treatment, but the facts prevailed. The initial goal was to "seal" the hole, much as is done for rhegmatogenous retinal detachment, and eliminate the cuff of subretinal fluid that surrounds the hole. When it was noted that many holes actually disappeared after surgery and patients obtained near normal vision, the skeptics again did not believe it. Fortunately, it is now accepted that complete disappearance of the hole frequently occurs.

PATHOGENESIS

It was widely believed that a posterior vitreous detachment pulled a full-thickness piece of tissue out of the macula, probably as a result of or during a saccade. Only in recent years has electron microscopy of the so-called operculum, which occurs in these cases, shown that few photoreceptors are present (2,3). Gass has published a definitive work, which seems to explain the pathogenesis (4,5). The central concept is that radial vitreous fibers remaining on the perimacular surface after apparent posterior vitreous separation contract and slowly tear the macula in a circumferential fashion. Many observers have noted that vitreous is attached to the optic nerve after an apparent posterior vitreous separation characterized by the presence of a prepapillary (Weiss) ring. Because of these observations, the event might better be termed *delamination of the posterior vitreous cortex*. The principal author has observed that the vitreous attached to the optic nerve is rarely contiguous with the remaining cortex attached to the inner margin of the hole. The principal author terms the so-called cuff of fluid, the *traction cuff*. Sjaarda has shown that using scanning laser ophthalmoscope (SLO) microperimetry extends the actual extent of fluid far beyond the margin of the cuff (6). The vitreous that is attached to the inner margin of the macular hole is rarely contiguous with the vitreous attached to the mid-peripheral retina. Terminology represents a serious problem in discussing these cases with vitreoretinal surgeons. Morris and Witherspoon have described peeling off the internal limiting membrane in a procedure they call *macular rhexis*. It is been known for years that pieces of ILM are avulsed when peeling epiretinal membranes. Many observers have observed whitening of the retina due to axoplasmic stasis if part of the ILM is peeled away from the retina. Many pathologists and clinicians, including the authors, believe that the material peeled in classic macular hole surgery can be residual vitreous cortex ILM, or epiretinal membrane. Blumenkranz has developed an attractive theory that layers of the ILM are delaminated by peeling, explaining the lack of axoplasmic stasis in cases with proven ILM in the removed tissue.

Some holes have no cuff, are elliptical, and are caused by typical epimacular membranes rather than vitreous. The authors refer to these holes as *secondary holes* and those described earlier as *primary* or *classic holes.*

Surgical success should be defined as disappearance of the hole and marked improvement in vision. This only occurs because few neuronal elements are missing and glial cells pull the macula back together.

INDICATIONS FOR MACULAR HOLE TREATMENT SURGERY

Freeman et al. have shown that smaller holes have the best prognosis. Size is much more important than duration with respect to closure rates. Most surgeons do not suggest repairing holes secondary to chronic macular edema from diabetic retinopathy, venous occlusive disease, or cystoid macular edema after cataract surgery, nor do they suggest such repair when secondary to uveitis. Traumatic macular holes involve a complex decision-making process because of the high likelihood of associated photoreceptor, retinal pigment epithelium, and optic nerve damage and because many will spontaneously close within 1 or 2 months. If there is good evidence that the macular hole is the only significant damage, these cases can be considered for surgery after a reasonable period of observation.

MACULAR HOLE PREVENTION

Arthur Willis first reported the concept of macular hole prevention by performing vitrectomy and peeling the posterior vitreous cortex away from the posterior retina. Michels and DeBuestros reported a series and initiated a randomized, multicenter trial. Freeman et al. completed the study and reported lack of efficacy for the technique. There is a significant incidence of retinal detachment after this surgery as well as a high rate of nuclear sclerosis progression. Charteris et al. reported that 50% of Stage I macular holes spontaneously disappear. The author (SC) has had the experience of advising surgery for a seemingly progressive Stage I hole on several occasions with the patient subsequently deciding against surgery. These patients were followed for several years and resolved without treatment. Progression from Stage I to Stage II with visual symptoms must be noted before surgery is recommended.

As only a few small series report an incidence of bilaterality greater than 12%, the concept of surgery on the normal contralateral eye of macular hole patients is unconscionable.

COMPLICATIONS OF PEELING VITREOUS FROM THE OPTIC NERVE

Hutton was the first to note permanent, postoperative peripheral field loss in macular-hole postsurgery patients. With screening field techniques, the incidence is more than 17%. Some have theorized that this is due to the gas bubble, which makes little sense, as it has not been observed in retinal detachment patients repaired using gas. Others have suggested that light toxicity causes this problem. This concept can be laid to rest by noting that the principal author has performed many vitrectomies for epimacular membrane with the same light and operating time and no visual field defects. The authors strongly believe that separating the vitreous from the optic nerve causes most of the damage. For this reason the principal author stopped separating the vitreous from the nerve in May 1995. There have been no cases of field loss in nearly 300 cases and the success rate is about 90%. Prolonged waiting to "dry" the macula in preparation for use of biologic modifiers may cause retinal drying, but the proof is not compelling at this time.

COMPLICATIONS OF INDUCED POSTERIOR VITREOUS SEPARATION

Varying rates of postoperative retinal detachment, some as high as 40%, have been reported after macular hole surgery. This is probably due to separation of the posterior vitreous cortex or movement of the bubble. In recent years, many surgeons scleral-depress the periphery and laser the holes that are frequently noted. Because the principal author noted that there usually was no connection between the residual cortex attached to the inner margin of the hole and the peripheral attached vitreous, no PVDs were intentionally created after May 1995. The incidence of retinal detachments seems to have decreased with no decrease in hole closure rates.

POSTOPERATIVE POSITIONING

Most surgeons recommend full-time or nearly full-time facedown positioning for the duration of a reasonably sized bubble (7). The authors believe in full-time, facedown positioning for 3 weeks. The patients are allowed to walk, work, read, watch TV's placed on the floor, ride in cars (not drive), and use the treadmill or stationary bicycle. A head-down position does not interfere with eating, showering, reading, or using the restroom. Facedown driving has consequences that extend beyond vitreoretinal surgery.

GAS OPTIONS

Several studies have shown that longer-duration, C_3F_8 bubbles produce higher closure rates than air or SF_6. The authors use C_3F_8 in all cases, as do most other surgeons (8–20).

BIOLOGIC MODIFIERS

Fibrin, serum, autologous platelet concentrate, thrombin, whole blood, cryo precipitates, and transforming growth factor beta (bovine, recombinant, and autologous) have been used to accelerate glial proliferation in the hole (21–23). Sterile endophthalmitis, uveitis, inflammatory PVR, and bacterial endophthalmitis have been reported after use of these agents. The authors and many other surgeons no longer use these agents because of unproven efficacy and the risk factors noted earlier. Freeman et al. showed no effect of serum in a controlled clinical trial. The principal author's method makes use of bleeding from the perimacular capillaries intentionally created with the MVR blade from the inner margin of the hole in large-hole or reoperation settings. Biologic modifiers may be necessary for very large holes.

SURGICAL TECHNIQUE FOR MACULAR HOLE TREATMENT

The authors recommend performing a core vitrectomy with no effort directed at removing vitreous from the optic nerve or mid-peripheral retina. All posterior vitreous cortex, ILM, and/or ERM attached to the margins of the macular hole are peeled with conformal forceps. The vitreous is trimmed down to the optic nerve, often after fluid/air exchange. No more than 100 mm Hg suction is used. No soft tip or metal cannulas are used. End-opening forceps such as the Tano diamond-dusted membrane peeler (Fig.11.1) has been found effective by some surgeons. The MVR blade is used to dissect the cortex/ERM/ILM away from the surface of the cuff (Fig. 11.2). The conformal end-opening forceps are the preferred technique at this time (Fig. 11.3). Cortical fibers usually remain

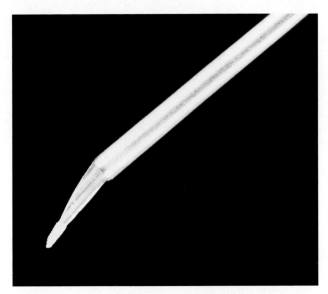

FIG. 11.1. Tano diamond-embedded flexible scraper.

attached to the inner margin of the macular hole and may stand up like fine hair at the inner margin of the hole. The cuff appearance will often disappear when the peeling process is complete. Vitreous fibers can be folded over and imbricated into the hole to act as a substrate (Fig. 11.4). A specific attempt is made to slightly damage the inner margin of the macular hole to stimulate glial activity if the ILM cannot be peeled. An attempt is also made to cause capillary bleeding by making scratches in the retina at the inner margin of the hole (Fig. 11.5) if the ILM is not peelable. This blood acts as an endogenous, safe

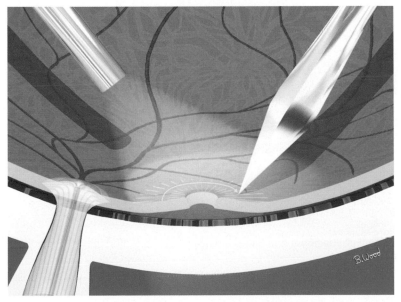

FIG. 11.2. The MVR blade is used to dissect the cortex/ERM/ILM away from the surface of the cuff, when peeling is not possible.

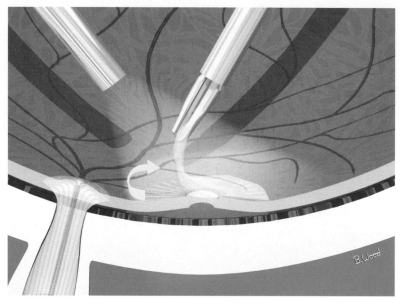

FIG. 11.3. The small, diamond-coated forceps are preferred for peeling the cortex/ERM/ILM in a circumferential fashion.

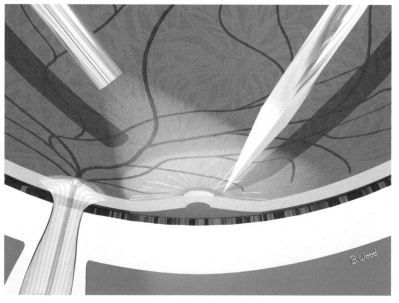

FIG. 11.4. Fine vitreous fibers can be folded over and imbricated into the hole to act as a substrate for capillary blood.

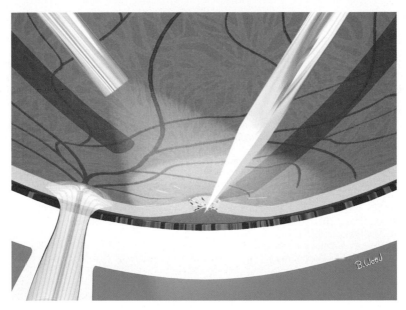

FIG. 11.5. Capillary bleeding is induced by scratching at the inner margin of the hole, and the blood acts as an endogenous, safe, biologic modifier.

biologic modifier. The intraocular pressure is lowered when initiating fluid/air exchange to increase bleeding into the hole. If vitreous/air interfaces demonstrate substantial domes of remaining vitreous, the vitreous cutter is inserted into the vitreous for further vitrectomy under air. Minimal traction is placed on the retinal surface with this maneuver. The Landers lens is used if the eye is phakic or pseudophakic.

RESULTS

Results have been reported as high as 100% for small series with cases selected for small, short-duration holes. The authors believe that 90% is a reproducible success rate with C_3F_8, 3 weeks of facedown positioning, and cortex/ERM/ILM peeling (24).

REFERENCES

1. Kelly NE, Wendel RT. Vitreous surgery for idiopathic macular holes: results of a pilot study. *Arch Ophthalmol* 1991;109:654–659.
2. Madreperla SA, McCuen BW 2nd, Hickinbotham D, et al. Clinicopathologic correlation of surgically removed macular hole opercula. *Am J Ophthalmol* 1995;120:197–207.
3. Ezra E, Munro PM, Charteris DG, et al. Macular hole opercula: ultrastructural features and clinicopathological correlation. *Arch Ophthalmol* 1997;115:1381–1387.
4. Gass JD. Idiopathic senile macular hole: Its early stages and pathogenesis. *Arch Ophthalmol* 1991;106:654–659.
5. Gass JD. Reappraisal of biomicroscopic classification of stages of development of a macular hole. *Am J Ophthalmol* 1995;119:752–759.
6. Sjaarda RN, Frank DA, Glaser BM, et al. Assessment of vision in idiopathic macular holes with macular microperimetry using the scanning laser ophthalmoscope. *Ophthalmology* 1993;100:1513–1518.
7. Tornambe PE, Poliner LS, Grote K. Macular hole surgery without face down positioning: a pilot study. *Retina* 1997;17:179–185.
8. Thompson JT. Kinetics of intraocular gases: disappearance of air, sulfur hexafluoride, and perfluoropropane after pars plana vitrectomy. *Arch Ophthalmol* 1989;107:687.

 9. Thompson JT. The absorption of mixtures of air and perfluoropropane after pars plana vitrectomy. *Arch Ophthalmol* 1992;110:1594.
10. Wong RF, Thompson JT. Prediction of the kinetics of disappearance of SF_6 and perfluoropropane intraocular gas bubbles. *Ophthalmology* 1988;95:609.
11. Chang S, Lincoff HA, Coleman DL. Perfluorocarbon gases in vitreous surgery. *Ophthalmology* 1985;92:651.
12. Peters MA, Abrams GW, Hamilton LH, et al. The nonexpansile concentration of perfluoropropane gas in the eye. *Am J Ophthalmol* 1985;100:831.
13. Han DP, Abrams GW, Bennett SR, et al. Perfluoropropane 12% vs 20%: effect on intraocular pressure and gas tamponade after pars plana vitrectomy. *Retina* 1993;13:302.
14. Smith RB, Carl B, Linn JG, et al. Effect of nitrous oxide on air in vitreous. *Am J Ophthalmol* 1974;78:314.
15. Van Slyke DD, Dillon RT, Margaria R. Studies of gas and electrolyte equilibria in blood. *J Biol Chem* 1934; 105:571.
16. Lincoff H, Weinberger D, Reppucci V, et al. Air travel with intraocular gas. I. The mechanism for compensation. *Arch Ophthalmol* 1989;107:902.
17. Lincoff H, Weinberger D, Stergiu P. Air travel with intraocular gas. II. Clinical considerations. *Arch Ophthalmol* 1989;107:907.
18. Aronwitz JD, Brubaker RF. Effect of intraocular gas on intraocular pressure. *Arch Ophthalmol* 1976;94:1191.
19. Del Priore LV, Michels RG, Nunez MA, et al. Intraocular pressure measurement after pars plana vitrectomy. *Ophthalmology* 1989;96:1353.
20. Charles S, Wang C. A motorized gas injector for vitreous surgery. *Arch Ophthalmol* 1981;99:1398.
21. Glaser BM, Michels RG, Kupperman BD, et al. Transforming growth factor beta-2 for the treatment of full thickness macular holes. A prospective randomized study. *Ophthalmology* 1992;99:1162–1173.
22. Ligget PE, Skolik SA, Horio B, et al. Human autologous serum for the treatment of full thickness macular holes: preliminary study. *Ophthalmology* 1995;102:1071–1076.
23. Thompson JT, Smiddy WE, Williams GA, et al. Comparison of recombinant transforming growth factor beta-2 and placebo as an adjuvant agent for macular hole surgery. *Ophthalmology* 1998; 105:700–706.
24. Thompson JT, Sjaarda RN, Lansing MB. The results of vitreous surgery for chronic macular hole. *Retina* 1997; 17:493–501.

12

Management of Subfoveal Choroidal Neovascular Membranes

In 1991 Thomas and Kaplan reported submacular surgery for subretinal neovascular membranes secondary to presumed ocular histoplasmosis syndrome (1). Subsequently these authors and many other surgeons applied their technique to idiopathic submacular membranes as well as membranes secondary to many other disease processes. In 1993 the principal author developed a simplified approach to submacular surgery, which will be described herein.

PATHOGENESIS OF SUBMACULAR MEMBRANES

Most submacular membranes initially have a neovascular component. It has been shown that VEGF plays a part in the neovascular phase of what ultimately becomes a fibrous scar. It is fortunate but somewhat surprising that laser photocoagulation can arrest further progression in approximately 50% of juxtafoveal cases. The notion of treating an evolving scar by making a scar is almost without precedent in medicine. The stimulus for membrane development is thought to be a defect in the retinal pigment epithelium (RPE)/Bruch's complex. The defect in so-called age-related macular degeneration probably occurs from apoptosis, which is genetically programmed cell death. Trauma, angioid streaks, laser photocoagulation, myopia, inactive choroiditis lesions such as histoplasmosis, and many other conditions can lead to this repair process as well. Although the initial article referred to removal of "neovascular" membranes, it is actually a scar that is removed. It is common for the scar (membrane) to be significantly larger than the "net" seen on the angiogram (Fig. 12.1).

Submacular hemorrhages have been surgically removed since the early 1990s. These cases have widely varying outcomes based on the underlying pathology and surgical trauma involved (2–4.) Some investigators have injected tissue plasminogen activator (TPA) under the retina at the time of surgery and wait approximately 45 minutes for apparent liquefaction of the clot before aspiration (5–8). Others inject TPA into the vitreous approximately 24 hours before surgical removal in an attempt to liquefy the blood clot (9). Recently it has been reported that TPA can be injected into the vitreous cavity in the office followed by a gas injection and face-down positioning (10). Hilel Lewis has shown that TPA does not cross the primate retina (11). This less invasive method was thought to displace the blood away from the macula; however, this has not been proven. The authors no longer recommend intravitreal TPA. There is no scientific evidence that pneumatic retinopexy displaces submacular blood away from the macula, and the authors no longer use this technique.

The presence or absence of submacular membranes is a major determinant of visual outcomes after each of these procedures, as is the complication rate. In March 1999,

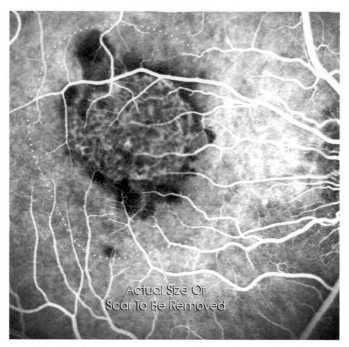

FIG. 12.1. Commonly, the scar to be removed is significantly larger than the neovascular net seen angiographically.

Harry Flynn and Cathleen McCabe reported a metaanalysis of all reported series of operated and nonoperated submacular hemorrhage cases (12). They found that one-third improved, one-third remained the same, and one-third became worse in *both* operated and nonoperated series. The authors have noted that a significant number of operated cases have completely blind eyes, which never occurs if surgery is not performed. In addition, few patients in the "improved" group improve by a functional class (e.g., from not reading to reading, or not driving to driving).

INDICATIONS FOR SUBMACULAR SURGERY FOR SUBFOVEAL MEMBRANES

Presumed photoreceptor and RPE viability are an absolute requirement when considering submacular surgery. The membrane acts as a diffusion barrier between the photoreceptors and the RPE, and leads first to degeneration of the outer segments and ultimately to degeneration of the inner segments. Free iron in the subretinal space for an extended period of time is toxic to the photoreceptor inner segments. Cases with membranes present for more than 6 months have almost no chance of visual improvement after membrane removal because of irreversible photoreceptor damage. Type I membranes seen in age-related macular degeneration (AMD) cases are under the RPE and cannot be removed without removing the overlying RPE. Type II membranes, as seen in idiopathic and histoplasmosis cases, are on the anterior surface of the RPE and can have a reasonable prognosis.

Age-related macular degeneration cases have a very poor visual prognosis after membrane removal. Approximately 20% of the AMD patients have improved vision, 60% are unchanged, and 20% become worse after submacular surgery. It is likely that eccentric fixation explains most cases of visual improvement. Poor vision after submacular surgery in these patients can be explained by several factors:

1. Diffuse, ongoing RPE disease.
2. High incidence of recurrences.
3. Photoreceptor and RPE damage from scar and hemorrhage.
4. Surgical removal of the RPE.
5. Absence of the choriocapillaris.

The membrane must be located between the retina and RPE, not under the RPE, to permit surgery without inadvertent removal of a segment of RPE. Most if not all AMD cases have Type I membranes, which are under the RPE. The authors have not performed submacular surgery on patients with AMD since 1994. Determination that the patient has AMD is not made by age alone but by the presence of drusen in the affected and/or other eye. A 50-year-old patient with advanced drusen has "AMD," but a 70-year-old patient with a unilateral membrane and no drusen in either eye probably has an idiopathic choroidal neovascular membrane (CNV) membrane.

Idiopathic cases have the best prognosis, whereas histoplasmosis is the most frequent indication in the central United States. Myopic patients with recent, medium to large well-defined lesions can benefit from submacular surgery. Selected angioid streaks and trauma cases are candidates for surgery as well.

SURGICAL SEQUENCE

A core vitrectomy is performed (Fig. 12.2) to facilitate passage of the instruments and to enable fluid/air exchange. No attempt is made to create a posterior vitreous detachment in submacular surgery cases (or macular holes). Many surgeons incorrectly believe that posterior vitreous detachment (PVD) is a required step, whereas in fact it probably increases the chance of retinal detachment and may damage the optic nerve. The principal author has had no rhegmatogenous detachments or retinotomy-related problems in a series of more than 250 cases in which no PVD was made.

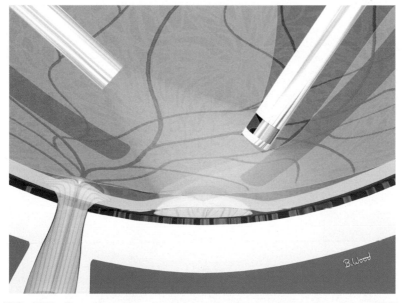

FIG. 12.2. Core vitrectomy is performed, with no attempt to create a PVD.

Thomas and Kaplan recommended injection of BSS under the retina to create a small retinal detachment before removing the membrane (1). The principal author observed that this step occasionally results in an acute hydraulic foveal hole. The author has learned that many other surgeons have experienced this problem as well and therefore has omitted the BSS injection step since 1992. In addition to preventing hydraulic rupture of the fovea, omitting BSS injection has the added advantage of preventing damage from shearing photoreceptors from the RPE in an area larger than the membrane.

A very small retinotomy is made with the MVR blade at the outer margin of membrane (Fig. 12.3), usually in the superotemporal quadrant. The retinotomy is made by teasing the nerve fibers apart along the orientation of the nerve fibers rather than cutting across the fibers. This concept is similar to making incisions along Langer's lines in facial plastic surgery. Diathermy is not applied to the retinotomy site because bleeding is not an issue, as retinal vessels are never transected. Diathermy causes an unnecessary nerve fiber layer defect and may stimulate scarring.

Diamond-tipped, end-opening Grieshaber forceps (see Fig. 10.4) are used to grasp the anterior surface of the outer margin of the membrane (Fig. 12.4). Forceps used with one or two blades under the membrane are more likely to strip the RPE or damage the choriocapillaris. Pics are never used because of the risk of RPE avulsion and bleeding from choriocapillaris trauma. The principal author developed end-opening, diamond-coated forceps membrane peeling and scissors segmentation/delamination of epiretinal membranes to reduce damage to the anterior retinal surface. Grasping of the anterior surface of submacular membranes with end-opening, diamond-coated forceps was developed to reduce damage to the RPE in an analogous manner to that developed for epiretinal membranes. The intraocular pressure is elevated to 60 mm Hg using the Accurus tamponade feature, air pump, or bottle height before removing the membrane to reduce bleeding. The membrane is rotated slowly to determine if there is excessive adherence to the retina or RPE. Excessive adherence is a common problem in patients with prior photocoagulation. Changing the direction of pulling can usually resolve this problem, although scissors are

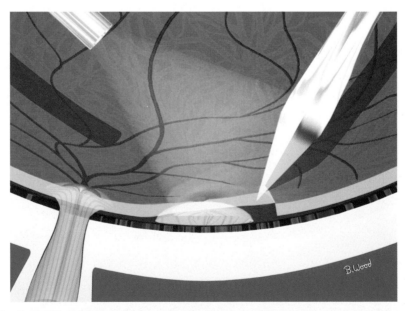

FIG. 12.3. A standard MVR blade is used to create a retinotomy, usually superotemporally. Tease the nerve fibers apart, with no cutting of the NFL or removal of retinal tissue.

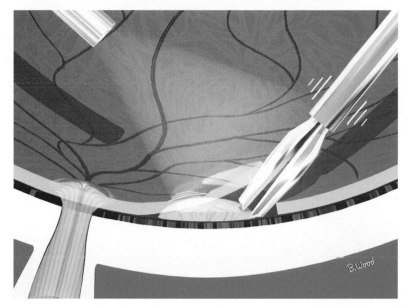

FIG. 12.4. Diamond-tipped end-opening forceps are used to grasp the anterior surface of the membrane. Rotate slightly to free up the membrane and to test for excessive adherence.

occasionally necessary to delaminate the membrane from the retina or RPE. The membrane should be removed very slowly to reduce retinal tearing and to enable close observation of the retina and RPE to prevent damage (Fig. 12.5). If the retina becomes more elevated during removal, the endoilluminator can be used to gently push the retina away from the membrane and toward the RPE. Suction should not be applied to the retinotomy because of the possibility of shearing damage to the photoreceptors and RPE.

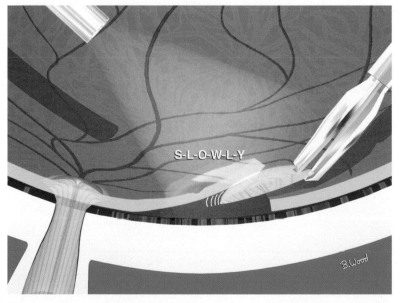

FIG. 12.5. Remove the membrane very slowly to reduce retinal tearing and to allow close observation of the retina and RPE to prevent damage.

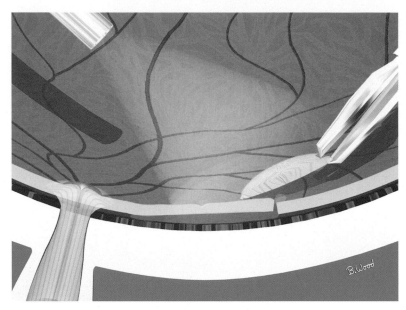

FIG. 12.6. Use the membrane to gently smooth the retinotomy margins into place and to express any subretinal fluid.

After the membrane is removed from the subretinal space, it is retained in the grasp of the forceps and used to gently push the retinotomy margins back together (Fig. 12.6) and express fluid from the subretinal space. The membrane is then moved to the anterior vitreous space and approximated to the port of the vitreous cutter. The membrane is then removed with the vitreous cutter (Fig. 12.7) using coaxial illumination from the operating microscope. Dragging the membrane through the peripheral vitreous and pars plana for

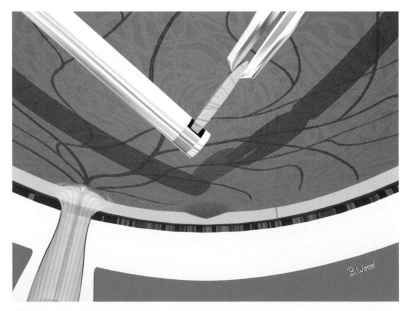

FIG. 12.7. Remove the membrane with the vitreous cutter, using the coaxial illumination from the operating microscope.

removal with the forceps may create vitreoretinal traction and subsequent retinal detachment. There is no need to submit the membrane to pathology, as the histologic appearance of these lesions is well known.

Fluid/air exchange is used for surface tension management for the retinotomy site to eliminate the need for laser retinopexy. Laser retinopexy creates a scotoma from nerve fiber layer damage and increases the chance of a new neovascular membrane at the laser site. The exchange is performed using the vitreous cutter for fluid egress and the Landers or equivalent high minus lens for visualization in phakic or pseudo-phakic eyes. The Accurus or equivalent air pump is used as an air source.

The intraocular pressure should be maintained at higher than normal levels during wound closure to prevent bleeding. Conjunctival closure and subconjunctival antibiotics and steroids are used in the manner described elsewhere in the text.

RESULTS

Underlying, ongoing pathology, surgical damage to the RPE and retina, as well as recurrent membranes determines the outcome. Careful case selection, as described earlier, is essential in producing better outcomes. The membrane recurrence rate has been reported from 25% (author's series) to 45%. An occasional patient will develop an extrafoveal recurrence and benefit from laser photocoagulation. Reoperation is indicated for a well-defined subretinal membrane in patients who had visual improvement after previous successful surgery.

TRANSPLANTATION OF RETINAL PIGMENT EPITHELIUM

Although tremendous advances have been made in the treatment of eye diseases, macular degeneration remains an enigma to ophthalmologists and their afflicted patients. It has been postulated that a contributing factor to the poor visual outcome following removal of choroidal neovascular membranes in macular degeneration patients is atrophy of the subfoveal choriocapillaris (13). Apparently, the area of atrophy can continue to enlarge 1 year after surgery. The stimulus for the choriocapillaris atrophy may be the failure of the RPE to repopulate the surgical bed (14). The extent of perfusion in the fovea is related to the visual prognosis and is therefore of great importance (15,16)

Unfortunately, tightly integrated RPE cells are removed along with subfoveal neovascular membranes in Age Related Macular Degeneration (ARMD) patients during submacular surgery. It has been shown in numerous studies that RPE removal will lead to choriocapillaris atrophy (17–22). While partial RPE regeneration may occur in some areas, other areas develop choriocapillaris atrophy and resultant disorganized photoreceptors. If one could insert new RPE cells during the submacular surgical procedure, perhaps the inevitable atrophy could be prevented, or at least minimized.

It is not difficult to imagine the inherent problems of RPE transplantation. Several questions quickly come to mind, including the following: Will transplanted RPE cells remain viable and if so, for how long? Where should these RPE cells be placed, intravitreal or subretinal? Will patients require lifelong immune suppression to prevent rejection? If RPE cells remain viable, will they function normally? Will they improve a patient's vision? Will they be more effective in atrophic ARMD patients than in exudative patients? For more than 25 years, researchers have been investigating these and the many other complex issues regarding RPE transplantation. Recent stories in the lay literature have caused an excitement among patients and therefore it is very important for physicians to be educated in order to counsel their patients effectively.

In 1975 researchers discovered that autotransplanted RPE cells underwent metaplasia after their injection into the vitreous cavity. The RPE cells first transformed into macrophages and then later into spindle-shaped cells with collagen production (23,24).

In 1989 physicians described a pars plana approach for transplantation of autologous RPE cells from a peripheral chorioretinal biopsy to prepared Bruch's membrane at the posterior pole of the same eye (25).

In 1991 Peyman reported his technique for RPE transplantation in two patients with extensive subfoveal scarring secondary to macular degeneration (26). His technique involved the preparation of a large retinal flap encompassing the macula and the arcades, removal of the submacular scar, and replacement of the RPE cells using either an autologous pedicle graft or homologous RPE cells and Bruch's membrane. One patient, who had undergone a pedicle graft, had an improvement of visual acuity from count fingers to 20/400 at 14 months. The other patient developed encapsulation of his homologous graft without any improvement in vision.

In 1992 scientists in Japan reported on the histology of transplanted RPE cells in New Zealand white rabbits (27). They found that by 1 week, the transplanted cells had formed a monolayer. By 3 weeks, grafted RPE cells had formed apical microvilli and tight junctions with adjacent cells. Their contact with Bruch's membrane appeared to be composed of basal infoldings that were well formed. Their findings demonstrated the functional appearance of the transplanted RPE cells. The same year, a group of researchers reported that RPE transplants stabilized retinal vasculature and prevented neovascularization in the Royal College of Surgeons (RCS) rat (28). Another study demonstrated that the transplantation of normal RPE cells reversed pathologic changes in the photoreceptors that had already occurred by the time of transplantation in the RCS rat (29).

In 1994 a Swedish group led by Algvere published their results on RPE transplantation in patients with exudative ARMD performed in Sweden with RPE harvested by investigators from Columbia University (30). Fetal RPE was placed beneath the neurosensory retina after the removal of submacular neovascularization in five patients with ARMD. The preoperative vision in all five patients was very poor. Surgical complications included cystoid macular edema and macular pucker. Microperimetry demonstrated that all five patients were able to fixate over the area of the RPE graft immediately after surgery, but an absolute scotoma developed in this region within several months. There is no evidence that the transplanted RPE cells survived in the subretinal space. It is noteworthy that these patients did not receive any immune suppression.

While progress was being made in transplantation techniques, the topic of rejection was also being studied. In 1997 Algvere's group published another study comparing the fate of fetal (13 to 20 weeks of gestational age) transplanted RPE cells in the subretinal space of five patients with fibrovascular membranes with those transplanted in four patients with atrophic ARMD (31). In patients with disciform lesions, all grafts were rejected over a 6-month period. In patients with nonexudative disease, however, three of four transplants showed little change in shape or size at 12 months. Visual acuity remained stable in these patients. The authors concluded that human RPE allografts are not invariably rejected in the subretinal space and that an intact blood/retinal barrier is likely to protect against rejection. More recent studies demonstrate a slow but significant effect of the systemic immune system in the subretinal space and therefore scientists are cautioning investigators against considering the subretinal space to be immunologically privileged (32).

The latest development in the field of RPE transplantation involves the cotransplantation of intact sheets of fetal retina with retinal pigment epithelium (33). Aramant and Seiler transplanted intact cografts into the subretinal space of RCS rats. After 6 to 7 weeks, transplanted photoreceptors, with the support of the cografted RPE cells, developed fully in organized parallel layers in the subretinal space. They concluded that such transplants have the potential to benefit retinal diseases with dysfunctional RPE and photoreceptors.

A tremendous amount of RPE transplantation research has been conducted and continues to be undertaken. Although this is an exciting area of research with tremendous potential benefits, we must remember that currently this remains an area of research, not treatment.

MACULAR TRANSLOCATION

Lindsey and Finklestein first reported macular translocation for the purpose of studying the relationship between the macula and the submacular RPE (34). The principal author developed the concept of macular translocation for the treatment of submacular CNV. Both retinal rotation and small flap translocation were developed and investigated in a Hanover pig model with the late Scott Langdon. It was determined that there was a high incidence of retinal detachment and PVR. This work was reported at the Bascom Palmer Eye Institute Annual Alumni meeting in 1987. The principal author stated at the meeting that this procedure should not be undertaken in humans because of retinal detachment and PVR risk. Machemer later reported performing this work in humans. Subsequently, deJuan, Tano, Toth, Lewis, Eckardt, and others began clinical studies. All this work confirmed the original concerns of the principal author concerning retinal detachment and PVR. In addition to retinal detachment and PVR, macular holes, new choroidal neovascular membranes at the BSS injection sites, hemorrhage, cycloversion, diploplia, phthisis, multiple reoperations, macular folds, and decreased or unchanged vision in spite of macular translocation were reported (35–38). The authors do not believe that this procedure is indicated because of the high incidence of complications.

deJuan developed a scleral resection method and later, an imbrication method called *limited macular translocation* (39). Complications associated with this method include retinal detachment, PVR, hemorrhage, macular hole, new CNV, phthisis, multiple reoperations, marked astigmatism, anisokoneia, diploplia, ptosis, enophthalmos, and failure to improve vision in spite of translocation. The authors do not believe that this method is indicated because of unacceptable complications. Hilel Lewis has developed an outpouching method using clips that may prove to be more effective than deJuan's technique of scleral imbrication.

NONSURGICAL TREATMENT OF SUBFOVEAL CHOROIDAL NEOVASCULAR MEMBRANES

Many medical and laser treatments have been advocated for subfoveal neovascular membranes. Most have been characterized by positive pilot studies ultimately followed by randomized clinical trials showing no efficacy. Examples of this sequence probably include alpha₁-interferon, thalidomide, brachytherapy, and radiation treatment. Angiostatic steroids and anti-VEGF agents have promise and are currently being investigated in well-constructed studies, although delivery system problems are significant.

Photocoagulation of juxtafoveal lesions has been shown to have a greater than 50% recurrence rate. Many patients present with subfoveal lesions; therefore laser treatment of these lesions was investigated in the MPS as well. It was shown that treated patients suffer an immediate loss of greater than three lines of vision but have slightly better vision after 18 months. Few physicians are comfortable with causing immediate loss of central vision, and only a small number treat in this manner.

Although a randomized trial of plasmapheresis has not been reported, there is no scientific rationale for this treatment, and it is unlikely that there is a beneficial effect. Unfortunately, many patients have been treated using this unproven, expensive treatment.

Peyman has advocated macular scleral buckling for AMD (40). The stated rationale is to displace some unknown toxic substances away from the macula. The authors are doubtful that this procedure will prove successful and are unaware of any reasonable rationale.

Acupuncture, magnetic treatment, and electrical treatment do not deserve comment. Criminals have preyed upon desperate patients for centuries and it is not surprising that high-tech fraud occurs where there is money to be made.

Laser treatment of drusen has been shown to cause faster disappearance of drusen than the spontaneous disappearance rate (41–43). The reader is reminded that drusen are "associated with" AMD; they do not "cause" AMD. Threshold treatment has been shown to result in higher CNV rates in two U.S. studies now investigating subthreshold treatment (44,45). Unfortunately, the Marta Figueroa data has shown no benefit with respect to choroidal neovascular event rates.

PHOTODYNAMIC THERAPY

Although the Macular Photocoagulation Study demonstrated the long-term benefits of laser photocoagulation for the treatment of subfoveal choroidal neovascularization (46), many ophthalmologists are reluctant to follow these guidelines. As doctors, practicing under the principle of "first do no harm," not to mention the litigious society we live in, it is difficult to intentionally worsen a patient's visual acuity in the hopes that 5 years later, the patient will be better off. Until recently, there has not been an alternative therapy for subfoveal lesions.

In October of 1999, the 1-year results of the Treatment of Age-Related Macular Degeneration with Photodynamic Therapy (TAP) Study Group were published (47). The multicenter, double-masked, placebo-controlled, randomized trial (TAP) investigated whether photodynamic therapy with verteporfin (Visudyne; Novartis Ophthalmics) could safely reduce the risk of vision loss in patients with subfoveal choroidal neovascularization caused by macular degeneration. Inclusion criteria included greatest linear dimension of lesion ≤5,400 μm, some "classic" component, best-corrected visual acuity of 20/40 to 20/200, and age ≥50. Lesions with retinal pigment epithelium tears (rips) were excluded. Verteporfin had been previously demonstrated to be an effective photosensitizer both *in vitro* and *in vivo* (48–52). Preclinical studies demonstrated that light-activated verteporfin could selectively occlude vessels of experimentally induced CNV in animal models with minimal effects on the surrounding and overlying retina and underlying choroid (53–55). Investigators believe that the mechanism of action is that the photosensitizer generates singlet oxygen and reactive oxygen intermediates that damage cellular components (56,57).

Visual acuity, contrast sensitivity, and fluorescein angiography outcomes were better in the verteporfin-treated eyes at every follow-up examination through the month 12 examination. Including all eyes that were followed, 61% assigned to the verteporfin group lost fewer that 15 letters of visual acuity (less than three lines of loss) compared with 46% in the placebo group. However, the subgroup analysis provided more conclusive results. When the area of classic CNV occupied 50% or more of the area of the entire lesion (predominantly classic), 67% versus 39% of patients in the placebo group lost less than 15 letters of vision. No statistical benefit in visual acuity was noted when the area of classic CNV was less than 50%. Hilel Lewis has reported that when the 100% classic subgroup of patients data are removed from the larger group with less than 100% classic, there is no longer a treatment benefit. The average patient required 3.4 treatments in the 1-year follow-up period due to the return of leakage on fluorescein angiography. Adverse ocular and systemic side effects were minimal, and included transient visual disturbances, injection site problems, transient photosensitivity reactions, and infusion-related low back pain.

Despite its high cost, limitation to predominantly classic lesions, and its apparently transient effect, photodynamic therapy is a welcome addition to the limited options available for the treatment of choroidal neovascularization in age-related macular degeneration. PDT should probably be thought of as a temporizing, stabilizing approach at this time. PDT may prove more efficacious in non-AMD subfoveal patients. PDT may be more effective when combined with one or more angiostatic agents.

TRANSPUPILLARY THERMOTHERAPY

Transpupillary thermotherapy (TTT) is a technique in which heat is delivered to the choroid and retinal pigment epithelium through the pupil using an IR diode laser to treat occult CNV. Occult CNV has been defined on an angiographic basis as either (a) fibrovascular retinal pigment epithelial detachment or (b) late-phase leakage of an undetermined source. Because the vast majority of patients with CNV present with occult lesions, the potential benefit of this treatment is enormous (58).

Since the 1860s, hyperthermia has been investigated as a potential anticancer treatment. The first use of transpupillary hyperthermia was reported in 1995 by Oosterhuis et al. (59) as an adjunct treatment of choroidal melanomas. More recently, Shields et al. (60,61) investigated the effectiveness of TTT alone on small choroidal melanomas. As opposed to cancer treatment, the goal of TTT is occlusion of neovascular vessels. Near-infrared irradiation is used as tissue penetration is high and absorption by ocular media is minimized.

In January of 1999, Reichel et al. (62) published a retrospective noncomparative case series of 16 eyes of 15 patients who presented with occult CNV. TTT was delivered using a modified infrared diode laser at 810 nm with an adjustable beam width of 1.2 mm, 2.0 mm, and 3.00 mm (Iris Medical Instruments, Mountain View, CA). Treatment began with one spot for 60 seconds such that no visible change or a barely detectable light-gray appearance was detected. Patients were seen 3 to 4 weeks later and treatment was repeated if there was no change in subretinal elevation on slit-lamp examination or when there was persistent leakage on late-phase fluorescein angiography.

Reichel reported that three eyes showed a two-or-more-line improvement in vision over a period of 6 to 25 months. Mean follow-up was 13 months. Visual acuity remained stable in nine eyes and the remaining four eyes showed a decline in visual acuity. They state there were no deleterious side effects, although others have noted development of significant reduced vision and the development of a pigmented scar.

A safe and effective treatment for occult CNV certainly would be a welcome addition to the field of ophthalmology; however, as the authors of the study point out, a randomized, prospective study would be necessary to evaluate the efficacy of this treatment modality.

DIETARY SUPPLEMENTATION

Oral antioxidants such as zinc, beta carotene, zeaxanthin, lutein, vitamin A, vitamin E, selenium, and others have been advocated for prevention of AMD, treatment of early stages of AMD, or atrophic (dry) AMD. The Age-Related Eye Study has provided an answer. Certain anti-oxidants combined with zinc have shown to have a 25% risk reduction rate. The Beaver Dam Eye Study looked at the dietary and smoking history of individuals with AMD compared with matched normals and concluded that spinach and, to a lesser extent, other dark leafy green vegetables slightly reduce the progression to AMD (63,64). Smoking was found to have a doubling effect on the incidence of AMD. The authors predict that some specific antioxidants may be proven to have minor value if given to individuals at genetic risk for AMD (drusen). It is likely that this effect will be greatest in patients who do not eat dark leafy green vegetables, other vegetables, whole grains, and fruit. Beta carotene has been shown to increase the risk of lung cancer in smokers in a Swedish study (65). At this time the authors counsel the children of patients with AMD, drusen patients, and patients with early AMD to stop smoking and eat spinach and other dark leafy green vegetables at least five times per week and to take anti-oxidants and zinc.

REFERENCES

1. Thomas MA, Kaplan HJ. Surgical removal of sub-foveal neovascularization in POHS. *AJO* 1991;111:1–7.
2. Steinhorst UH, Theischen M, Winter R. Subretinal lavage: a technique of continuous irrigation for removal of traumatic submacular hemorrhage. *Ophthalmologica* 1997;211:399–401.
3. Capone A. Submacular surgical procedures. *Int Ophthalmol Clin* 1995;35:83–93.
4. Ibanez HE, Williams DF, Thomas MA, et al. Surgical management of submacular hemorrhage, *Arch Ophthalmol* 1995;113:62–69.
5. Humayun M, Lewis H, Flynn HW Jr, et al. Management of submacular hemorrhage associated with retinal arterial macroaneurysms. *Am J Ophthalmol* 1998;126:358–361.
6. Claes C, Zivojnovic R. Efficacy of tissue plasminogen activator in subretinal hemorrhage removal. *Bull Soc Belge Ophthalmol* 1996;261:115–118.
7. Hawkins WR. Intraocular fibrinolysis of submacular hemorrhage with TPA and surgical drainage. *Am J Ophthalmol* 1994;118:559–568.
8. Lim JI, Drews-Botsch C, Sternberg P Jr, et al. Submacular hemorrhage removal. *Ophthalmology* 1995;102:1393–1399.
9. Chaudhry NA, Mieler WF, Han DP, et al. Preoperative use of tissue plasminogen activator for large submacular hemorrhage. *Ophthalmic Surg Lasers* 1999;30:176–180.
10. Johnson MW. Pneumatic displacement of submacular hemorrhage. *Curr Opin Ophthalmol* 2000;11:201–206.
11. Kamei M, Misono K, Lewis H. A study of the ability of TPA to diffuse into the subretinal space after intravitreal injections in rabbits. *Am J Ophthalmol* 1999;128:739–746.
12. McCabe CM, Flynn HW, McLean WC, et al. Nonsurgical management of macular hemorrhage secondary to retinal artery macroaneurysm. *Arch Ophthalmol* 2000;118:780–785.
13. Castellarin A, Nasir M, Sugino IK, et al. Decreased choriocapillaris perfusion following surgical excision of choroidal neovascular membranes in age-related macular degeneration. *Br J Ophthalmol* 1997;81:481–489.
14. Castellarin A, Nasir M, Sugino IK, et al. Progressive choriocapillaris atrophy after surgery for age-related macular degeneration. *Retina* 1998;18:143–149.
15. Akduman L, Del Priore LV, Desai VN, et al. Perfusion of the subfoveal choriocapillaris affects visual recovery after submacular surgery in the presumed ocular histoplasmosis syndrome. *Am J Ophthalmol* 1997;123:90–96.
16. Pollack JS, Del Priore LV, Smith ME, et al. Postoperative abnormalities of the choriocapillaris in exudative age-related macular degneration. *Br J Ophthalmol* 1996;80:314–318.
17. Korte GE, Reppucci V, Henkind P. RPE destruction causes choriocapillaris atrophy. *Invest Ophthal Vis Sci* 1984;25:1135–1145.
18. Kuwabara T, Ishikawa Y, Kaiser-Kupfer MI. Experimental model of gyrate atrophy in animals. *Ophthalmology* 1981;88:331–334.
19. Takeuchi M, Itagaki T, Takahashi K, et al. Changes in the intermediate stage of retinal degeneration after intravitreal injection of ornithine. Nippon Ganka Gakkai Zasshi. *Acta Soc Ophthalmol Jpn (Tokyo)* 1993;97:17–28.
20. Valentino A, Kaplan HJ, Del Priore LV, et al. Retinal pigment epithelium repopulation in monkeys after submacular surgery. *Arch Ophthalmol* 1995;113:932–938.
21. Del Priore LV, Kaplan HJ, Hornbeck R, et al. Retinal pigment epithelium debridement as a model for the pathogenesis and treatment of macular degeneration. *Am J Ophthalmol* 1996;122:629–643.

22. Del Priore LV, Hornbeck K, Kaplan HJ. Debridement of the pig retinal epithelium *in vivo. Arch Ophthalmol* 1995;113:939–944.
23. Mueller-Jensen K, Machemer R, Azarnia R. Autotransplantation of retinal pigment epithelium in intravitreal diffusion chamber. *Am J Ophthalmol* 1975;80:530–537.
24. Mueller-Jensen K, Mandelcorn MS. Membrane formation by autotransplanted retinal pigment epithelium. *Mod Probl Ophthalmol* 1975;15:228–234.
25. Lane C, Boulton M, Marshall J. Transplantation of retinal pigment epithelium using a pars plana approach. *Eye* 1989;3:27–32.
26. Peyman GA, Blinder KJ, Paris CL, et al. A technique for retinal pigment epithelium for age-related macular degeneration secondary to extensive subfoveal scarring. *Ophthalmic Surg* 1991;22:102–108.
27. Yamaguchi K, Yamaguchi K, Young RW, et al. Vitreoretinal surgical technique for transplanting retinal pigment epithelium in rabbit retina. *Jpn J Ophthalmol* 1992;36:142–150.
28. Seaton AD, Turner JE. RPE transplants stabilize retinal vasculature and prevent neovascularization in the RCS rat. *Invest Ophthalmol Vis Sci* 1992;33:83–91.
29. Lavail MM, Li L, Turner JE, et al. Retinal pigment epithelial cell transplantation in RCS rats: normal metabolism in rescued photoreceptors. *Exp Eye Res* 1992;55:555–562.
30. Algvere PV, Berglin L, Gouras P, et al. Transplantation of fetal retinal pigment epithelium in age-related macular degeneration with subfoveal neovascularization. *Graefes Arch Clin Exp Ophthalmol* 1994;232:707–716.
31. Algvere PV, Berglin L, Gouras P, et al. Transplantation of RPE in age-related macular degeneration: observations in disciform lesions and dry RPE atrophy. *Graefes Arch Clin Exp Ophthalmol* 1997;235:149–158.
32. Zhang X, Bok D. Transplantation of retinal pigment epithelial cells and immune response in the subretinal space. *Invest Ophthalmol Vis Sci* 1998;39:1021–1027.
33. Aramant RB, Seiler MJ, Ball SL. Successful cotransplantation of intact sheets of fetal retina with retinal pigment epithelium. *Invest Ophthalmol Vis Sci* 1999;40:1557–1564.
34. Bressler NM, Finklestein D, Sunness JS, et al. Retinal pigment epithelial tears through the fovea with preservation of good visual acuity. *Arch Ophthalmol* 1990;108:1694–1697.
35. Macular translocation. American Academy of Ophthalmology. *Ophthalmology* 2000;107:1015–1018.
36. Lewis H, Kaiser PK, Estafanous M. Macular translocation for subfoveal choroidal neovascularization in ARMD: a prospective study. *Am J Ophthalmol* 1999;128:135–146.
37. Ohji M, Fujikado T, Saito Y, et al. Foveal translocation: a comparison of two techniques. *Semin Ophthalmol* 1998;13:52–62.
38. Ninomiya Y, Lewis JM, Hasegawa T, et al. Retinotomy and foveal translocation for surgical management of subfoveal choroidal neovascular membranes. *Am J Ophthalmol* 1996;122:613–621.
39. de Juan E Jr, Vander JF. Effective macular translocation without scleral imbrication. *Am J Ophthalmol* 1999;128:380–382.
40. Peyman GA, Conway MD, Recasens MA, et al. Use of a macular buckle in the treatment of exudative age-related macular degeneration. *Ophthalmic Surg Lasers* 1999;30:619–630.
41. Figueroa MS, Regueras A, Bertrand J. Laser photocoagulation to treat macular soft drusin in ARMD. *Retina* 1994;14:391–396.
42. Wetzig PC. Photocoagulation of drusen-related macular degeneration: a long-term outcome. *Trans Am Ophthalmol Soc* 1994;92:299–303.
43. Olk RJ, Friberg TR, Stickney KL, et al. Therapeutic benefits of infrared (810 nm) diode laser macular grid photocoagulation in prophylactic treatment of nonexudative ARMD. *Ophthalmology* 1999;106:2082–2090.
44. The Choroidal Neovascularization Prevention Trial Research Group. Choroidal neovascularization in the Choroidal Neovascularization Prevention Trial. *Ophthalmology* 1998;105:1364–1372.
45. Choroidal Neovascularization Prevention Trial Research Group. Laser treatment in eyes with large drusen: short-term effects seen in a pilot randomized clinical trial. *Ophthalmology* 1998;105:11–23.
46. Macular Photocoagulation Study Group. Laser photocoagulation of subfoveal neovascular lesions in age-related macular degeneration: results of a randomized clinical trial. *Arch Ophthalmol* 1991;109:1220–1231.
47. Treatment of Age-Related Macular Degeneration with Photodynamic Therapy (TAP) Study Group. Photodynamic therapy of subfoveal choroidal neovascularization in age-related macular degeneration with verteporfin. *Arch Ophthalmol* 1999;117:1329–1345.
48. Schmidt-Erfurth U, Hasan T, Gragoudas E, et al. Vascular targeting in photodynamic occlusion of subretinal vessels. *Ophthalmology* 1994;101:1953–1961.
49. Allison BA, Waterfield E, Richter AM, et al. The effects of plasma lipoproteins on *in vitro* tumor cell killing and *in vivo* tumor photsensitization with benzoporphyrin derivative. *Photochem Photobiol* 1991;54:709–715.
50. Schmidt-Erfurth U, Hasan T, Schomacker K, et al. *In vivo* uptake of liposomal benzoporphyrin derivative and photothrombosis in experimental corneal neovascularization. *Lasers Surg Med* 1995;17:178–188.
51. Schmidt-Erfurth U, Bauman W, Gragoudas E, et al. Photodynamic therapy of experimental choroidal melanoma using lipoprotein-delivered benzoporphyrin. *Ophthalmology* 1994;101:89–99.
52. Young LH, Howard MA, IIu LK, et al. Photodynamic therapy of pigmented choroidal melanomas using a liposomal preparation of benzoporphyrin derivative. *Arch Ophthalmol* 1996;114:186–192.
53. Miller JW, Walsh AW, Kramer M, et al. Photodynamic therapy of experimental choroidal neovascularization using lipoprotein-delivered benzoporphyrin. *Arch Ophthalmol* 1995;113:810–818.
54. Kramer M, Miller JW, Michaud N, et al. Liposomal benzoporphyrin derivative verteporfin photodynamic therapy: selective treatment of choroidal neovascularization in monkeys. *Ophthalmology.* 1996;103:427–438.

55. Husain D, Miller JW, Michaud N, et al. Intravenous infusion of liposomal benzoporphyrin derivative for photo-dynamic therapy of experimental choroidal neovascularization. *Arch Ophthalmol* 1996;114:978–985.
56. Weishaupt KR, Gomer CJ, Dougherty TJ. Identification of singlet oxygen as the cytotoxic agent in photo-inactivation of murine tumor. *Cancer Res* 1976; 36:2326–2329.
57. Photodynamic effect of hematoporphyrin on blood microcirculation. *J Pathol Bacteriol* 1963; 86:99–102.
58. Freund KB, Yannuzzi LA, Sorenson JA. Age-related macular degeneration and choroidal neovascularization. *Am J Ophthalmol* 1993;115:786–791.
59. Oosterhuis JA, Journee-de Korver HG, Kakebeeke-Kemme HM, et al. Transpupillary therapy in choroidal melanomas. *Arch Ophthalmol* 1995;113:315–321.
60. Shields CL, Shields JA, DePotter P, et al. Transpupillary thermotherapy in the management of choroidal melanoma. *Ophthalmology* 1996;103:1642–1650.
61. Shields CL, Shields JA, Cater J, et al. Transpupillary thermotherapy for choroidal melanoma: tumor control and visual results in 100 consecutive cases. *Ophthalmology* 1998;105:581–590.
62. Reichel E, Berrocal AU, Michael IP, et al. Transpupillary thermotherapy of occult subfoveal choroidal neovas-cularization in patients with age-related macular degeneration. *Ophthalmology* 1999;106:1908–1914.
63. VandenLangenberg GM, Mares-Perlman JA, Klein R, et al. Association between antioxidant and zinc intake and the 5-year incidence of early age-related maculopathy in the Beaver Dam Eye Study. *Am J Epidemiol* 1998; 148:204–214.
64. Klein R, Klein BE, Moss SE. Relationship of smoking to the incidence of age-related maculopathy. The Beaver Dam Eye Study. *Am J Epidemiol* 1998;147:103–110.
65. De Luca LM, Ross SA. Beta-carotene increases lung cancer incidence in cigarette smokers. *Nutr Rev* 1996;54: 178–180.

13
Trauma

Vitreous surgery techniques have greatly improved the management of ocular trauma. Work-related activities, home maintenance, automobile and motorcycle accidents, fireworks, hunting, violence, and recreational activity create a continued threat of severe ocular injury. The vast range of objects and velocities implicated in ocular trauma leads to the wide spectrum of injuries seen (1,2). In this chapter the emphasis is on several stereotypic subgroups.

WOUND-RELATED CELLULAR MIGRATION/PROLIFERATION

Any interruption of tissue results in proliferation of the interrupted cell groups. Planar cell groups respond to loss of contact inhibition by a migration/proliferation of the cells adjacent to the interruption. Misalignment of the proliferating plane may result in reduplication of the original tissue layer. Migration/proliferation ceases when contact inhibition is restored by continuity of the new cell group, with similar cells representing the margin of defect. This new structure can be called a membrane; however, it is actually a reparative extension of previously normal tissues. The widely used term *fibrovascular ingrowth* implies that wound-related cellular proliferation originates from extraocular tissues. The severe proliferation that occurs in blunt trauma after choroidal rupture is clinically indistinguishable from fibrovascular ingrowth. There is little direct evidence of extraocular origin for most cases of wound-related cellular proliferation. Because the reparative mechanism stems from tissue disruption and destruction, the additional damage of retinopexy should be avoided in most instances.

SUBSTRATES FOR PROLIFERATION

Cellular proliferation occurs on preexisting support substrates such as the cornea, retina, vitreous, lens, and iris. The vitreous has been referred to as a "scaffold" (3,4), but this is a relative misnomer since a scaffold is not a structural element but a temporary support for workers. The word *substrate* can better describe the manner in which cellular migration and proliferation occur on the vitreous collagen matrix. More accurately, it is critical to recognize that proliferation usually occurs along the anterior and posterior vitreous cortex, although a foreign object can make a path through the vitreous along which apparent transvitreal proliferation can occur (8). As the retina is an ideal substrate for proliferation, it is not necessary to implicate the vitreous when periretinal cellular migration and proliferation occur.

TIMING OF VITRECTOMY

Immediate vitrectomy in penetrating ocular trauma cases should be avoided unless certain types of intraocular foreign bodies (IOFBs) are present. Arterial bleeding, choroidal swelling, leaking wounds, striate keratopathy, and lack of preparation add to the difficulty of immediate vitrectomy (5,6). More important, penetrating trauma frequently occurs in the young patient not having a posterior vitreous detachment (PVD). Without adequate vitreoretinal separation, iatrogenic retinal breaks, difficult surgery, and postoperative contraction of residual vitreous can ensue (5,6).

Typically, the hemorrhage and inflammation that accompany trauma induce a PVD in 7 to 14 days, allowing safer, more effective vitreous surgery. Cellular proliferation starts at 10 to 14 days, making this the ideal time to intervene (3,5,7,9). If the retina can be seen, these cases can be watched at weekly intervals and vitrectomy can be avoided if cellular proliferation does not occur. Cases with opaque media require vitrectomy at this 10- to 14-day point because further delay could lead to cellular proliferation, which is initially invisible by ultrasound. Decreased vitreous mobility observed on ultrasound examination indicates hypocellular collagen contraction and/or early cellular proliferation.

INTRAOCULAR FOREIGN BODIES

Vitreous surgery allows excellent visualization, prevention of postoperative transvitreal proliferation, and removal of blood, lens materials, and organisms if present. Bronson or giant magnet foreign-body removal has virtually disappeared in the last decade because of the widespread availability of vitreous surgery training, technology, techniques, and diamond-coated forceps (Fig. 13.1). Intraocular magnets can be used to pick up foreign bodies for transfer to diamond-coated forceps and removal (10–16).

Inert Versus Toxic Foreign Bodies

Most iron- and copper-containing foreign bodies should be removed immediately (17,18). Stainless steel, aluminum, and lead foreign bodies are much less toxic and can be tolerated in selected cases. Indication for removal of these less toxic materials must be individualized on a clinical basis. Occasionally, iron- and copper-containing foreign bodies will be overlooked and only discovered after they have become encapsulated. If no

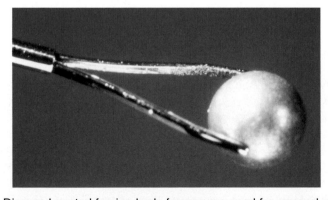

FIG. 13.1. Diamond-coated foreign-body forceps are used for removal of all IOFBs.

evidence of toxicity is seen in these cases, frequent follow-up should be undertaken rather than surgery. Clinical examination of adjacent structures (cornea, iris, and lens) is probably a better indication of toxicity than electroretinography. Plastic materials can be left in place in selected cases. Submacular and intraoptic nerve foreign bodies should be managed on an individual basis because of the hazards of removal. Any exogenous biologic material such as vegetable matter should be removed immediately because of the risk of infection and inflammation. Endogenous cilia and bone fragments are usually well tolerated and need not be removed unless vitrectomy is performed for other reasons or they appear to be the cause of inflammation.

Timing of Surgery

All large, toxic, biologic, or sharp IOFBs should be removed as soon as the patient can be taken to the operating room. This approach decreases secondary mechanical trauma, rapid toxicity, and endophthalmitis. Plastic, glass, and lead shotgun pellets can be observed until vitrectomy is indicated for other reasons. Although late-night vitreous surgery creates logistical and cost problems, it decreases the risk of endophthalmitis and toxic damage and should be undertaken if indicated.

Surgical Sequence and Techniques

Wound Repair

Any visible corneal or scleral wound should be sutured before proceeding with the vitrectomy. Running shoelace monofilament nylon sutures distribute stress evenly, are elastic and well tolerated, and may be rapidly placed. Silk sutures are inelastic and lead to wound leaks during the vitrectomy, whereas absorbable sutures are inelastic and not permanent. Interrupted sutures can cause striate keratopathy and take longer to place. Small sutures (10-0) are used for central cornea, 9-0 for midcornea, and 8-0 for peripheral cornea or sclera.

Surgical judgment should guide the decision-making process concerning excision of prolapsed tissue. Viable-appearing iris or ciliary body in a very recent injury can be irrigated and repositioned. Any sign of infection or necrosis indicates excision. Retinopexy should not be used anterior to the muscle ring (ora serrata) and should be applied only to definite retinal breaks located posteriorly. Excessive and unnecessary retinopexy leads to greater wound-related cellular proliferation and inflammation. Endolaser retinopexy should be applied only to specific breaks identified during vitrectomy.

A posterior wound should be explored only if pressure on the globe can be completely avoided. The vitreous and retina can be prolapsed from a posterior wound by surgical manipulation. If vitrectomy is completed first, the location of the wound will be known, and the eye can be softened and filled with air/gas before proceeding with posterior wound repair in the rare instance that it is thought necessary. Most posterior wounds are self-sealing and wound closure does not decrease the incidence of wound-related cellular proliferation. Retinopexy increases the incidence of wound-related cellular proliferation and should be avoided.

Conjunctival Incisions

A 1-mm-wide, limbus-based, 360° flap is required for scleral buckling and some posterior wound explorations. A temporal 60°, 1- to 2-mm-wide limbus-based flap for the active instruments and infusion cannula can be combined with a 30° superonasal incision for the endoilluminator if scleral buckling is not anticipated.

Sclerotomies

The incision for the vitrectomy instrument, infusion cannula, and endoilluminator should be made in the usual position, 3 mm posterior to the limbus if the lens is to be removed or 4 mm posterior to the limbus if not. Extra care must be taken to avoid choroidal infusion in trauma cases because hypotony and choroidal edema are frequently present.

The incision for the foreign-body removal should usually be the superotemporal vitrectomy instrument incision, enlarged after the vitreous is removed using a diamond or disposable knife.

Lens Removal

If the lens is clear, it should be allowed to remain unless a very large foreign body requires translimbal removal. Many small, localized traumatic cataracts do not progress and therefore may not require removal. The vitrectomy instrument should be used for anterior vitrectomy if any vitreous is in the anterior chamber or capsular bag. The fragmenter is faster than vitrectomy instruments for lensectomy but should never be applied to the vitreous. If vitreous enters the capsular bag, it should be removed with a vitrectomy instrument and the lensectomy should be completed with the fragmenter. In most cases the capsule should be removed with the diamond-coated forceps.

Vitrectomy

The vitreous may be clear or have significant hemorrhage in acute IOFB cases, but in either instance it must be completely removed. The first goal is to remove enough vitreous to remove all vitreous attachments to the foreign body. Although it is tempting to remove the foreign body as soon as it is seen, it is far better to complete the vitrectomy first. A big advantage of the vitrectomy approach is the avoidance of removal-induced vitreous traction. The need for a relatively complete vitrectomy before foreign-body removal is absolute.

Foreign-Body Removal

It is not recommended that an extraocular magnet be used in conjunction with vitrectomy; the advantage of a slow, controlled removal without vitreous traction would be lost. Some surgeons have recommended intraocular magnets, but the authors have not used these devices because of the availability of the diamond-coated forceps. When all the vitreous around the IOFB has been removed, the superotemporal incision is enlarged to accommodate the largest outside diameter of the diamond IOFB forceps.

Moderately Sized Foreign Bodies

After the foreign body is grasped in the forceps and brought to the anterior vitreous area, its size can be better assessed. If the foreign body will not fit safely through the wound but is not larger than 6 mm in its smallest diameter, the scleral wound should be enlarged with a knife (Fig. 13.2). It is best to plug the other sclerotomy so that the sur-

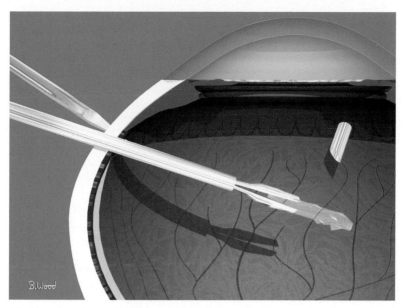

FIG. 13.2. Use free hand to enlarge wound to allow removal of foreign body <6 mm in diameter.

geon's hand is free to enlarge the wound. A knife at the opposite end of the circumferential sclerotomy from the shank of the forceps should be used to extend the sclerotomy while stabilizing the other end of the wound with the shank of the forceps. Using this approach, it is not necessary to release the grasp of the foreign body and a large, leaky incision need not be present while searching for and picking up the IOFB.

Cylindrical Foreign Bodies

Long, cylindrical, small-diameter foreign bodies such as wire frequently lie tangential to the retinal surface. The initial pick-up of the foreign body will then result in the IOFB being perpendicular to the shank of the forceps. If it were removed with this orientation, the scleral opening would have to be unnecessarily large. It is therefore best to use a second 20-gauge diamond-tipped forceps to bimanually transfer or regrasp the foreign body to permit removal along the long axis of the IOFB (Fig. 13.3).

Large Foreign Bodies

If the foreign body is brought to the anterior vitreous and appears too large to be removed through the pars plana, translimbal removal should be performed (Fig. 13.4).The grasp on the foreign body need not be lost, as the lens is removed with the fragmenter in the surgeon's other hand. A cataract-type limbal section is then initiated with a blade, again in the surgeon's other hand. The infusion system prevents hypotony during the initial incision but will cause iris prolapse as the wound is enlarged with the scissors. If the pupil is large and iridectomy is not required, the infusion should be turned off to avoid iris prolapse. If an iridectomy is required, the infusion-induced iris prolapse can be used to the surgeon's advantage, permitting ab-externo iridectomy with

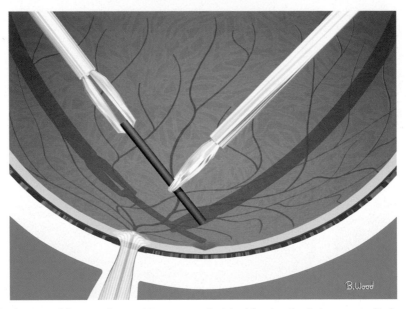

FIG. 13.3. A second forceps is used to grasp cylindrical foreign body to remove it along its long axis.

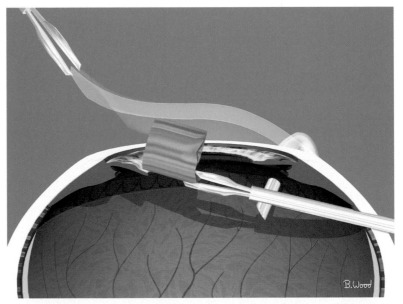

FIG. 13.4. Large foreign bodies should be removed through a limbal incision, without re-grasping in the anterior chamber.

one hand. When the wound is completed, the IOFB should be passed retrograde through the wound without attempting to regrasp the foreign body in the anterior chamber. The wound should then be closed with a running shoelace, 8-0 nylon suture.

Encapsulated Foreign Bodies

The fibrous capsule must be incised to safely remove an encapsulated IOFB (Fig. 13.5). The vitrectomy should be completed first and all vitreous traction to the foreign body site should be severed. The capsular incision should be performed with 20-gauge scissors (Fig. 13.6). A cruciate incision will allow the IOFB to be completely free before the IOFB forceps are used to remove the fragment (Figs. 13.7 and 13.8). Standard removal techniques as described earlier are used, depending on the size of the foreign body. Subretinal IOFBs are removed with diamond-coated forceps (Fig. 13.9).

After the IOFB has been removed, the wound should be closed with a running shoelace 8-0 nylon suture, leaving a 20-gauge size opening around a scleral plug.

The vitrectomy should then be completed, removing any fibrin, capsular material, or hemosiderin left from the removal process. In acute cases in young people, it may not be possible to remove a portion of the posterior vitreous cortex (PVC) on the macula and optic nerve; however, all connections between these areas and to the peripheral retina must be severed. Theoretically, it would be beneficial to remove the entire PVC, but this is impossible in many young people without damaging the optic nerve or retina. Any subsequent cellular proliferation along these remaining portions of PVC can be managed, if necessary, at a later date.

Subretinal surgery is occasionally required, but most of these membranes are highly vascular and should be left in place.

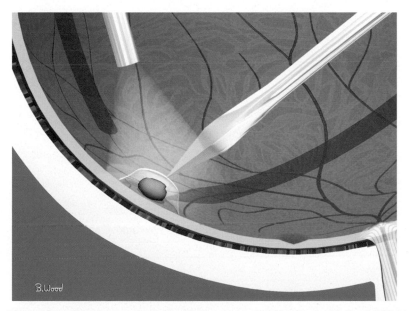

FIG. 13.5. After vitreous removal, the fibrous capsule is incised with the MVR blade.

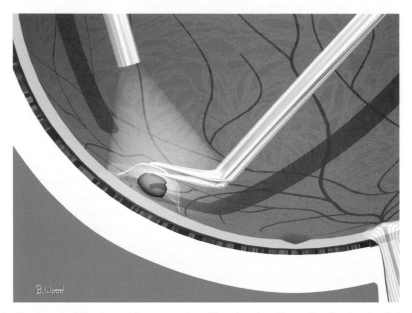

FIG. 13.6. Removal of the top of the capsule with scissors allows the foreign body to be freed before removal.

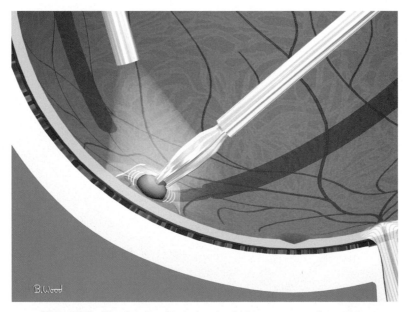

FIG. 13.7. The foreign body is wiggled to remove all traction.

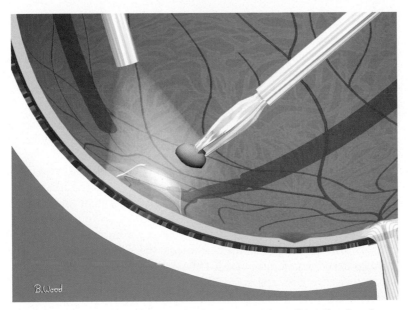

FIG. 13.8. The foreign body is removed with the forceps after all traction has been removed.

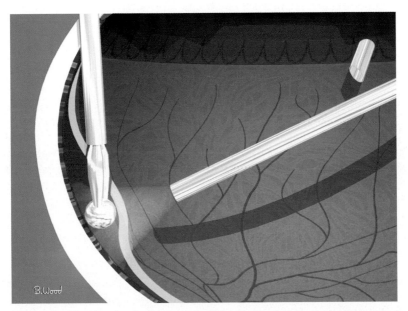

FIG. 13.9. Subretinal foreign bodies are removed with the foreign-body forceps via a retinal break.

Retinopexy

Laser retinopexy should only be performed if a definite retinal break is seen, not for prophylaxis along trauma contact and wound sites. If the break is located contiguous with the optic nerve, papillomacular bundle, or macula, it is not treated, since breaks in these areas almost never result in detachment, and retinopexy in these areas can decrease central vision.

Surface Tension Management

Internal fluid/air exchange and subsequent air/gas exchange should be used if a definite retinal break is present. Internal drainage of subretinal fluid (SRF) should follow internal fluid/air exchange if detachment exists. Post reattachment endolaser retinopexy can then be used to treat the break(s).

Although perfluorocarbon (PFC) liquids have been recommended for IOFB removal and management of coexisting retinal detachment, the principal author has not found these agents to be necessary in most cases. The concept is to float up the IOFB and SRF, but PFC liquids increase cost and are difficult to remove completely. PFC liquids are needed if a giant break is present.

Air/gas exchange with C_3F_8 after post reattachment endolaser retinopexy should be used for small to moderate retinal defects.

Large retinal defects or especially severe trauma should be managed by air/silicone exchange without retinopexy. The purpose of postoperative surface tension management is to prevent aqueous humor from passing through nonvisible retinal defects, new traction-induced breaks, and defects that are intentionally untreated. Retinopexy avoidance is an excellent approach for the prevention of PVR.

Scleral Buckling

Segmental buckling can be used for peripheral breaks but is unnecessary for posterior breaks. Circumferential segmental explants are preferable to radial buckles in all instances. The authors no longer utilize prophylactic encircling bands. Vitreous traction from initial IOFB impact, egress of the foreign body, or vitreous removal creates a relatively high incidence of dialyses and aphakic-like retinal breaks. These can be difficult to recognize at the time of surgery, thus emphasizing the need for a careful search and air/silicone exchange in difficult cases. Late traction from vitreous incarceration in the sclerotomies plays a role in postoperative detachment as well.

Antibiotic/Steroid Therapy

Subconjunctival antibiotic therapy against both Gram-positive and Gram-negative organisms should be utilized. Subconjunctival repository steroids such as triamcinolone should be used to decrease postoperative fibrin formation and scarring.

DOUBLE PENETRATING INJURY

High-velocity objects from shotgun and explosive injuries typically enter the eye anteriorly and exit posteriorly, creating two ocular wounds. Low-velocity injuries such as hammering metal on metal typically cause IOFBs (5,17–25).

Initial Repair

Any corneal or anterior scleral wound should be closed as soon as the patient is seen, and any visible wound should be closed before attempting further exploration. Great care must be taken to avoid tissue prolapse from surgical manipulation. Running shoelace monofilament nylon sutures should be utilized as described earlier. Posterior exploration should be accomplished only to the extent that it can be done without exerting any pressure on the globe.

Timing of Vitrectomy

Vitrectomy should be performed between 7 and 14 days unless angle closure from lens swelling or endophthalmitis is an issue. Ultrasonic evidence of retinal detachment does not necessarily indicate early vitrectomy. Delay for 7 to 14 days permits PVD to occur, decreases choroidal swelling, decreases bleeding, and provides better corneal clarity.

Surgical Sequence and Techniques

Lens Removal

Clear lenses or small, localized cataracts should be allowed to remain. Any central, posterior subcapsular opacity warrants lensectomy because this will almost invariably progress after vitrectomy. Wounds at the ciliary body/pars plana level permit wound-related cellular proliferation to proceed along the anterior vitreous cortex/lens interface, creating a cyclitic membrane. Although prophylactic lens removal is not indicated, these cases must be watched weekly postoperatively for any evidence of cyclitic membrane growth. The aspirating fragmenter technique should be utilized again, with care taken to avoid vitreous in the fragmenter. The vitrectomy instrument should be used to remove any vitreous in the anterior chamber or capsular bag as well as for capsular removal. Iris surgery should be performed only if absolutely necessary to see posteriorly; overzealous removal creates postoperative inflammation and glare.

Vitrectomy

The AVC should be removed to decrease the chance of cyclitic membrane formation unless the trauma is very posterior and the anterior retina and vitreous are normal. An opening should then be made through the PVC nasally or in any area known to have attached retina. Vacuum cleaning/extrusion may be necessary through this initial opening to remove free blood products in the sub-PVD space. When an adequate view of the retina is obtained, vitrectomy can proceed by enlarging this opening in a circumferential fashion. If retinal detachment is present, extremely low suction force should be used. If a retinal break is seen, vitrectomy should be continued with intermittent drainage of SRF. Layer-by-layer removal of the vitreous increases the chance of retinal breaks and is more time-consuming than the full-thickness, circumferential method described earlier.

All vitreous attached to the exit wound should be removed if it can be accessed without further damage to the retina. The vitreous applied to the surface of the wound should be allowed to remain because its removal can create bleeding, retinal breaks, wound leaks, and enhancement of cellular proliferation (Fig. 13.10). At the 14-day point, it is extremely unusual for an exit wound to leak. As in vitrectomy for diabetes, the goal of cone truncation is to eliminate the anteroposterior traction, which is the critical element in successful management of these cases.

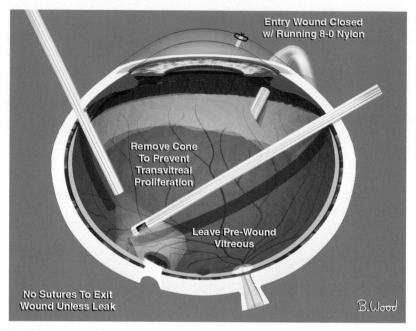

FIG. 13.10. Cone truncation removes anteroposterior traction and prevents transvitreal proliferation.

Surface Tension Management

Fluid/air exchange is utilized as in other clinical situations when a retinal break is present. Internal drainage of SRF followed by fluid/air exchange and completion of SRF drainage should be performed if detachment is present. Air can also be utilized to confine bleeding and to help seal leaky wounds by a surface tension effect. The use of PFC liquids, gas, and silicone was described earlier.

Retinopexy

Laser endophotocoagulation is used only if retinal breaks are apparent. Most posterior exit wounds do not give rise to retinal detachment, and retinopexy serves only to increase wound-related cellular proliferation.

Scleral Buckling

The authors no longer use prophylactic encircling bands. This change was made because buckles increase operating time, postoperative pain, refractive error, strabismus, and cost, and may intrude into the sclera.

CORNEAL/SCLERAL LACERATION

The great variability of corneal/scleral lacerations makes generalization difficult, but certain principles merit discussion. Microsurgery has advanced the success rate in these cases, as has vitrectomy technology.

Wound Repair

As discussed previously, running monofilament sutures are best for closing corneal/scleral lacerations. Running sutures distribute stress evenly, stimulate less vascularization, leak less, and are placed rapidly. All knots should be buried if interrupted sutures are used.

The scleral portion should be closed by sequential suturing, exploration, and further suturing. Unless extremely large pieces of sclera are absent, primary closure is preferable to scleral grafting. As these cases frequently develop wound-related cellular proliferation, scleral resection-like shortening that occurs from primary closure of a defect can be beneficial.

Timing of Lens Removal

Many factors relate to the question of whether lens removal should occur at the time of primary surgical repair or later. Hypotony-induced choroidal edema, striate keratopathy, and miosis make safe lens removal difficult at the time of initial wound repair. Arterial bleeding is also common, as is surgical-induced corneal stromal swelling. Delayed lensectomy can be easier because the lens imbibes water, sliding endothelial cells have closed the cornea, the pupil may dilate better, and arterial bleeding has ceased. If ideal circumstances permit lensectomy at the time of primary repair, this, of course, would avoid two trips to the operating room.

Role of Posterior Vitrectomy

Lacerations anterior to the ora serrata (muscle ring) do not create a need for posterior vitrectomy in the early stages. These cases must be observed very frequently for evidence of vitreous "orientation" and loss of vitreous mobility. Taut vitreous with stress lines directed toward a wound is associated with a high incidence of retinal detachment. If this condition coexists with opaque media, frequent ultrasound examinations, including the periphery, are necessary to rule out retinal detachment. In virtually all instances of taut vitreous with hypocellular vitreous contraction, vitrectomy will be necessary. If the vitreous is clear, the retina must be observed frequently for signs of detachment and/or cellular proliferation. True vitreous "organization" is a late sign and should not be permitted to occur.

COMPLICATIONS

Infection

Immediate surgical repair with subconjunctival antibiotic prophylaxis and removal of all necrotic exteriorized tissue leads to a surprisingly low incidence of endophthalmitis. If suspected endophthalmitis does occur, it should be managed as described elsewhere in this book.

Corneal Opacification

Corneal bloodstaining and large central opacities contraindicate the conventional approach to vitrectomy because of the visibility requirements. If ultrasound reveals retinal detachment, a special keratoprosthesis (26) could be utilized to permit vitrectomy. This device allows visualization without a fundus contact lens and permits replacement with the original bloodstained cornea or a donor button if permanent opacity is suspected. The principal author prefers, however, to trephine the cornea, perform the entire procedure "open-sky" (Fig. 13.11); that is, lens (remnant) removal, vitrectomy, IOFB removal, epi- and sub-

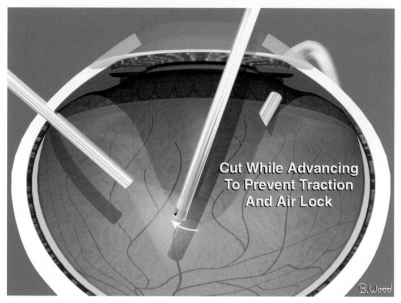

FIG. 13.11. Open-sky vitrectomy is preferred over the temporary epikerato-prosthesis if corneal opacity prevents retinal visualization.

retinal dissection, instillation of silicone oil through the corneal opening, and suturing of the donor button. This approach is faster than use of the temporary epikerato-prosthesis. It allows removal of very large IOFBs, gentle dissection of epiciliary tissue, bimanual surgery, subretinal dissection, aspiration of all intraocular fluid, and easy instillation of silicone. Although endolaser can easily be used open sky, many of these cases are candidates for retinopexy avoidance using medium- to long-term silicone.

Glaucoma

Erythroclastic (hemolytic) glaucoma can be managed effectively by vitrectomy (27) if medical management fails. *Phakogenic glaucoma* is a general term that includes phakolytic and lens-induced pupillary block. If unresponsive to medical treatment, these forms of glaucoma can be managed effectively by vitrectomy as well. Other forms of traumatic glaucoma are well beyond the scope of this book.

REFERENCES

1. Goldblum D, Frueh BE, Koerner F, et al. Eye injuries caused by cow horns. Retina, 1999;19:314–317.
2. Hamanaka N, Ikeda T, Inokuchi N, et al. A case of intraocular foreign body due to graphite pencil complicated by endophthalmitis. *Ophthalmic Surg Lasers* 1999;30:229–231.
3. Cleary PE, Minckler DS, Ryan SJ. Ultrastructure of traction retinal detachment in rhesus monkey eyes after a posterior penetration ocular injury. *Am J Ophthalmol* 1980;90:829.
4. Cleary PE, Ryan SJ. Experimental posterior penetrating eye injury in the rabbit 11. Histology of wound, vitreous, and retina. *Br J Ophthalmol* 1979;63:312.
5. Ryan SJ, Allen AW. Pars plana vitrectomy in ocular trauma. *Am J Ophthalmol* 1979;88:483.
6. Ryan SJ. Results of pars plana vitrectomy in penetrating ocular trauma. *Int Ophthalmol* 1978;1:5.
7. Ryan SJ. Guidelines in the management of penetrating ocular trauma with emphasis on the role and timing of pars plana vitrectomy. *Int Ophthalmol* 1979;1:105.
8. Cleary PE, Ryan SJ. Vitrectomy in penetrating eye injury: results of a controlled trial of vitrectomy in an experimental posterior penetrating eye injury in the rhesus monkey. *Arch Ophthalmol* 1981;99:287.

9. deJuan E, Sternberg P, Michels RG, et al. Timing of vitrectomy after penetrating ocular injuries. *Ophthalmology* 1984;91:1072.
10. Chiquet C. Intraocular foreign bodies: factors influencing final visual outcome. *Acta Ophthalmol Scand* 1999; 77:321–325.
11. Coday MP. Nailing down the diagnosis: imaging intraocular foreign bodies. *Arch Ophthalmol* 1999;117:548.
12. De Souza S, Howcroft MJ. Management of posterior segment intraocular foreign bodies. *Can J Ophthalmol* 1999;34:23–29.
13. Chiquet C, Zech JC, Gain P, et al. Visual outcome and prognostic factors after magnetic extraction of posterior segment foreign bodies in 40 cases. *Br J Ophthalmol* 1998;82:801–806.
14. Kozielec GF, To K, et al. Penetrating eye injury from a metal wedge. *Ophthalmic Surg Lasers* 1999;30:59–60.
15. Azad R, Sharma YR, Mitra S, et al. Triple procedure in posterior segment intraocular foreign body. *Indian J Ophthalmol* 1998;46:91–92..
16. Pavlovic S, Schmidt KG, Tomic Z, et al. Management of intra-ocular foreign bodies impacting or embedded in the retina. *Aust N Z J Ophthalmol* 1998;26:241–246.
17. Michels RG. Surgical management of non-magnetic intraocular foreign bodies. *Arch Ophthalmol* 1975;93:1003.
18. Michels RG. Closed vitrectomy in trauma: selected intraocular foreign bodies. In: Freeman HM, ed. *Vitreous surgery and advances in fundus diagnosis and treatment.* New York: Appleton-Century-Crofts, 1977:335–344.
19. Hutton WL, Snyder WR, Vaiser A. Vitrectomy in the treatment of ocular perforating injuries. *Am J Ophthalmol* 1976;81:733–739.
20. Mandelcorn MS. Results after vitrectomy for trauma. *Can J Ophthalmol* 1977;12:34.
21. Benson WE, Machemer R. Severe perforating injuries treated with pars plana vitrectomy. *Am J Ophthalmol* 1976;81:728.
22. Michels RG. Early surgical management of penetrating ocular injuries involving the posterior segment. *South Med J* 1976;69:1175.
23. Conway BP, Michels RG. Vitrectomy techniques in the management of selected penetrating ocular injuries. *Ophthalmology* 1978;85:560.
24. Michels RG, Conway BP. Vitreous surgery techniques in penetrating ocular trauma. *Trans Ophthalmol Soc UK* 1978;98:472.
25. Abrams GW, Topping TM, Machemer R. The effect of vitrectomy on intraocular proliferation following perforating injuries in rabbit eyes. *Arch Ophthalmol* 1978;96:521.
26. Landers MB, Foulks G, Landers DM, et al. Temporary keratoprosthesis for pars plana vitrectomy. *Am J Ophthalmol* 1981;91:615.
27. Brucker AJ, Michels RG, Green WR. Pars plana vitrectomy in the management of blood-induced glaucoma with vitreous hemorrhage. *Ann Ophthalmol* 1978;10:1427.

14
Endophthalmitis

A broad definition of endophthalmitis includes any severe intraocular inflammation. Toxic substances, necrotic tumors, noninfectious uveitis, and infarction can create the clinical picture of vitritis, hypopyon, and ocular pain.

Infectious endophthalmitis can be of bacterial, fungal, or parasitic etiology. Vitreous surgery reduces the number of organisms, reduces inflammatory components, enhances the penetration and diffusion of antibiotics, and aids in identification of the pathogen. Late complications related to cellular proliferation on the vitreous matrix are reduced as well.

Early diagnosis and treatment is of paramount importance when managing a patient with endophthalmitis. It is strongly recommended that all ocular surgery postoperative patients be examined on the first postoperative morning as well as immediately if the patient complains of pain or decreased vision. If the operating surgeon cannot personally examine the patient, immediate and definite arrangements should be made with another qualified physician. The welfare of the patient is always the surgeon's responsibility. Once endophthalmitis is suspected, one should examine the patient often and take definitive action when indicated. While the more common signs of endophthalmitis are well known by physicians, one should also be cognizant of less frequent signs. These include chemosis, lid edema, membrane formation on the intraocular lens (IOL), and retinal hemorrhages.

ETIOLOGIC SUBGROUPS

Endogenous Endophthalmitis

Endogenous endophthalmitis accounts for a minority of cases (1). Predisposing conditions include immune deficiency, immune suppression, diabetes mellitus, chronic renal failure, IV drug abuse, and patients receiving hyperalimentation. These patients can develop endophthalmitis without prior ocular disease. Such cases may be bilateral, increasing both the impact on the patient and the management difficulties. Systemic workup and therapy play an extensive role in the management of these patients and require infectious disease consultation. Metastatic infection accounts for approximately 8% of endogenous bacterial endophthalmitis. At times, vitrectomy is indicated in this patient group but is quite difficult because of the associated anesthesia risk and the potential bilaterality of the disease.

Exogenous Endophthalmitis

Ocular trauma (2,3) accounts for approximately 20% of bacterial endophthalmitis (4,5). Ocular surgery (6–8) accounts for the vast majority (approximately 70%), as it facilitates the introduction of organisms into the eye. Management of trauma cases usually requires vitreous surgery and may involve removal of intraocular foreign bodies. Although conventional surgical wisdom suggests removal of any implanted materials if infection occurs, this logic does not apply to the IOL. Removal of an IOL, especially in an endophthalmitis case, has an extremely high risk of iris avulsion, endothelial trauma, intraocular bleeding, choroidal expulsive hemorrhage, and retinal detachment. Vitrectomy with intraocular antibiotics without implant removal can be successful in a high percentage of cases. This is probably because the smooth surface of the lens implant coupled with the high fluid throughput of vitrectomy removes all organisms on the lens surface.

Fortunately, the incidence of acute postoperative endophthalmitis remains relatively low. Extracapsular cataract surgery with or without an IOL insertion carries an incidence of 0.072%. Vitrectomy (0.051%) and penetrating keratoplasty (0.11%) involve a much smaller risk than insertion of a secondary IOL (0.30%). The most frequent organisms include coagulase-negative staphylococcus, *Staphylococcus aureus, Streptococcus* species, and Gram-negative bacteria.

Delayed-onset postcataract surgery endophthalmitis is most often caused by *Propionibacterium* acnes, coagulase-negative staphylococcus, or candida. In the setting of *Propionibacterium* acne endophthalmitis, inflammatory plaque and associated capsule must be removed at a minimum; in most instances the intraocular lens must be removed as well (9).

The incidence of trauma-related endophthalmitis varies with or without the presence of a retained foreign body. Following a penetrating injury, the incidence of endophthalmitis ranges from 3.2% to 7.4%. With a retained foreign body, the incidence jumps to between 6.9% and 7.3% (metallic – 7.2%, nonmetallic – 7.3%, organic – 6.3%). The most frequent organisms include *Bacillus* species, *Staphylococcus* species, and *Streptococcus* species.

Organisms of the *Streptococcus*, coagulase-negative *Staphylococcus*, and *Hemophilus* species are the most common in filtering bleb-related cases. Immediate vitrectomy intervention is mandatory in these often rapidly deteriorating cases.

ANTERIOR CHAMBER VERSUS VITREOUS ASPIRATION

Vitreous taps have a much higher incidence of positive cultures than anterior chamber taps (10). Both types of taps risk pain, wound disruption, intraocular hemorrhage, retinal detachment, and delayed therapy. Because of these problems, many clinicians recommend performing the tap in the operating room. Vitreous samples obtained at the time of therapeutic vitrectomy probably have higher yields and are safer than vitreous taps. The authors do not use taps to manage most cases. Busy office and operating room schedules and the concern about contamination of other cases can lead to a delay between suspected diagnosis and the performance of the tap. The rapid progression of this disease does not warrant any delay in the onset of therapy. Taps should only be done if they are accomplished immediately and with the intent of not performing vitreous surgery at that time. Suspicion of the operating room environment, IOL, or surgical materials as an etiologic agent demands an epidemiologic approach to the work-up. In general, the goal should be to initiate treatment immediately.

TIMING OF VITRECTOMY

Vitreous surgery is not required for every case of infectious endophthalmitis. Patients with acute postoperative endophthalmitis and vision of hand motion or better may be treated with tap and injection of intravitreal antibiotics alone, as shown by the Endophthalmitis Vitrectomy Study (EVS) study (11). If the vision is worse than hand motion, vitreous surgery should be undertaken immediately, regardless of the hour of the day or night.

Advanced cases with corneal decompensation cannot have vitreous surgery under safe conditions because of the visualization requirements. Open-sky vitrectomy would be fraught with complications and is not recommended. Immediate intracameral antibiotics offer the best hope in this poor-prognosis group and in patients with medical problems preventing surgical intervention.

EVS findings, do not apply to endophthalmitis, which are endogenous, delayed postoperative, traumatic, or filtering bleb-related cases.

SURGICAL SEQUENCE AND TECHNIQUES

The operating room should be alerted to prepare for a dirty case with all appropriate isolation and postsurgical cleanup precautions. This should not be used as an excuse for delay of therapy, however. At times, it is best to operate in a nonophthalmic operating room with only the minimal equipment required for the case.

General anesthesia is vastly superior to local anesthesia in these cases because the inflamed orbit makes retrobulbar block hazardous and ineffective. Intravenous antibiotics should be started at this time if a presurgical medical treatment plan has not been utilized.

If a cataract wound, surgical wound, or ruptured filtering bleb is present, it must be closed before initiation of vitreous surgery. Absorbable sutures should be oversewn or replaced with 8-0 or 9-0 monofilament nylon sutures. Careful attention to a tight wound before vitrectomy can decrease subsequent problems.

Trans–Pars Plana Versus Translimbal Approach

Because many endophthalmitis cases can and should be handled by predominantly anterior-segment surgeons, the limbal approach is possible. Unfortunately, this approach prevents adequate visualization for posterior vitrectomy and causes more corneal and iris trauma. Translimbal vitrectomy should be reserved for the novice surgeon, only in a true emergency. Translimbal vitrectomy is virtually impossible in patients with posterior-chamber IOLs, which represents the biggest subgroup of endophthalmitis cases.

Infusion Cannula Versus End-Irrigating Endoilluminator

In most posterior vitrectomies, the separate infusion cannula is preferable to an end-irrigating endoilluminator. With the separate infusion there is less turbulence and fluid throughput as well as enhanced surgical flexibility. The 6-mm infusion cannula may be preferable to the 4-mm in endophthalmitis cases because of the thickened choroid. However, the thickened choroid, the difficulty in visualizing the pars plana infusion cannula, and the need for speed all point to the use of the end-irrigating endoilluminator in the most severe endophthalmitis cases.

Vitrectomy

The vitrectomy instrument should be used with the lowest possible suction force, preferably with proportional suction control to reduce the chance of tearing necrotic retina and iris. Utilize the highest possible cutting rate and never pull the cutter away from the retina while suction is being applied. The anterior vitreous cortex should be removed first, with special care taken to avoid iris contact and peripheral vitreoretinal traction. The iris tissue can be quite necrotic and may be easily shredded or avulsed. On occasion, hypotony will lead to oozing from iris vessels, requiring bipolar diathermy. If a fibrin membrane covers the anterior surface of the intraocular lens, it can be removed through a peripheral iridectomy constructed with the vitreous cutter. Limbal incisions frequently leak, causing hypotony and miosis.

Endophthalmitis is one of the rare situations in which only a "core" vitrectomy should be done to avoid traction on the potentially necrotic retina. The dense initial vitreous aspirate should be removed for smear, culture, and sensitivity testing (12,13). Blood culture bottles have been shown by Joondeph and Flynn et al. to be superior to inoculating culture plates and tubes in the operating room (14). The endoilluminator is essential to adequate visualization. Vacuum cleaning (extrusion) and membrane peeling should never be utilized in these cases because of the necrotic retina. If there is severe retinal necrosis, the retina will appear white and rough-surfaced with the vessels appearing dull. Such retinas are extremely prone to retinal breaks and can be seen to move with the probe several millimeters away from the retina, even with the mild pulsatile suction force of the vitrectomy instrument.

USE OF ANTIBIOTICS

Intracameral Antibiotics

Intraocular antibiotics should be used in virtually all cases (15). There currently is less disagreement in the literature about safe doses of intraocular antibiotics than in previous years. Because of the risk of retinal toxicity, the lowest published effective dose should be used. Intraocular antibiotics should always be used if an IOL is present. Antibiotics diluted in the infusion fluid are not recommended because of the toxicity question and the difficulty in assessing total retinal dose with this method. Vancomycin 1.0 mg/0.1 mL and ceftazidime 2.25 mg/0.1 mL are the most commonly used agents today. D'Amico et al. have shown that pharmacists mix antibiotics more accurately than nurses and that nurses are far more accurate than physicians (16). Many toxicity cases are probably due to incorrect concentrations and/or volumes being injected. Intraocular dexamethasone 0.4 mg/0.1mL has been recommended by many investigators and has been shown to produce better outcomes (17).

The infusion system should be removed and the 8-0 nylon suture utilized to close all but one temporal wound after vitrectomy is completed. An 8-0 nylon monofilament suture should be preplaced in this wound but not tied. The antibiotic should then be injected slowly in the midvitreous cavity through this wound with a 25-gauge blunt cannula and the suture pulled up as the needle is removed. If two or three separate injections are utilized, as is usually the case, these can be applied sequentially in the same wound with this method. Mixing the antibiotics in the same syringe is poor practice and results in dilution and possibly precipitation.

Subconjunctival Antibiotics and Steroids

After conjunctival closure, subconjunctival antibiotics should be injected. Vancomycin 25 mg and ceftazidime 100 mg are the most widely used agents at the time of this writing. Detailed discussion of antibiotic options is left to other publications because of their rapidly changing status. It is recommended that an antibiotic that is primarily for Gram-positive organisms and effective on penicillinase producers be combined with an antibiotic that is primarily for Gram-negative organisms. Substances released from inflammatory cells, as well as bacteria, cause severe tissue destruction and inflammation. The inflammation suppression role of steroids is thought to far outweigh the potential enhancement of infection. If the case is strongly thought to be fungal in origin, then steroids should probably be omitted.

Topical Antibiotics

Topical antibiotics and steroids should be used in all cases, primarily to inhibit potential, associated lid, cul-de-sac, bleb, and wound infections (18). Care should be taken to prevent cross contamination by doctors, nurses, and technicians taking of care of other patients.

RESULTS

The causative organisms and pretreatment delay constitute the most important factors in therapeutic success. If cases with mild pathogens that could have been managed with subconjunctival and systemic antibiotics are operated upon, the success rate appears to improve. Even with the best management, a significant percentage of these eyes will be lost because of unnecessary surgery. In view of the overall poor prognosis in endophthalmitis cases, major emphasis should be placed on *prevention*. Meticulous preparation of the operative field, including a drape that covers the lashes and lid margins, Betadine preparation, microscope draping, use of the highest-quality infusion fluids (Alcon BSS, BSS Plus) and extreme care if tubing or any other instruments with a lumen or cavity are re-sterilized. Subconjunctival antibiotics should be used at the end of vitrectomy cases, which should decrease the incidence of this dreaded complication.

COMPLICATIONS

Corneal edema, glaucoma, and cataract can be seen after otherwise successful endophthalmitis management with or without vitrectomy. Prompt therapy is probably the single most important factor in prevention of these nonspecific complications.

Retinal breaks and detachment related to retinal necrosis and surgically induced retinal traction occurs in at least 10% of the cases. Postoperative follow-up should emphasize peripheral retinal examination by indirect ophthalmoscopy because of the relatively high frequency of retinal breaks.

REFERENCES

1. Romero CF, Rai MK, Lowder CY, et al. Endogenous endophthalmitis: case report and brief review. *Am Fam Physician* 1999;60:510–514.
2. Brinton GS, Topping TM, Hyndiuk RA, et al. Post-traumatic endophthalmitis. *Arch Ophthalmol* 1984;102:547.
3. Forster RK. Endophthalmitis. In: Duane TD, ed. *Clinical ophthalmology,* Vol. 4. New York: Harper & Row, 1981:1–20.
4. Abu el-Asrar AM. Post-traumatic endophthalmitis: causative organisms and visual outcome. *Eur J Ophthalmol* 1999;9:21–31.
5. Meredith TA. Post-traumatic endophthalmitis. *Arch Ophthalmol* 1999;117:520–521.
6. Forster RK. Etiology and diagnosis of bacterial post-operative endophthalmitis. *Ophthalmology* 1978;85:320.
7. Schmitz S, Dick HB, Krummenauer F, et al. Endophthalmitis in cataract surgery: results of a German study. *Ophthalmology* 1999;106:1869–1877.
8. Solomon A, Ticho U, Frucht-Pery J, et al. Late onset bleb associated endophthalmitis following glaucoma filtering surgery with or without antifibrotic agents. *J Ocul pharmacol Ther* 1999;15:283–293.

9. Clark WL, Kaiser PK, Flynn HW Jr, et al. Treatment strategies and visual acuity outcomes in chronic postoperative *Propionibacterium* acnes endophthalmitis. *Ophthalmology* 1999;106:1665–1670.
10. Cottingham AJ, Forster RK. Vitrectomy in endophthalmitis; results of study using vitrectomy, intraocular antibiotics, or a combination of both. *Arch Ophthalmol* 1976;94:2078.
11. Endophthalmitis Vitrectomy Study Group. Results of the endophthalmitis vitrectomy study. A randomized trial of immediate vitrectomy and of intravenous antibiotics for the treatment of postoperative bacterial endophthalmitis. *Arch Ophthalmol* 1995;113:1479–1496.
12. Frederick AR. A modification of the Ocutome setup to permit the sterile collection of intraocular specimens. *Ocutome Fragmatome Newsletter* 1978;3:2.
13. Smith RE: A technique for collecting uncontaminated specimens for culture during vitrectomy for endophthalmitis. *Ocutome Fragmatome Newsletter* 1978;3:2.
14. Joondeph BC, Flynn HW Jr, Miller D, et al. A new culture method for infectious endophthalmitis. *Arch Ophthalmol* 1989;107:1334–1337.
15. Peyman GA, Vashine DW, Crouch ER, et al. Clinical use of intravitreal antibiotics to treat bacterial endophthalmitis. *Trans Am Acad Ophthalmol Otolaryngol* 1974;8:862.
16. D'Amico DJ, Caspers-Velu L. Comparative toxicity of intravitreal aminoglycoside antibiotics. *Am J Ophthalmol* 1985;100:264–275.
17. Park SS, Vallar RV, Hong CH, et al. Intravitreal dexamethasone effect on vancomycin elimination in endophthalmitis. *Arch Ophthalmol* 1999;117:1058–1062
18. Bannerman TL, Rhoden DL, McAllister SK, et al. The source of coagulase-negative staphylococci in the Endophthalmitis Vitrectomy Study. A comparison of eyelid and intraocular isolates using pulsed-field gel electrophoresis. *Arch Ophthalmol* 1997;115:357–361.

15

Retinopathy of Prematurity

Continuous improvement in outcomes cannot be accomplished by simply going forward with the techniques and technologies that led to success in the past. The Cryotherapy for Retinopathy of Prematurity (ROP) Study is a significant success story, but progress cannot end there. The scientific validity of laser photocoagulation for ROP has become reasonably accepted by using retrospective studies comparing the outcomes to cryotherapy data (1–15). Laser treatment causes less pain, results in minimal arrhythmias, and prevents conjunctival damage, unlike cryotherapy (1,2,8,11,12,16,18). Laser therapy was initially performed using an argon laser (514 nm) delivered by means of a beam-steering attachment on the operating microscope. This method was generally performed in the operating room. The invention of the laser indirect ophthalmoscope (LIO) delivery system enabled treatment without an operating microscope. Diode lasers are approximately 10,000 times more efficient than argon ion lasers, eliminating the need for water-cooling, large enclosures, and special electrical power (230 V AC, three-phase, 60 Amp/phase). The diode laser enabled lightweight, portable LIO-based systems to be used in the newborn intensive care unit (NICU). The near infrared wavelengths of typical diode lasers (~810 nm) are primarily absorbed in the melanin pigment of the choroid and retinal pigment epithelium rather than hemoglobin. This absorption spectrum reduces uptake in the tunica vasculosa lentis and the formation of secondary thermal anterior subcapsular cataracts.

Clinical trials are always based on the reasonable notion that a set of physicians, practicing at the state of the art, can disagree on the most effective management. The issue may be whether the treatment is effective compared with the natural history of untreated patients or an alternative treatment. Further, this set of investigators must agree on a small, finite number of groups for randomization. It is critical to all randomized trials to determine standardized entrance criteria for randomization. The minimum pathology required for treatment in the context of the study is often referred to as "threshold." If most investigators are concerned about treatment complications or skeptical about treatment efficacy, the "threshold" will require relatively advanced pathology. On the contrary, if the known treatment complications are minimal and there is optimism concerning efficacy, the threshold for randomization will require less advanced disease. It is seldom possible to have a cohort large enough to compare several different degrees of severity as indications for treatment. Unless "early" versus "late" treatment is studied, utilization of the treatment timing "recommended" by the study is an arbitrary decision. Large-scale, expensive, randomized trials are essential but can have the unintended consequence of limiting further progress because of the perception that departure from the study *entrance* criteria is not ethical. The major emphasis that malpractice attorneys place on ROP amplifies this rigid adherence to "guidelines" that were intended to be study entrance criteria.

INCREASING OXYGEN SATURATION

Gagnon suggested that increasing the oxygen saturation to nearly 100% when "threshold" is reached reduces the rate of progression to Stages IV and V (17). A report by Seiberth et al. found "the incidence of threshold ROP may be significantly reduced when supplemental oxygen is given when ROP reaches Stage 3" (18). This study based results of an historic control group of 545 preterm infants born between 1991 to 1993 compared with an experimental group of 510 preterm infants born between 1994 and 1996. A significant difference in the development of threshold ROP was found between the control group (average oxygen saturation) and the experimental group (target oxygen saturation of ≥98%).

A randomized controlled study called the Supplemental Therapeutic Oxygen for Prethreshold Retinopathy of Prematurity (STOP-ROP) was designed to determine the efficacy and safety of supplemental therapeutic oxygen for infants with *prethreshold* ROP to reduce the probability of progression to threshold ROP and the need for peripheral retinal ablation (19). This multicenter study was funded by the National Eye Institute, the National Institute for Child and Human Development, and the National Institute for Nursing Research. According to the guidelines of this study, preterm infants with birth weights of less than 1,250 g were screened for ROP at regular intervals. When an infant developed Stage 1 or Stage 2 disease in Zone 1 without Plus disease, Stage 2 disease in Zone 2 with Plus disease, or Stage 3 disease in Zone 2 with less than five contiguous or less than eight total clock hours of Stage 3 disease (with or without Plus disease), they were considered "prethreshold." If these prethreshold patients were already on supplemental oxygen, they were considered eligible for enrollment in the study. After informed consent was obtained, the infant was either randomized to "conventional oxygen oximetry" with a target transcutaneous reading between 89% and 94% or to "supplemental oxygen oximetry" with a target range of 96% to 99% for at least 2 weeks, and until both eyes were at study endpoints. A favorable ophthalmic endpoint was regression of the ROP into Zone 3 for at least two consecutive weekly examinations or full retinal vascularization. An unfavorable ophthalmic outcome was defined as reaching threshold criteria for laser or cryotherapy in at least one eye as defined by the CRYO-ROP study (20). Examiners were blinded to each patient's enrollment status. Infants were then followed with weekly funduscopic examinations. Secondary outcomes of the study included retinal detachment and other ophthalmic outcomes as well as pulmonary status, growth, and interim illnesses.

Six hundred forty-nine infants were enrolled from 30 centers over a 5-year period. ROP progression rates were lower with supplemental oxygen than with conventional oxygen, but the difference was not statistically significant. Use of supplemental oxygen did not cause additional progression of prethreshold ROP but did not significantly reduce the number of infants requiring peripheral ablative surgery. A subgroup analysis did suggest a benefit of supplemental oxygen among infants who had prethreshold ROP without plus disease, but this finding requires additional study. Supplemental oxygen increased the risk of adverse pulmonary events, including pneumonia and/or exacerbations of chronic lung disease and the need for oxygen, diuretics, and hospitalization at 3 months of corrected age. While the risk/benefit of supplemental oxygen for each infant needs to be individually assessed by clinicians, supplemental oxygen, as used in this study, can be given without the fear of exacerbating active prethreshold ROP.

THE QUESTION OF EARLIER LASER OR CRYOTHERAPY

The authors believe that it will be demonstrated that laser (or cryo) treatment before "threshold" will prove to have less complications and better outcomes than utilization of the currently accepted "threshold." Several reports have reached this conclusion. Spencer et al. (21) and Ben-Sira et al. (22) reported favorable anatomic outcomes in eyes treated with cryo for 3 to 7 clock hours of Stage 3 disease with plus disease. These treatments were limited to the area immediately anterior to the Stage 3 disease. The observation that treatment of less severe cases of ROP may require smaller treatment areas of avascular retina was also noted by Nissenkorn et al. (23). Although it is logical to argue that the treatment of ROP at an earlier point than "threshold" will necessarily expose more infants to the complications of treatment, it also follows that it may be possible to offset these risks by performing a more limited treatment commensurate with the extent of the disease at the time the decision to treat is made.

The point at which limited treatment, performed earlier than "threshold," would result in better visual outcomes versus the side effects of treatment would be difficult to ascertain, as risk assessment and side effects of treatment would depend entirely on the experience of the examiner. Fleming et al. reported results with diode laser therapy for "earlier than threshold" ROP that indicated improved results could be obtained with laser if treatment was initiated before the development of "threshold" disease (24).

The principal author and Chris Devine surveyed 76 physicians who either treat or perform screening examinations for ROP (25). Of the 34 respondents, 91% believe that a trend toward "earlier than threshold treatment" already exists. Of those physicians who perform laser or cryotherapy for ROP, 78% of respondents indicated that they treat earlier than threshold at least under certain conditions. The most frequently cited condition under which they would treat before "threshold" was for Zone 1 ROP, prethreshold ROP with contralateral "threshold" ROP, and severity of plus disease. Of all respondents, 48% reported that they felt that threshold criteria resulted in too many infants either receiving treatment too late or not receiving treatment when it would have proven beneficial because they did not meet "threshold" criteria. Overall, 42% of respondents reported that they felt threshold criteria represented the best balance between outcomes and side effects. Respondents commenting "uncertain" to the preceding categories accounted for 10%.

Clearly, the results of the CRYO-ROP study indicate that up to 47.1% of treated patients have an unfavorable outcome at 5.5 years of follow-up (26). Although some of these patients may have had a poor outcome regardless of treatment type or timing, one should consider, in light of the previously mentioned studies, that there might be a significant number of individuals who suffered a poor outcome as a result of receiving treatment "too late." An unknown percentage of patients not receiving any treatment because they never reached "threshold" disease may also have suffered poor outcome. It seems plausible that there is a subgroup in the CRYO-ROP study that had a poor outcome due to the treatment itself, which might have been reduced by a more limited treatment earlier in the course of the disease. One attempt to minimize the number of poor outcomes could be the judicious use of a limited "earlier than threshold treatment."

Specifically, the use of cryotherapy or laser indirect ophthalmoscopy to the areas of avascular retina adjacent to Stage 3 disease of less than "threshold" disease appears to be a reasonable approach grounded in the work noted earlier. Laser therapy may be preferable in most cases, as it has fewer ophthalmic and medical side effects than cryotherapy. Some recent studies conclude that laser photocoagulation provides better long-term structural outcome and visual acuity than cryotherapy (27). In cases in which the tunica vasculosa lentis is still patent and prominent, cryotherapy or lower laser power settings may prove more beneficial by reducing the risk of cataracts (28). If a more limited treatment is to be applied, patients must be followed more closely to ensure an adequate treatment response.

SURGICAL ANATOMY

Current clinical practice frequently describes the anatomic picture of ROP with incorrect terms such as *disorganized retina, retrolental mass,* and *inoperable retinal detachment.* A better understanding of the pathoanatomy permits more accurate preoperative evaluation and surgery (Fig. 15.1). As in other disease entities, cellular migration and proliferation occur on retinal or vitreous surfaces. Cellular proliferation at the posterior vitreous cortex (PVC)/retinal interface creates adherence between these layers and curved planar contraction. As retinal detachment develops, this interface folds upon itself, creating apparent retinal/retinal adherence. Marked adherence of PVC to equatorial retina pulls the equatorial retina anteriorly, creating a marked concavity of the thin preequatorial retina, often mistaken for a dialysis.

Anteriorly, proliferation occurs along the anterior vitreous cortex (AVC)/lens interface, creating the well-known retrolental membrane. This is often incorrectly described as a retrolental mass, when in fact it is a thin planar structure composed of displaced, contracted, normal tissue. Most vessels seen at this interface are actually retinal vessels translocated centrally because of the posterior interface contraction and resultant closed-cone traction retinal detachment. As the PVC/retinal interface moves anteriorly, it comes into contact with the AVC/lens interface, creating a four-layer complex that can be referred to as a retrolental membrane complex.

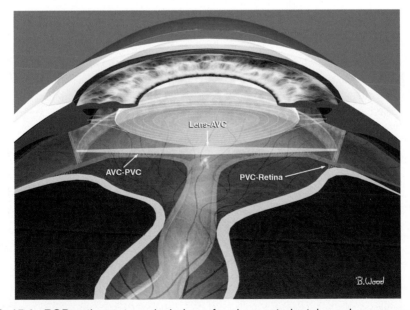

FIG. 15.1. ROP pathoanatomy includes a four-layer retrolental membrane complex.

PREOPERATIVE EVALUATION

Office Technique

Every attempt should be made for the infant to remain cradled in a normal position in the parent's arms rather than restrained. Eyelids should only be retracted if absolutely necessary. Because of poor vision, these children usually squeeze their lids closed in response to physical stimulation of the lids. Under no circumstances should any form of sedation be utilized in the office environment because of the increased risk of cardiac and respiratory arrest. The best method is to look quickly and frequently as the child moves about without restraint.

Examination Under Anesthesia

Examination under anesthesia should only be undertaken if a form of therapy has a reasonable chance of being performed at the same time. Anesthesia should not be used for a work-up just because of a protocol- or report-driven mentality. Parents must be provided with preexamination information about surgical options, including no surgery, lensectomy only, or lensectomy/vitrectomy, and in many instances, surgery on either or both eyes.

Electrophysiologic Testing

The electroretinogram (ERG) is always nonrecordable in total retinal detachment (29,30). Almost all patients with an opaque retrolental complex have a total or nearly total detachment. The ERG is useless in evaluating these children, and anesthesia time should not be utilized for this purpose. There is no evidence that the visual evoked potential (VEP) is of any predictive value in patients who have light perception. Light perception can be determined by blinking and head movements in response to light without requiring expensive, inconclusive VEP testing and/or ERG. Sector scan, real-time contact ultrasonography can be valuable, primarily in evaluation of the opaque cornea and the rare patient with a totally opaque retrolental complex. Ultrasound examination can be performed quite well in the office and does not require sedation or anesthesia. The closed-cone traction retinal detachments are frequently misinterpreted as "stalks" or "disorganized fibrotic tissue." Knowledge of the anatomy and surgical experience result in more accurate ultrasonographic diagnoses.

Many patients are said to have iris neovascularization (rubeosis) when, in fact, they have persistent anterior tunica vasculosa lentis and/or dilated iris stromal vessels. These patients can develop corneal edema and glaucoma secondary to corneal/iris contact from a pupillary block mechanism. Persistence of posterior tunica vasculosa lentis might also play a role in the development of the retrolental complex.

There is often thick yellow-brown material in the subretinal space, some of which is of hematogenous origin. In late cases, it can be replaced by dense, honeycomb-like plaques, dendritic elements, and cholesterol crystals.

Management of Pupillary Block Glaucoma

Pupillary block glaucoma and corneal edema from iris contact usually occur at 3 to 4 months of age, which is often too early for definitive vitreoretinal surgery, since anti-VEGF or angiostatic agents are unavailable This problem can be recognized by the parents' noting lid edema and tearing, and by daily inspection of the eye with a penlight. If this is noted, chamber deepening, lensectomy, and sector iridectomy can save the anterior segment and allow vitrectomy at a later date.

Timing

Although some surgeons advocate surgical intervention for Stage 4-A disease, scleral buckling or vitrectomy has not been proven to be efficacious. Dilated iris and retinal vessels indicate activity of the disease and are relative contraindications to surgery. Similarly, an exudative component to the retinal detachment as indicated by retinal convexity and subretinal exudate indicates the need to delay surgery. Surgery on active cases appears to cause a higher reproliferation rate.

Another advantage of delaying surgery is the reduction in anesthesia risks associated with greater body weight and better pulmonary function. If there is any question about the medical condition, surgery should be delayed; successful operations have been performed on 18-month-old patients. There is an inherent compromise: early operations are associated with better visual function and more straightforward surgical anatomy; however, these cases pose a greater anesthesia risk and have a higher incidence of reproliferation.

Risk Analysis

Because of the current success rate and high medical risk, and because only ambulatory vision is achieved in successful cases, care must be taken to secure informed consent. Competent anesthesiologists experienced in anesthesia for neonates must be included in the preoperative planning. Preoperative evaluation and postoperative medical management require an experienced neonatologist or experienced pediatrician.

SURGICAL SEQUENCE AND TECHNIQUES

Combined Examination Under Anesthesia

If the office examination was inadequate in determining the need for surgery, mask insufflation anesthesia with indirect ophthalmoscopy should confirm the need for surgery and indicate the eye with the best prognosis or determine the need for bilateral surgery. Because of the relationship between anesthesia and morbidity/mortality, there is no time for retinal drawings, ultrasound "for documentation," or prolonged photographic procedures. If the need for surgery is confirmed, the patient should be intubated, prepped, draped, and operated upon.

Surgical Management of Stage IV

Several years ago a group of leading ROP surgeons convened to develop a randomized trial to compare scleral buckling with the natural history of Stage IV retinopathy of prematurity. A study was designed and a grant application submitted to the National Eye Institute. Unfortunately, the study was not funded and the question concerning efficacy of scleral buckling in ROP remains unanswered. The principal author has not performed scleral buckling in ROP for more than 18 years because of the serious complications and lack of proof of efficacy. Complications of scleral buckling include death from arrhythmias, intrusion of the buckle into the sclera, and conjunctival damage. The encircling buckles must be severed or removed, which requires a second operation at a later date to avoid intrusion into the eye.

The authors do not perform vitrectomy on Stage IV-A cases. Many of these cases stabilize and the macula never detaches. Anesthesia risks and the potential creation of retinal breaks, progressive glial proliferation, and cataract formation argue against surgery when the traction retinal detachment is extramacular.

The authors only operate on Stage IV-B cases if there is elevation of a broad area of the macula. Surgery on a thin, knife-edge-like fold through the macula will not result in attaching more photoreceptors or increasing vision. Unfortunately, many surgeons operate on these cases apparently because they are less difficult and have reasonable outcomes.

Trese has recommended "lens-sparing" vitrectomy in Stage IV and Stage V cases (31,32). In our experience, it is seldom possible to save the lens and perform adequate peripheral dissection in most Stage V and many Stage IV-B cases. Placement of the sclerotomies more posteriorly to save the lens may result in creation of peripheral retinal breaks and dialyses. Very little data have been presented to support advocacy of lens sparing.

Vitrectomy for Stage V

Despite laser photocoagulation, cryotherapy, and scleral buckling, a considerable number of low-birth-weight infants develop end-stage retinopathy of prematurity (ROP). Surgery for the Stage V narrow or closed-cone traction retinal detachment was impossible until, in 1977, the principal author developed a transciliary body vitreous surgical approach with scissors delamination (33–37). The principal author has operated on more than 1,300 eyes with Stage V ROP since 1977. Although there are some anatomically successful cases, the visual outcomes are universally poor (15% to 20% improved), and there is a high incidence of reproliferation (45%). Relatively poor outcomes emphasize the need for prevention and early intervention in this tragic disorder (38).

Summary of Indications for Surgery

Because of the certainty of severe amblyopia, significant anesthesia risk, and relatively poor prognosis, unilateral Stage 5 cases should not be operated upon, whereas unilateral Stage 4B cases are an open question. Stage 4-A peripheral detachments, which by definition do not affect the macula, should not be operated on. Stage 4-B cases with a broad area of elevation, not just a "knife-edge" fold through the macula, are ideal cases for surgery. The principal author had operated on the largest series of Stage 5 cases but stopped do so in 2000 after analysis of long-term success rates. Six-month follow-up data revealed a 17% anatomic success rate, but long-term data demonstrated a 10% anatomic success rate because of frequent reproliferation and glaucoma. Long-term visual success rates no longer justify surgery for Stage 5, in the principal author's opinion. A handful of patients achieve hand motion vision, which does not enable better functioning. A few cases that achieved finger counting or better vision ultimately lost this vision from reproliferation, glaucoma, or the trophic effects of an ectopic macula, as reported by Tasman.

Entry Site

Limbal entry creates striate keratopathy, regional corneal edema, wound leaks, and poor access to the preequatorial traction (39). Pars plana entry introduces the instruments into the subretinal space and creates an obligatory dialysis and rhegmatogenous component. Ciliary body entry approximately 0.5 mm posterior to the limbus is the safest approach. This entry into the iris root frequently requires sector iridectomy at this site or passage anterior to the iris. All incisions should be made with a single puncture using the 20-gauge shank, 1.4-mm blade, lancet-tip, microvitreoretinal (MVR) blade. A 30° bent, 20-gauge, blunt-tipped infusion cannula (May) is utilized at a site slightly superior to the middle of the medial rectus. Bimanual technique allows small incisions, mobility of the globe, and interchangeability between the nasal and temporal instruments. Coaxial illumination from the microscope without a fundus contact lens can be used because of the anterior location of the retina/ERM. Stage 4-B cases require an end-irrigating endoilluminator and fundus contact lens. Standard sew-on infusion cannulas tend to strike the lid margins and rotate posteriorly into the subretinal space. Full-function probes and cannula systems are too large for these small eyes. Recently, end-irrigating endoilluminators have been used in lieu of the angulated infusion cannula. This approach allows the microscope light to be turned off and a contact lens used for better visualization.

Endocapsular Lensectomy

As discussed earlier, the lens is removed in most cases. The sclerotomies are made between the ciliary sulcus and the iris root. The 30°, 20-gauge, blunt, hand-held, infusion cannula (May) or the Alcon end-irrigating, endoilluminator is used for infusion in all cases.

The principal author has previously reported the method of endocapsular lensectomy. Penetration of the equatorial lens capsule with the infusion cannula is utilized (Fig. 15.2). The vitreous cutter is used to create a circular rhexis in the posterior capsule (Fig. 15.3). Cortical clearing hydrodissection is used to facilitate a rapid and safe lensectomy

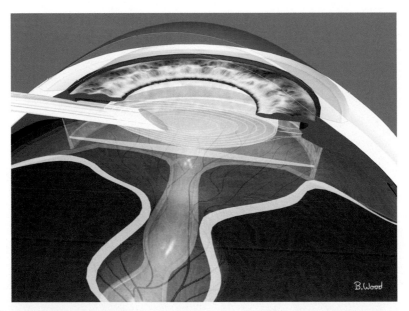

FIG. 15.2 Lensectomy is initiated by penetrating the equatorial lens capsule with the infusion cannula.

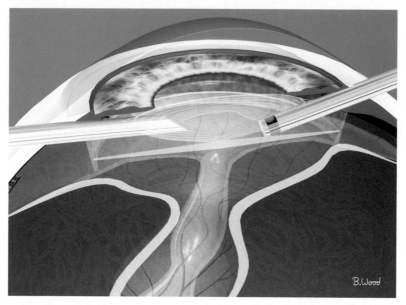

FIG. 15.3. A circular rhexis is created in the posterior lens capsule with the vitreous cutter.

(Fig. 15.4). Aspiration and cutting with the vitreous cutter is used to mobilize the cortex after removal of the nucleus (Fig. 15.5). Care is taken to avoid damage to the anterior capsule. After all cortex is removed, the capsule is removed with the Griesehaber, diamond-coated, end-opening, 612.12 forceps using a circular zonulorhexis movement (Fig. 15.6). Care is taken to avoid traction on the peripheral retina and contact with the iris.

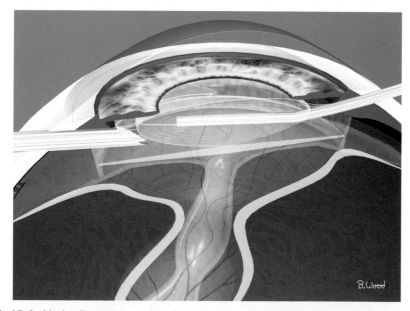

FIG. 15.4. Hydrodissection and hydrodelineation facilitate a safe, rapid lensectomy.

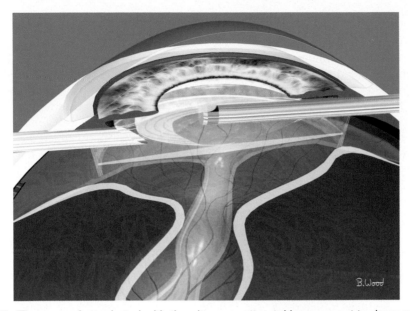

FIG. 15.5. The cortex is aspirated with the vitreous cutter, taking care not to damage the anterior capsule.

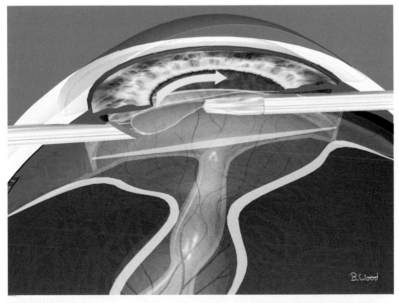

FIG. 15.6. The capsule is removed in a circular zonulorhexis fashion with the end-opening forceps.

Inside-Out Segmentation

The principal author developed scissors segmentation of epiretinal membranes more than 20 years ago. Segmentation is defined as making so-called vertical cuts in epiretinal membranes dividing the structure into multiple epicenters, relieving tangential traction. Segmentation is essential for ROP surgery because the epiretinal membranes are too adherent to permit membrane peeling (stripping). The initial segmentation cut should be made in the center of the hypocellular contracted confluence of the anterior and posterior vitreous cortex (funnel). This frontal plane structure was formerly called the retrolental membrane. Multiple (four to eight) pie-shaped radial cuts extending over the equatorial ridge are made through the epiretinal membrane extending down to the retinal surface (Fig. 15.7). Inside-out segmentation is safer than outside-in because the central retina is much thicker and stronger than the peripheral retina, and scissors cause an unavoidable "push-out" force as they close.

Inside-Out Delamination

The principal author developed scissors delamination to enable complete removal of epiretinal membranes by shearing the glial attachments between the retina and the membrane. Inside-out delamination is used to detach the aforementioned pie-shaped segments of epiretinal membrane from the retinal surface (Fig. 15.8). Circumferential scissors cuts can then be used to detach the pie-shaped segments from the pars plana (Fig. 15.9). The freed-up segments can then be removed from the eye with the vitreous cutter using high suction with the port safely away from the retina.

Drainage of Subretinal Fluid

Drainage of subretinal fluid is performed only if a retinal break is identified or apparent subretinal fluid in the vitreous cavity is noted. Fluid/air exchange followed by air/gas

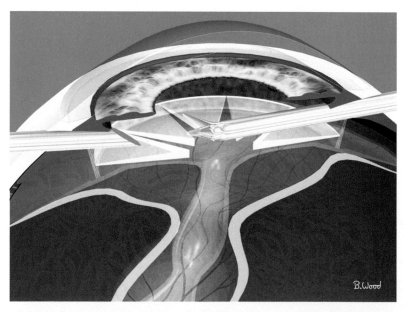

FIG. 15.7. Multiple radial cuts are made in the epiretinal membrane, working from inside out.

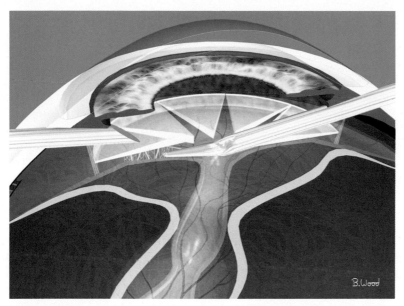

FIG. 15.8. Inside-out scissors delamination is used to detach the membrane segments from the retina.

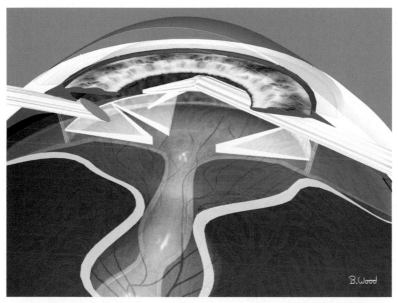

FIG. 15.9. Circumferential scissor cuts detach the delaminated segments from the pars plana.

C_3F_8 exchange must then be performed. Extreme care must be taken to avoid iatrogenic retinal breaks in ROP cases because the retina becomes structurally mature in the detached position and then has insufficient surface area to cover the RPE until long-term collagen remodeling takes place.

Internal drainage of subretinal fluid (SRF) should be performed very carefully because structural rigidity of the retina often prevents complete reattachment, and subretinal air or gas will follow the needle into the subretinal space via the internal drainage cannula. Foot-pedal control by the proportional suction system of a 25-gauge 5/8-inch needle placed obliquely through the equatorial sclera is the safest and most efficient method of drainage. A marked transretinal pressure gradient should be avoided because it can cause relief tears of the retina. Frequently, SRF will pass from the subretinal space to the supra-nonpigmented epithelial region.

Fluid/Air or Fluid/Gas Exchange

The authors never use fluid/air exchange unless a retinal break is observed or created during vitrectomy. If a break is noted, fluid/air exchange is performed simultaneously with direct transscleral drainage or internal drainage of subretinal fluid. If reattachment is accomplished, laser endophotocoagulation is used to surround the breaks with confluent treatment.

Surface Tension Management

Perfluorocarbon liquids are inappropriate in ROP cases because extreme retinal foreshortening, retinal stiffness, and retinal breaks all increase the likelihood of the PFC liquid entering the subretinal space. Silicone appears to cause increased proliferation at the silicone/retinal interface by sequestration of cytokines and cells. The only purpose of silicone surface tension management is rhegmatogenous confinement, which is not required if care has been taken to avoid retinal breaks. If large breaks occur, inward curling of the edge and subretinal silicone is a frequent problem.

Simultaneous, Bilateral Vitreous Surgery

The principal author developed the concept of simultaneous bilateral surgery 10 years ago and has now performed bilateral surgery in more than 100 patients. The author has had no endophthalmitis cases in ROP surgery and only three cases in more than 16,000 (0.02%) adult vitrectomies. Although the author has had no deaths in the largest series of ROP surgery, the predicted anesthesia risk exceeds the statistical risk of endophthalmitis. The total operating time on simultaneous bilateral cases has not exceeded 70 minutes. This approach cuts in half the anesthesia risk and cost.

Scleral Buckling

Delamination of the equatorial PVC (ERM) combined with circumferential dissection of preequatorial plate (anterior loop) traction eliminates the need for scleral buckling. The problem of scleral intrusion of the buckle is thus avoided.

Scleral buckling increases iris/retinal adherence by pushing equatorial sclera and retina centrally and anteriorly toward the capsule remnants and posterior iris surface. Scleral buckling necessitates rectus muscle traction sutures, with attendant traction-induced bradycardia. Sufficient quantities of anticholinergic agents to block this reflex can cause tachycardia and postoperative pulmonary problems.

Wound Closure

At the end of the dissection, and possibly the use of air/gas, a 22-gauge tapered, flexible intravenous cannula (Jelco) is substituted for the infusion cannula. Two passes of an 8-0 monofilament nylon shoelace suture are placed around the cannula, three loops are made, and the knot is pulled up as the assistant withdraws the cannula; in this way normal intraocular pressure is maintained.

Simplified Surgery

No cannulas, open-sky methods, iris retractors, pics, silicone, liquid perfluorocarbon liquids, wide-angle visualization, or viscoelastics are utilized in vitreous surgery for retinopathy of prematurity. The delamination scissors are used for all segmentation and delamination. Use of a limited number of techniques and technologies reduces operating time, cost, and error. Faster surgery permits safe simultaneous, bilateral surgery.

Summary

As in the management of diabetic retinopathy, prevention is the key to better outcomes for patients with retinopathy of prematurity. Continuous monitoring of the oxygen saturation with real-time feedback control of inspired oxygen may result in better outcomes. It is hoped that the Stop-ROP study will guide the neonatologist/ophthalmologist team to better protocols and that pre-"threshold" diode laser treatment will also improve outcomes.

REPROLIFERATION

A significant number of cases that have had complete delamination of all epiretinal membrane redetach from recurrent proliferation. Factors that influence reproliferation include residual lens material, blood, surgical disruption of the retinal surface, retinopexy, and surface tension agents. Iris/retinal adherence is a frequent configuration, but localized or widespread reproliferation on the retinal surface is common. The principal author almost never reoperates on these cases because of the very poor prognosis. If good vision was obtained and then redetachment accompanied by visual loss occurs, the author would consider reoperation.

VISUAL REHABILITATION

Residual SRF is pumped out very slowly by the RPE because of osmotic and other reasons, often requiring 2 to 6 months for maximal reattachment. Only when reattachment occurs can slow regeneration of rod and cone outer segments begin. Experimental retinal detachment studies have shown a rough correlation between the duration of retinal detachment and recovery period. After reattachment occurs, full retinoscopic correction (18 to 30 D) should be worn full-time, even without evidence of visual behavior. Full visual recovery can take as long as 2 to 3 years postoperatively because of the factors mentioned earlier and because of slow central nervous system development. The parents and consulting physician should be informed of this slow recovery so as to encourage full-time use of aphakic correction.

REFERENCES

1. Algawi K, Goddin M, O'Keefe M. Refractive outcome following diode laser versus cryotherapy for eyes with retinopathy of prematurity. *Br J Ophthalmol* 1994;78:612.
2. Barron DF, Sivulich KA. Laser therapy as a treatment for retinopathy of prematurity. *Pediatr Nurs* 1994;20:90.
3. Goggin M, O'Keefe M. Diode laser for retinopathy of prematurity-early outcome. *Br J Ophthalmol* 1993;77:559.

4. Hammer ME, Pusteri JB, Hess JB, et al. Threshold retinopathy of prematurity: transition from cryopexy to laser treatment. *Retina* 1995;15:486.
5. Hunter DG, Repka MX. Diode laser photocoagulation for threshold retinopathy of prematurity: a randomized study. *Ophthalmology* 1993;100:238.
6. Knight-Nanan DM, O'Keefe M. Refractive outcome in eyes with retinopathy of prematurity treated with cryotherapy or didode laser: 3-year follow-up. *Br J Ophthalmol* 1996;80:998.
7. Laws F, Laws D, Clark D. Cryotherapy and laser treatment for acute retinopathy of prematurity: refractive outcomes, a longitudinal study. *Br J Ophthalmol* 1997;81:12.
8. Ling CS, Fleck BW, Wright E, et al. Diode laser treatment for retinopathy of prematurity: structural and functional outcome. *Br J Ophthalmol* 1995;79:637.
9. McNamara JA, Tasman W, Brown GC, et al. Laser photocoagulation for states 3+ retinopathy of prematurity. *Ophthalmology* 1991;98:576.
10. McNamara JA, Tasman W, Vander JF, et al. Diode laser photocoagulation for retinopathy of prematurity: preliminary results. *Arch Ophthalmol* 1992;110:1714.
11. Seiberth V, Linderkamp O, Vardarli I, et al. Diode laser photocoagulation of stages 3+ retinopathy of prematurity. *Ophthalmology* 1996;93:182.
12. Seiberth V, Linderkamp O, Vardarli I, et al. Diode laser photocoagulation of stages 3+ retinopathy of prematurity. *Graefes Arch Clin Exp Ophthalmol* 1995;233:489.
13. White E, Repka MX. Randomized comparison of diode laser photocoagulation versus cryotherapy for threshold retinopathy of prematurity: 3-year outcome. *J Pediatr Ophthalmol Strabismus* 1997;34:83.
14. Yang CM. Diode laser photocoagulation for retinopathy of prematurity. *J Formos Med Assoc* 1995;94:56.
15. Yang CM, Chen MS, Tsou, et al. Comparison of cryotherapy and laser photocoagulation in stage III retinopathy of prematurity. *J Formos Med Assoc* 1997;96:734.
16. Laatikainen L, Mattila J, Karna J. Combined use of argon laser photocoagulation and cryotherapy in the treatment of retinopathy of prematurity. *Acta Ophthalmol Scand* 1995;73:333.
17. Edmond D, Lachance C, Gagnon J, et al. Arterial partial pressure of oxygen required to achieve 90% saturation of hemoglobin in very low birth weight newborns. *Pediatrics* 1993;91:602.
18. Seiberth V, Linderkamp O, Vardarli I, et al. Supplemental oxygen in acute retinopathy of prematurity stage 3. Session II, poster 27. Presented at AAO annual meeting, San Francisco, CA, 1997.
19. Supplemental therapeutic oxygen for prethreshold retinopathy of prematurity (STOP-ROP), a randomized, controlled trial. Primary outcomes. *Pediatrics* 2000;105:295–310.
20. National Eye Institute: CRYO-ROP Study. Potomac, MD, National Eye Institute, 1993.
21. Spencer R, Hutton WL, Snyder WB, et al. Limiting applications of cryotherapy for severe retinopathy of prematurity. *Ophthalmic Surg* 1992;23:766.
22. Ben-Sira I, Nissenkorn I, Weinberger D, et al. Long-term results of cryotherapy for active stages of retinopathy of prematurity. *Ophthalmology* 1986;93:1423.
23. Nissenkorn I, Axer–Siegel R, et al. Effect of partial cryoablation on retinopathy of prematurity. *Br J Ophthalmol* 1991;75:160.
24. Fleming TN, Runge PE, Charles ST. Diode laser photocoagulation for prethreshold, posterior retinopathy of prematurity. *Am J Ophthalmol* 1992;114:589.
25. Charles S, Devine C. Retinopathy of Prematurity. *Ophthalmol Clin North Am* 1998;11:517-524.
26. Multicenter trial of cryotherapy for ROP: Snellen visual acuity and structural outcome at 5½ years after randomization. *Arch Ophthalmol* 1996;114:417.
27. Paysse EA, Lindsey JL, Coats DK, et al. Therapeutic outcomes of cryotherapy versus diode laser photocoagulation for threshold ROP. *J AAPOS* 1999;3:234–240.
28. Seiberth V, Linderkamp O, Vardarli I, et al. Diode laser photocoagulation for threshold retinopathy of prematurity in eyes with tunica vasculosa lentis. *Am J Ophthalmol* 1995;119:748.
29. Foulds WS, Ikeda H. The effects of detachment of the retina on the induced and resting ocular potentials in the rabbit. *Invest Ophthalmol* 1966;5:93.
30. Hamasaki DI, Machemer R, Norton EWD. Experimental retinal detachment in the owl monkey. VI: The ERG of detached and reattached retina. *Graefes Arch Clin Exp Ophthalmol* 1969;177:212.
31. Maguire AM, Trese MT. Lens-sparing vitreoretinal surgery in infants. *Arch Ophthalmol* 1992;110:284.
32. Ferrone PJ, Harrison C, Trese MT. Lens clarity after lens-sparing vitrectomy in a pediatric population. *Ophthalmology* 1997;104:273–278.
33. Charles S. Vitreous surgery for retinopathy of prematurity (ROP). Presented at Retinopathy of Prematurity Conference, Washington, DC, December 4–6, 1981.
34. Charles S. Delamination advised for treating stage V retrolental fibroplasia. *Ophthalmol Times* 1982;7:11.
35. Charles S. Vitreous surgery for retrolental fibroplasia. In: Jakobiec FA, Sigelman J, eds. *Advanced techniques in ocular surgery,* Chapter 27. Philadelphia: WB Saunders, 1984.
36. Charles S. Vitrectomy with ciliary body entry for retrolental fibroplasia. In: McPherson A, ed. *Retinopathy of prematurity,* Chapter 20. Philadelphia: BC Decker, 1986.
37. Charles S. Vitrectomy for retrolental fibroplasia: case reports. Presented at The Fourteenth Annual Scientific Meeting of The Retina Society. San Francisco, CA, September 19, 1981.
38. Seaber JH, Machemer R, Elliot D, et al. Long-term visual results of children after initially successful vitrectomy for stage V retinopathy of prematurity. *Ophthalmology* 1995;102:199–204.
39. Lightfoot D, Irvine AR. Vitrectomy in infants and children with retinal detachments caused by cicatricial retrolental fibroplasia. *Am J Ophthalmol* 1982;94:305.

16

Pediatric Traction Retinal Detachments

Diverse disease processes may create traction retinal detachments in the pediatric age group. Special approaches are required to manage these difficult problems. These young patients have many years ahead of them and require the most aggressive attempts at restoration of vision. Patients in the pediatric age group having retinal detachments of several years' duration can have remarkable visual recovery, and this emphasizes the need to proceed with such cases. In contrast, the very young patient, especially with retinopathy of prematurity (see Chapter 9), is a high-risk patient requiring careful assessment of the risk/benefit ratio of surgery. From the ocular standpoint, unilateral disease in the pre-6-year-old has an extremely high incidence of amblyopia, diminishing the visual impact of successful surgery.

PERSISTENT HYPERPLASTIC PRIMARY VITREOUS, PERSISTENT FETAL VASCULATURE

Persistent hyperplastic primary vitreous is also known as persistent fetal vasculature. It is usually a unilateral phenomenon accompanied by a smaller eye (1). The almost uniform incidence of amblyopia means that these cases should be operated on early and, in most cases, to prevent long-term traction detachment or a flat chamber (2,3). This condition is usually recognized early in life and the patient should be operated upon if a traction detachment is recognized, the cataract is sufficient to cause visual loss and amblyopia, or there is shallowing of the anterior chamber secondary to pupillary block. Nothing is known about the pathogenesis of this disorder other than its relationship to the persistence of the hyaloid artery system (1). Bilateral cases in males are usually associated with Norrie syndrome. Norrie cases should not be operated on because the retina is dysplastic and the vitreoretinal interface cannot be delineated at surgery.

Surgical Sequence and Techniques

A temporal 60° and superonasal 30° conjunctival and Tenon's capsule incision is made 1 mm posterior to the limbus, because of the anterior placed sclerotomy sites. A microvitreoretinal (MVR) blade sclerotomy is made just behind the iris plane above the medial rectus. This usually is 1.5 to 2.5 mm posterior to the limbus. A blunt 20-gauge, 30°, bent cannula or end-irrigating endoilluminator is used for infusion through this site. If the original MVR blade is used to make a central discission in the opaque pupillary or retrolental membrane, this site can later be utilized to visualize the infusion cannula. After the infusion cannula is introduced, a similar incision is made just above the lateral rectus for the vitrectomy instrument. The vitrectomy instrument is introduced into the lens substance, except in the rare instance that there is a clear lens. If the lens is clear, occasionally it is possible to introduce just the scissors through the pars plana without infusion and to transect the membrane behind the lens, which can allow the traction detachment to resolve. More commonly, the lens is cataractous or a large retrolental membrane is present, requiring lens removal. The vitrectomy instrument is used to remove the retrolental membrane centrally, being careful not to amputate a ciliary process and thus cause bleeding. After a large opening is made, almost to the tips of the ciliary processes, the right angle, 20-gauge scissors are introduced and are used to cut between ciliary processes in order to segment the ring. If this is not done, the circumferential traction will keep the ciliary processes extended.

As the anterior portion of the stalk extending posteriorly is resected, bleeding will frequently occur from the remnants of the hyaloid artery system. This should be treated with bipolar diathermy using a disposable bipolar endoilluminator (see Chapter 4). Although the stalk can be resected midway in the vitreous cavity, it is usually necessary to delaminate the posterior termination of the stalk away from the retinal surface. Care should be taken to avoid the retina, which can be pulled up into the central portion of the stalk around the optic nerve area. If there is a small "tabletop" traction detachment surrounding the optic nerve, the standard infusion cannula may be placed to allow the endoilluminator and scissors to be used to delaminate the membrane. Alternatively, the end-irrigating endoilluminator can be used. In most cases, this is unnecessary. After the procedure is completed, the wounds are closed in the customary manner with running shoelace 8-0 nylon sutures. The conjunctival incisions are closed with 6-0 plain gut sutures.

Results

Anatomic results are excellent in this group, well over 95%. Bleeding and postoperative retinal detachment are exceedingly rare.

Amblyopia is such a frequent accompaniment of this disorder that aggressive treatment by early surgery, early contact lens fitting, and patching of the other eye are necessary. On occasion, a patient will achieve an excellent visual result, but amblyopia is more common. If aggressive contact lens fitting and patching are not done, amblyopia is the uniform result (2).

TOXOCARA CANIS

The parasite *Toxocara canis* can migrate from the choroidal vessels through the choroid and retina into the vitreous cavity (4). As it migrates through the eye, it creates an intense inflammatory reaction, which may simulate endophthalmitis or severe uveitis. After this initial phase, a fibrous proliferation, more extensive than that seen with vascular retinopathy, enters the eye. It may come from both the posterior entrance site of the parasite and the pars plana exit site. If this membrane, created by the inflammatory reaction, does not cause traction detachment, it is not necessary to operate. If there is a small traction detachment away from the macula, this also can be followed by observation, or occasionally can be treated by scleral buckling alone.

These cases have a high incidence of late rhegmatogenous detachment secondary to longstanding traction. Although scleral buckling can reattach some of these detachments, vitreous surgery with resection of the stalk is beneficial in certain cases. Occasionally, the macula will become detached in the relatively early stages of this disease in a nonrhegmatogenous fashion. When this occurs, vitrectomy is necessary.

Surgical Sequence and Techniques

The conventional 60° temporal and 30° superonasal conjunctival and Tenon's capsule incisions are made 1 mm posterior to the limbus. The sclerotomies are made 2 mm posterior to the limbus if the lens is clear. The vitrectomy instrument is introduced super-otemporally and the endoilluminator, superonasally. The vitreous is usually conically shaped and the posterior vitreous cortex (PVC) is continuous with the tract. Although a casual examiner would think that this tract progresses through the vitreous cavity, in fact, posterior vitreous detachment usually occurs with the proliferation on the vitreous surface. If resection of the dense tract alone is performed, the clear vitreous may cause the traction detachment to remain. For this reason the vitrectomy is completed first and then attention is directed to the stalk. Care should be taken to avoid a steep radial fold of retina underlying the stalk, which is present in many cases. Scissors segmentation and delamination techniques should be utilized to allow release of retinal traction. The principles are similar to those used for traction detachments from diabetic retinopathy, although the proliferation is much more dense and localized. Bleeding may occur from this stalk and can be treated with bipolar diathermy, paying close attention to avoid the retina and optic nerve.

Scleral buckling is not utilized in these young patients because of the possibility of later intrusion of the encircling element. If a rhegmatogenous component is present, it must be managed by internal drainage of subretinal fluid, fluid/gas exchange, and laser endophotocoagulation.

Results

The visual outlook depends primarily upon the involvement of the macula in the full-thickness chorioretinal destructive process. If the macula is secondarily detached but has not been invaded by the parasite, excellent visual recovery is possible. Fortunately, recurrence of postoperative inflammation is not a problem in these cases.

NEW APPROACHES

A recent report on the use of cyanoacrylate glue in the repair of retinal detachment associated with posterior retinal breaks in infants and children reported favorable results (5). Although this is a preliminary and limited study, this approach may offer another option in the management of difficult pediatric cases.

Several reports have commented on the use of silicone oil in the management of complicated pediatric retinal detachments (6–8). Although the anatomic success rate appears to be acceptable, the final visual acuity and high incidence of complications suggest that the role of silicone oil in the pediatric population requires further evaluation.

REFERENCES

1. Yanoff M, Fine BS. *Ocular pathology: a text and atlas.* Hagerstown, MD: Harper & Row, 1975:698.
2. Gass JDM. Surgical excision of persistent hyperplastic primary vitreous. *Arch Ophthalmol* 1970;83:163.
3. Smith RE, Maumenee AE. Persistent hyperplastic primary vitreous. *Trans Am Acad Ophthalmol Otolaryngol* 1974;78:911.
4. Hogan MJ, Kimura SJ, Spencer WH. Visceral larval migrans and peripheral retinitis. *JAMA* 1965;194:1345.
5. Hartnett ME, Hirose T. Cyanocrylate glue in the repair of retinal detachment associated with posteror retinal breaks in infants and children. *Retina* 1998;18:125–129.
6. Scott IU, Flynn HW, Azen SP, et al. Silicone oil in the repair of pediatric complex retinal detachments: prospective, observational, multi-center study. *Ophthalmology* 1999;106:1339–1407.
7. Moisseiev J, Vidne O, Treister G. Vitrectomy and silicone oil injection in pediatric patients. *Retina* 1998;18: 221–227.
8. Biedner B, Rothkoff L, Klemperer I, Silicone oil for complicated retinal detachment in the pediatric population. *Eur J Ophthalmol* 1996;6:451–453.

=========== 17 ===========

Inadvertent Penetration of the Eye

Inadvertent penetration of the globe can occur in association with many ocular procedures. Most, if not all, of these incidents can be prevented with strict attention to technique. The keys to prevention are awareness of the factors likely to cause penetration and constant vigilance. Many factors are associated with inadvertent penetration of the eye. They include patient movement, posterior staphylomas, myopic eyes, and poor technique (1–3).

OFFICE INJECTIONS

Subconjunctival injection in the lower fornix is safer than sub-Tenons (infra-Tenons) or so-called periocular injection. Subconjunctival injection under the bulbar conjunctiva is potentially dangerous. Myopic eyes are more likely to be penetrated than emmetropic or hyperopic eyes because of greater ocular length, thin sclera, and staphylomas. Injections should be performed with the patient supine. Viscous lidocaine provides better anesthesia than drops. Both physicians' hands should be braced against the patient's facial bones, with the needle entering laterally and nearly parallel to the lid margins. If the needle is directed toward the apex of the orbit, the globe can be penetrated if the patient moves forward.

PRESURGICAL ANESTHESIA

Topical and intraocular anesthesia is rapidly increasing in popularity for cataract surgery. Although some straightforward core vitrectomy procedures can be performed with topical anesthesia, the extraocular muscles must be blocked for macular and complex surgery. Peribulbar anesthesia using a blunt, curved, flexible cannula and small conjunctival incision is theoretically safer than multiple injections into the anterior orbital tissue. The patient should be directed to position the eye in the primary position during retrobulbar injection. Grizzard has shown that this position minimizes displacement and increased tension on the optic nerve, which increase the risk of penetration of the nerve (4).

Oversedation is a significant cause of patient motion and inadvertent penetration of the eye during the administration of anesthesia. Explanation is frequently better than sedation, especially for elderly patients. There is no evidence that blunt, so-called retrobulbar needles are safer than the standard, sharp, 25 or 27-gauge needles used by the authors. Sharp needles require less force than blunt needles and are therefore less likely to advance suddenly or cause pain and patient movement.

TOXICITY

Intraocular Gentamycin and other aminoglycoside antibiotics are very toxic to the retina (5–7). Lidocaine is apparently relatively safe, but Wydase has been shown to be very toxic to the retina (8). Randomized trials have not conclusively demonstrated beneficial effect of Wydase (9,10). The authors never use Wydase and suspect that many surgeons are unaware of the lack of evidence of efficacy and potential hazards and use this agent on a "routine" basis.

RECOGNITION

Corneal edema occurs instantaneously when the intraocular pressure is elevated to very high levels. Some surgeons have reported that the patients experience marked pain, anxiety, and/or nausea if intraocular injection or penetration of the eye occurs. Hypotony is a variable and somewhat delayed finding in these cases. Hemorrhage into the orbital tissue, eye wall, or eye can occur if a scleral laceration or double penetrating injury occurs.

IMMEDIATE ACTION

The fundus should be *immediately* inspected with the indirect ophthalmoscope by the operating surgeon if there is any suspicion of inadvertent penetration. If a penetration is recognized, elective anterior segment surgery should be canceled in most instances and a vitreoretinal surgeon should be contacted immediately. An immediate indirect ophthalmoscopic examination of the fundus can determine if there has been a single or double penetration and if the macula, posterior pole, optic nerve, or retinal vessels have been damaged. Although some surgeons recommend immediate vitrectomy if an aminoglycoside antibiotic is injected into the eye, the diffusion rate is very rapid and it is highly likely that retinal damage will occur before a vitrectomy can be accomplished. The laser indirect ophthalmoscope (LIO) is ideal to treat the penetration site(s) before diffusion of vitreous hemorrhage can occur. Cryopexy is less desirable than LIO because it requires pressure on the eye and a conjunctival incision, and probably causes more reparative scarring. Exploration of the sclera and suturing of the scleral penetration sites is not indicated in these cases.

DELAYED VITRECTOMY

Although some surgeons recommend immediate vitrectomy, the authors believe that it is better to delay vitrectomy and find vitrectomy unnecessary in most cases. Indications for vitrectomy include the development of a tract, retinal detachment, or formation of an epimacular membrane. Vitreous hemorrhage should be observed frequently for the development of hypocellular collagen contraction as evidenced by decreased vitreous mobility. Ultrasonic imaging can determine the presence of hypocellular collagen contraction or retinal detachment. Scleral buckling is seldom, if ever, indicated.

SURGICAL INDICATIONS

If vitreous hemorrhage persists more than 10 days, hypocellular collagen contraction as evidenced by decreased vitreous mobility, or a fibrous tract or retinal detachment occurs, vitrectomy is indicated. If the eye is no light perception (NLP) from optic nerve damage, surgery is not indicated. Surgery is not usually indicated for removal of subretinal blood and never indicated for intravitreal anesthetic agents.

SURGERY APPROACH

Standard vitrectomy methods for trauma are used as previously described. Retinopexy around the penetration sites is only indicated if a retinal break is observed. Exploration of the site, cryopexy, or scleral buckling is not required.

REFERENCES

1. Edge R, Navon S. Scleral perforation during retrobulbar and peribulbar anesthesia: risk factors and outcome in 50,000 consecutive injections. *J Cataract Refract Surg* 1999;25:1237–1244.
2. Ginsburg RN, Duker JS. Globe perforation associated with retrobulbar and peribulbar anesthesia. *Semin Ophthalmol* 1993;8:87–95.
3. Modarres M, Parvaresh MM, Hashemi M, et al. Inadvertent globe perforation during retrobulbar injection in high myopes. *Int Ophthalmol* 1997–1998;21:179–185.
4. Grizzard WS, Kirk NM, Pavan PR, et al. Perforating ocular injuries caused by anesthesia personnel. *Ophthalmology* 1991;98:1757.
5. Campochiaro PA, Lim JI. Aminoglycoside toxicity in the treatment of endophthalmitis. The aminoglycoside toxicity study group. *Arch Ophthalmol* 1994;112:48–53.
6. Peyman GA. Aminoglycoside toxicity. *Arch Ophthalmol* 1992;110:446.
7. Campochiaro PA, Conway BP. Aminoglycoside toxicity: a survey of retinal specialists. Implications for intraocular use. *Arch Ophthalmol* 1991;109:946–950.
8. Gottlieb JL, Antoszyk AN, Hatchell DL, et al. The safety of intravitreal hyaluronidase: a clinical and histologic study. *Invest Ophthalmol Vis Sci* 1990;31:2345–2352.
9. Bowman RJ, Newman DK, Richardson EC, et al. Is hyaluronidase helpful for peribulbar anaesthesia? *Eye* 1997; 11:385–388.
10. Crawford M, Kerr WJ. The effect of hyaluronidase on peribulbar block. *Anaesthesia* 1994;49:907–908.

18

Management of Suprachoroidal Hemorrhage

Suprachoroidal hemorrhage is a devastating complication of intraocular surgery. This complication is very difficult to anticipate, prevent, and manage (1–5) (Fig. 18.1). Intraoperative management is complex, as is the decision to intervene in the postoperative period. These cases are also called *choroidal hemorrhages* because blood dissects into the spongy choroidal tissue. They are termed *expulsive hemorrhages* if the choroid and retina are forced out of the eye by high pressure in the suprachoroidal space.

INCIDENCE OF SUPRACHOROIDAL HEMORRHAGE

The incidence of suprachoroidal hemorrhage in extracapsular cataract surgery and phakoemulsification is approximately 0.15%; filtering procedures, 0.15%; penetrating keratoplasty, 0.56%; vitrectomy, 0.41%. In the principal author's vitrectomy series the incidence was 0.03% (5/16,000). Small-incision cataract surgery does not necessarily reduce the incidence of this complication, as the intraocular pressure (IOP) must be reduced to

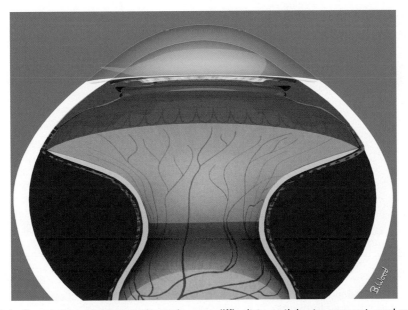

FIG. 18.1. Suprachoroidal hemorrhage is very difficult to anticipate, prevent, and manage.

atmospheric pressure during intraocular lens (IOL) insertion. Clearly, the duration of low intraocular pressure is less with phakoemulsification than with intracapsular surgery. Small-incision surgery with self-sealing wounds construction facilitates rapid wound closure and normalization of the intraocular pressure. Filtering procedures remain a common cause of this complication. Late hemorrhages are common if antimetabolites are used, producing a sustained, very low intraocular pressure.

PATHOGENESIS AND PREVENTION

A key factor in the pathogenesis of suprachoroidal hemorrhages is a high transarterial wall pressure gradient due to acute lowering of the intraocular pressure to atmospheric pressure in the presence of hypertension. The bleeding is probably due to shearing of vessels traversing the suprachoroidal space caused by scleral stretch. Penetration of the eye is a frequent and often unrecognized cause of suprachoroidal hemorrhage. Hypertension and arterial disease are probably factors in the pathogenesis. Patients should be normotensive during cataract, penetrating keratoplasty, secondary intraocular lens, and filtering procedures. Always paralyze the patient, if general anesthesia is being used to prevent hemorrhage secondary to "bucking on the tube."

COMPLICATIONS OF SUPRACHOROIDAL HEMORRHAGE

Bad outcomes in nonexpulsive cases are usually not directly due to the hemorrhage but are secondary to retinal detachment from hypocellular collagen contraction and adherence of vitreous to anterior structures (iris, wound, capsule) (Fig. 18.2). Many patients suffer optic nerve damage secondary to the acute increase in intraocular pressure or possibly intrasheath pressures.

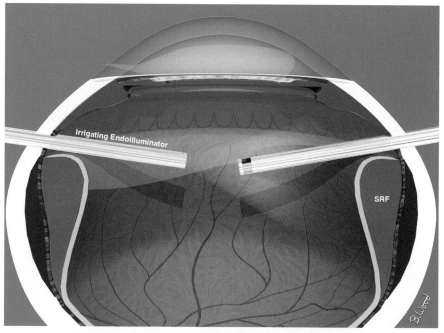

FIG. 18.2. Retinal detachment arises from hypocellular collagen contraction and adherence of the vitreous to anterior structures.

ACUTE MANAGEMENT

It is not advisable to open the anterior chamber to implant, reposition, or replace the intraocular lens if a suprachoroidal hemorrhage occurs. It is better not to cut down on the sclera if a hemorrhage occurs; instead, the focus should be on closing the wound with 8-0 nylon sutures as rapidly as possible. Viscoelastic can occasionally be used to reposition the iris. The surgeon should close the wound and delay surgery until inflammation is gone, if a suprachoroidal hemorrhage is recognized.

INDICATIONS FOR SURGERY

Rhegmatogenous or traction retinal detachment secondary to hypocellular collagen contraction and adherence of vitreous to anterior structures is the most common indication for vitrectomy. A flat chamber is also an indication for surgical intervention. An arbitrary duration of the suprachoroidal hemorrhage is often cited as an indication for vitrectomy. The authors disagree with this indication and use the indications described earlier. Appositional (kissing) suprachoroidal hemorrhage is not an absolute indication for surgery. There is no scientific evidence for retinal detachment due to retinal/retinal adherence. There is usually a layer of vitreous interposed between the retinal surfaces.

SURGICAL MANAGEMENT OF SUPRACHOROIDAL HEMORRHAGE

The infusion should be initiated with the long, hand-held, angulated, blunt cannula (May) (see Fig. 2.3) or the end-irrigating endoilluminator. The suprachoroidal hemorrhage usually drains through each pars plana sclerotomy during the early part of the vitrectomy (Fig. 18.3).

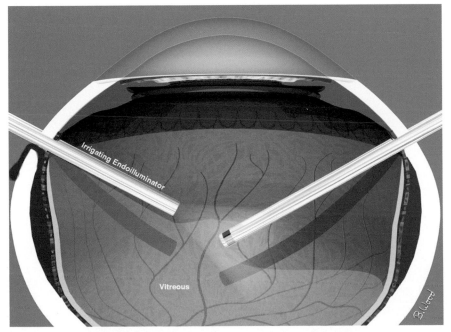

FIG. 18.3. Scleral cutdowns are not required for drainage, as the hemorrhage drains through the sclerotomies during vitrectomy.

Scleral cutdowns are not required to drain the blood and may cause severe, acute bleeding. Manipulation of the sclera with a scleral depressor breaks up clots, allowing faster egress of blood through the standard pars plana sclerotomies. Removal of all the blood is unnecessary, as the blood acts as a scleral buckle and will slowly absorb in the postoperative course.

MANAGEMENT OF ASSOCIATED RETINAL DETACHMENT

Silicone is usually preferred to gas in conjunction with vitrectomy. The purpose of silicone surface tension management is rhegmatogenous confinement for unrecognized retinal breaks and subsequent retinal breaks secondary to collagen contraction and epiretinal membrane formation.

SUMMARY

As in many medical problems, prevention followed by early recognition and conservative management is the key to reducing bad outcomes from suprachoroidal hemorrhage.

REFERENCES

1. Chu TG, Green RL. Suprachoroidal hemorrhage. *Surv Ophthalmol* 1999;43:471–486.
2. Glazer LC, Williams GA. Management of expulsive choroidal hemorrhage. *Semin Ophthalmol* 1993;8:109–113.
3. Beatty S, Lotery A, Kent D, et al. Acute intraoperative suprachoroidal haemorrhage in ocular surgery. *Eye* 1998; 12:815–820.
4. Tabandeh H, Sullivan PM, Smahliuk P, et al. Suprachoroidal hemorrhage during pars plana vitrectomy: risk factors and outcomes. *Ophthalmology* 1999;106:236–242.
5. Wirostko WJ, Han DP, Mieler WF, et al. Suprachoroidal hemorrhage: outcome of surgical management according to hemorrhage severity. *Ophthalmology* 1998;105:2271–2275.

= 19 =

Management of Venous Occlusive Disease

Venous occlusive disease is encountered relatively frequently in vitreoretinal practice. Randomized, multicenter trials have been conducted to evaluate various therapeutic options. In general terms, many patients with branch retinal vein occlusion (BRVO) do reasonably well without treatment, whereas others respond to focal/sector laser treatment. In contrast, central retinal vein occlusion (CRVO) patients have a worse visual prognosis than BRVO, and PRP serves only to manage neovascular complications. Systemic medical therapy has not been demonstrated to be efficacious for the CRVO or BRVO patient.

An occasional BRVO or CRVO patient requires vitrectomy to remove vitreous hemorrhage and/or treat a traction retinal detachment. These patients usually require sector or panretinal photocoagulation during vitrectomy. The traction retinal detachment (TRD) patients are managed similarly to diabetic TRD patients.

LASER TREATMENT OF CENTRAL RETINAL VEIN OCCLUSION

Anastomosis between the retinal venous circulation and choroidal circulation has been postulated as a therapeutic strategy for CRVO. Constable et al. have used a high-power argon laser to make a fistula between a branch vein and the underlying choroids (1). His method teaches intentional penetration of a vein using an explosive power level. Many investigators have observed vitreous or subretinal hemorrhage, epiretinal membranes, subretinal scars, and traction retinal detachment (2–4). The authors discontinued this approach in 1998 because of the high complication rate. Brian Leonard developed an alternative approach to address certain complications (presented at the Retina Society meeting in Washington, DC, in September 1998). According to his method, full-power (2 to 3 watts) green laser should be applied *near* the vein but not on the vein. In addition, Leonard recommends using a 1-second duration rather than the usual 100-ms duration. Avoiding the vein with the laser dramatically reduces hemorrhage, as does using the long-duration pulse. Leonard reports approximately a 75% success rate in creation of an angiographically demonstrable anastomosis. It appears that intraretinal hemorrhage and edema clear much more rapidly, but the real issue is whether the visual results are better than in untreated patients. Leonard has a randomized trial under way to answer this question. The apparent mechanism in creation of an anastomosis is via the healing process of the laser-produced rupture in Bruch's membrane.

SURGICAL TREATMENT OF CENTRAL RETINAL VEIN OCCLUSION

Several investigators have suggested using microcannulas to cannulate the central retinal vein (5). It is the authors' opinion that this strategy is unlikely to benefit the patient because of the high probability of damage to the vascular endothelium. Others have suggested mechanical techniques for creation of an anastomosis between a retinal vein and the choroidal circulation (6). It is likely that this micropuncture approach would have higher complications than laser anastomosis, and there is no reason to believe that a surgical approach would be mechanically superior to a laser approach.

SURGICAL TREATMENT OF BRANCH RETINAL VEIN OCCLUSION

The principal author reported surgical decompression of BRVO using microscissors combined with an MVR blade in 1988 (7). This procedure has also been called *sheathotomy*. After several cases, a conclusion was reached that even though mechanical decompression could be accomplished in most instances, with apparent accelerated clearing of hemorrhage and edema, it did not seem to facilitate visual improvement. Opremcak reintroduced the procedure, using a bent MVR blade, in 1998 and his data seems to indicate that approximately one-third of the patients had improved vision, one-third were the same, and one-third became worse (8). It does not appear that the outcomes are better than the natural history of the disease, and the authors have significant concern about patients made worse by the procedure. A randomized trial is under way that, it is hoped, will answer the questions of safety and efficacy.

REFERENCES

1. McAllister IL, Constable IJ. Laser-induced chorioretinal venous anastomosis for treatment of non-ischemic central retinal vein occlusion. *Arch Ophthalmol* 1995;113:456–462.
2. Atkan SG, Subasi M, Akbatur H, et al. Problems of chorioretinal venous anastomosis by laser for treatment of nonischemic central retinal vein occlusion. *Ophthalmologica* 1998;212:389–393.
3. McAllister IL, Douglas JP, Constable IJ, et al. Laser-induced chorioretinal venous anastomosis for nonischemic central retinal vein occlusion: evaluation of the complications and their risk factors. *Am J Ophthalmol* 1998;126: 219–229.
4. Browning DJ, Rotberg MH. Vitreous hemorrhage complicating laser induced chorioretinal anastomosis for central retinal vein occlusion. *Am J Ophthalmol* 1996;122:588–589.
5. Weiss JN. Treatment of central vein occlusion by injection of tissue plasminogen activator into a retinal vein. *Am J Ophthalmol* 1998;126:142–144.
6. Fekrat S, de Juan E Jr. Chorioretinal venous anastomosis for central retinal vein occlusion: transvitreal venipuncture. *Ophthalmolic Surg Lasers* 1999;30:52–55.
7. Osterloh MD, Charles S. Surgical decompression of branch vein occlusions. *Arch Ophthalmol* 1988;106: 1469–1471.
8. Opremcak EM. Surgical decompression of branch retinal vein occlusion via arteriovenous crossing sheathotomy: a prospective review of 15 cases. *Retina* 1999;19:1–5.

20

Complications

Most complications of vitreous surgery, after an initial surgical learning phase, result from biologic problems associated with specific disease states. Implicit in the discussion of management of complications is their recognition. The importance of frequent follow-up of the complex vitreous surgery patient cannot be overemphasized. In some cases, the primary ophthalmologist, less familiar with vitreous surgery, will not initiate appropriate action if complications occur. It is therefore quite important for the surgeon to follow the patient with a general ophthalmologist. Every attempt should be made to educate colleagues in the recognition and management of these complications, but the primary responsibility rests with the surgeon.

CORNEAL COMPLICATIONS

Poor epithelial adherence can persist for weeks if the epithelium is removed at the time of vitrectomy (1–4). Care during the preparation, frequent irrigation of the cornea with BSS, and shorter operating times dramatically reduce the need to remove the epithelium. The principal author removes the epithelium in fewer than 2% of cases. When necessary, the epithelium should be mobilized rather than scraped. The rounded blade used for mobilization should never touch Bowman's membrane. The defect should be made the same size as the pupil, avoiding the peripheral cornea. Some surgeons use Gelfoam, tear substitutes, or viscoelastics during surgery, but the authors have not found these to be necessary or efficacious. Bandage contact lenses or pressure patches are unnecessary in the typical postoperative management. In the rare cases requiring epithelial removal, the epithelium is healed within several days following vitrectomy and is always healed on the 2-week office visit. If the patient develops a recurrent epithelial defect, cessation of topical medications and taping the lid closed for 12 to 24 hours will usually be sufficient. A rare patient will require a therapeutic soft contact lens. Infection of the corneal epithelial defect may occur in conjunction with soft-lens usage.

With decreased turbulence, less fluid throughput, better lens removal techniques, and better irrigating fluids, endothelial cell damage is much less common after vitrectomy. If those patients with previous surgical trauma, glaucoma, or inherited endothelial dystrophies are excluded, postoperative corneal edema should not happen. Prolonged contact of the gas or silicone bubble can damage the corneal endothelium and must be avoided by proper postoperative positioning. Epithelial edema can be managed by topical hyperosmotic medications, although this is largely symptomatic treatment. Fortunately, sliding of endothelial cells and the regaining of function of the remaining cells cause clearing of corneal edema in most cases. If corneal edema persists and the eye is required for the patient's visual function, penetrating keratoplasty should be performed.

Precipitates on the endothelium are frequently interpreted as evidence of inflammation, whereas in many cases they represent pigment released from iris and retinal pigment epithelium or erythroclasts.

INFLAMMATION

Most cells in the anterior chamber are erythroclasts released either from the vitreous lamella or as a result of intraoperative or postoperative bleeding. If no retinopexy is performed, vitrectomy results in little inflammation. Iris trauma in conjunction with vitreous surgery results in inflammation and should be avoided. Retained nucleus appears to play a greater role in postoperative inflammation than does persistent cortex. All cases of iris neovascularization and most cases of retinal detachment have protein release in the anterior chamber, which is visible as "flare." Treatment of the basic disease process by reattachment of the retina or panretinal photocoagulation (PRP) is more effective than topical steroids in reducing the flare due to neovascularization. Angiostatic and anti–vascular endothelial growth factor (anti-VEGF) compounds may prove to be effective in these cases. Topical and intraoperative subconjunctival, long-acting steroids are used in all patients who are not steroid glaucoma responders. This is primarily because any severe inflammation can result in the development of a cyclitic membrane, periretinal membranes, and, ultimately, phthisis bulbi. Steroids do not appear to significantly retard healing of any of the ocular structures and should be used to reduce inflammation. The authors never prescribe systemic steroids for primary ocular conditions. Inflammation not responsive to frequent topical steroids is treated with repeated subconjunctival triamcinolone.

IRIS NEOVASCULARIZATION

The cause and treatment of iris neovascularization has been extensively discussed in Chapter 6. Occasionally, iris neovascularization will appear when retinal detachments with severe periretinal proliferation are operated on unsuccessfully. Other than the suppression of the associated inflammation, there is no specific treatment for this form of iris neovascularization if the retinal detachment is inoperable. However, as a rule, it does not go on to cause neovascular glaucoma (NVG) and will involute. If PRP causes involution of iris neovascularization, the large vessels will not disappear because of rheologic considerations. The examiner must concentrate on the presence of capillary activity and endothelial budding on the iris surface rather than on the more impressive large vessels. Peripheral anterior synechiae and ectropion uveae are late changes and never disappear, even when capillary involution occurs. Although some clinicians have emphasized the difficulty in differentiating iris neovascularization from dilation of preexisting stromal vessels, as a rule this is not a difficult problem.

GLAUCOMA

Increased intraocular pressure (IOP) from varied mechanisms is an all too frequent complication of vitreous surgery. A high incidence of suspicion and frequent follow-up is a necessity for recognizing and managing this dreaded complication (5).

Erythroclastic (Hemolytic) Glaucoma

Erythroclastic (hemolytic) glaucoma was quite frequent after vitrectomy before vacuum-cleaning/extrusion techniques and intraoperative coagulation methods were utilized (6).

This type of glaucoma is transient and self-limited. The vast majority of cases can be treated with ocular hypotensive medications such as topical carbonic anhydrase inhibitors, beta-blockers, alpha-agonists, and other agents. Extreme caution should be used in the administration of systemic hyperosmotic agents to diabetic patients. The authors never use these agents because of the risk of stroke, myocardial infarction, and ketoacidosis. Extreme caution should be taken to prevent the intraocular pressure from staying above 30 mm Hg in the patient with vascular disease, systemic hypotension, and poor retinal perfusion.

Air/Gas Pupillary Block

When air/gas is utilized in the vitrectomized, aphakic, or pseudophakic patient, the surface tension effect of the bubble can seal the pupil, just as it does a retinal break, resulting in a transiris pressure gradient. The continued production of aqueous then forces the iris forward against the cornea, closing the angle and elevating the intraocular pressure. This can be prevented by proper postoperative positioning and typically occurs when the instructions to patients are disregarded. In most cases, reinforcement of the instructions given to the patient with assistance from the office and nursing staff can reverse this pupillary block immediately. If it is unrecognized for several days, the iris can become adherent to the cornea, requiring reoperation with a chamber-deepening procedure through the pars plana. Iridectomies do not prevent this complication and are not required in most vitrectomy procedures.

Neovascular Glaucoma

The treatment of NVG can be separated into components. The basic process underlying the iris neovascularization must be treated by PRP and/or retinal reattachment to reduce VEGF. If the pressure is highly elevated, this must be managed aggressively. Timolol, brimonidine, and lantanoprost are effective in many of these patients in combination with a topical carbonic anhydrase inhibitor. In others these medications appear to have little effect. If medical management is unable to achieve pressure control in the region below 35 mm Hg, endocyclophotocoagulation can be combined with endopanretinal photocoagulation. Filtering procedures usually fail unless there is near complete involution of neovascularization and inflammation. Patients without light perception are usually taken off their pressure drops and treated only with topical steroids and pain medications. High intraocular pressure destroys the pain fibers to the eye just as they destroy the optic nerve and eliminate the need for enucleation. Enucleation is only necessary if there is risk of systemic infection from endophthalmitis, certain tumors, or a cosmetic appearance that cannot be managed with a scleral shell.

CYCLOCRYOTHERAPY

In-office cyclocryopexy is usually reserved for NLP cases. Cyclocryotherapy may cause phthisis bulbi, but it can be used for diseases that will result in phthisis bulbi without cyclocryotherapy. In the vitrectomized aphakic eye, there is no matrix in the pupillary plane along which a cyclitic membrane can develop unless fibrin is present. It is important to use large doses of periocular steroids in conjunction with cyclocryotherapy. Cyclocryotherapy can be performed on bare sclera so as to cause more predictable destruction of the ciliary processes as well as less postoperative conjunctival and Tenon's capsule damage and discomfort. If the cryopexy is used at −80°C and confluent treatments held for 1 minute, the effect appears to be reasonably predictable. It is better to use 180° treatment and additional treatment only in reoperation situations. If the cryopexy is directed over the ciliary body with only minimal anterior extension, there is less damage to the remaining functioning trabecular meshwork. If the iceball reaches the limbus, this means it is reaching the trabecular meshwork internally and has extended too far. At this point, the probe should be reapplied and treatment directed more posteriorly. Ultrasound or transscleral 1,064-nm laser cyclodestructive procedures may be effective in lieu of cyclocryotherapy in these cases. Endocyclophotocoagulation is more effective and has fewer complications than cryo, laser, or ultrasound, but it requires intraocular surgery.

FILTERING PROCEDURES FOR NEOVASCULAR GLAUCOMA

Trabeculectomies (7), valve, and filtering shunt procedures (8–12), and pars plana filtering procedures (13) have been utilized with moderate success in selected patients with NVG. There are no data to indicate which of these procedures is most efficacious, although it is probable that setons with large surface areas are the best option. It appears that in the filtering procedures, there is a dynamic dilutional effect whereby VEGF is decreased due to increased fluid throughput. Because of this the iris neovascularization may involute rapidly and neovascularization may appear in the bleb.

Extensive PRP to cause involution of iris vessels should precede filtering procedures whenever possible. Frequent topical or subconjunctival steroids should be used to suppress inflammation before and after filtering procedures.

Steroid Glaucoma

Steroid glaucoma can usually be managed by topical medications and only rarely requires glaucoma surgery. In rare situations, the plaque of subconjunctival steroids may be excised if, after several weeks, the pressure is difficult to control. This has been shown by Mandell to result in reversibility of the glaucomatous process (14). The efficacy of steroids is so great in the postvitrectomy patient that they should be universally used, accepting that a small incidence of steroid glaucoma will occur.

Open-Angle Glaucoma

Open-angle glaucoma can be exacerbated by transpars plana vitrectomy. It appears that this type of open-angle glaucoma is secondary to the trauma suffered by the trabecular meshwork from infusion fluid, cells, cytokines, protein, and debris. In this way it is comparable to the metabolic trauma suffered by the endothelium from infusion fluid and other intraocular agents. Open-angle glaucoma can usually be managed by topical medications but may require surgery.

ENDOPHTHALMITIS

Endophthalmitis was relatively frequent in the early days of vitrectomy at some institutions; it now fortunately has become an infrequent complication. The principal author has had three cases of endophthalmitis in more than 16,000 vitrectomies. The better equipment, shortened operating times, and better irrigating solutions have probably contributed to the rarity of endophthalmitis now seen after vitrectomy. The authors recommend the use of subconjunctival antibiotics with coverage for both Gram-positive and

Gram-negative bacteria as the final step in surgery. Even though these agents will only infrequently play a role, the devastating effect of endophthalmitis should be prevented at all costs. The authors are currently using tobramycin and Ancef. If endophthalmitis does occur in the postvitrectomy patient, there is no need to perform further vitrectomy. A needle may be placed through the pars plana into the vitreous cavity and fluid aspirated for culture and sensitivity testing. This same needle can then be used for intraocular antibiotic injection. Some have recommended the use of antibiotics routinely in the infusion fluid. The question about toxicity of these substances, especially with cumulative dosing, coupled with the relative infrequency of endophthalmitis makes this approach unnecessary and possibly dangerous.

RETINAL COMPLICATIONS

Cystoid Macular Edema

Removal of the vitreous causes minimal if any inflammation or cystoid macular edema (CME). Postvitrectomy inflammation is caused primarily by iris trauma, retinopexy, retinal trauma, laser treatment, agents injected into the eye, and residual lens material. Vitrectomy can reduce or eliminate CME by debulking inflammatory factors in the vitreous. Vitrectomy, especially when combined with aphakia, decompartmentalizes the eye-facilitating egress of cells, proteins, and cytokines through the trabecular meshwork. Oral nonsteroidal antiinflammatory agents as well as subconjunctival and topical steroids have a beneficial effect on postvitrectomy inflammation and cystoid macular edema (15).

Vascular Occlusion

The elevation of IOP associated with vitrectomy can create vascular occlusion and permanent visual loss. Strict attention to intra- and postoperative intraocular pressure is required to prevent this severe complication. Children and adults with low blood pressure are at high risk for retinal and optic nerve ischemia from elevation of the IOP.

Retinal Breaks and Detachment

Retinal breaks may precede vitrectomy, occur at the time of vitrectomy, or appear in the postoperative course (16). Any breaks present at the time of vitrectomy should have been identified and treated. but on occasion surgical difficulties prevent this. Retinal breaks occurring at the time of vitrectomy can be divided into two groups: those caused by direct retinal trauma and those related to vitrectomy traction. Any time that instruments are brought near the retinal surface, the potential exists for creating a retinal break. A retinal tear can be made with any intraocular instrument, although it is most frequently found as a result of epiretinal membrane (ERM) dissection. When the vitreous is removed, there is obligatory traction on the retina from the suction force on the vitreous fiber framework. This mechanism is similar to that of an aphakic retinal detachment occurring after vitreous loss at cataract surgery. With this form of detachment, there are small breaks at the posterior edge of the vitreous base. These are frequently difficult to recognize at the time of vitrectomy or are only of partial thickness at that time, becoming full thickness later. Thus there is a built-in incidence of aphakic-like retinal detachment as a result of vitreous removal by any method. More direct trauma to the peripheral retina occurs from the entry of instruments through the pars plana. Large instruments with abrupt increases in diameter can cause dialyses, whereas small instruments can push the vitreous base in front of them and create dialyses or small breaks as well.

Late retinal breaks occur from several mechanisms. Trauma to the retina at the time of vitrectomy may result in partial-thickness retinal loss with subsequent retinal break formation. Postoperative traction can occur from residual vitreous, particularly that incarcerated in the sclerotomies. Any form of periretinal proliferation can cause retinal shortening and retinal breaks from tangential traction. In some cases, large retinal breaks occur without any evidence of traction or surgical trauma. These are seen in the context of ischemic retinopathies and appear to be due to retinal necrosis from vascular occlusive disease.

Nonrhegmatogenous Retinal Detachment

Periretinal migration and proliferation from glial, retinal pigment epithelial, or wound-related cellular proliferation can lead to elevation of the retina without a rhegmatogenous component. Required ERM peeling, segmentation, and delamination elicits a reparative effort with further proliferation, causing retinal elevation. Residual ERM can contract also, creating nonrhegmatogenous retinal elevation. If these elevated areas are small, they can be observed without surgical intervention. At times, vitreous will unintentionally be left, causing residual traction on the retina. If extramacular retina is elevated, it can be observed postoperatively for an extensive period with much the same criteria as those used at the time of the original surgery. Nonrhegmatogenous macular elevation or any elevation accompanied by iris neovascularization should indicate the need for reoperation with scissors segmentation and delamination methods. At times, circumferential segmental scleral buckling is required.

Management of Retinal Detachment

Rhegmatogenous detachment repair after vitrectomy almost always requires gas or silicone for surface tension management. Because vitreous removal markedly decreases the viscosity of the vitreous fluid, a very small break will rapidly result in total retinal detachment. With the use of the surface tension effects of air/gas, these cases can be reattached more expeditiously and safely. In most instances, the procedure is set up for full vitrectomy with the customary incisions, the endoilluminator, cutter, and tools. Any residual vitreous traction is removed and the visualization is improved by removal of any blood or debris. If ERM is causing retinal foreshortening, peeling, segmentation, and delamination are utilized. After removal of the causative traction, internal drainage of subretinal fluid (SRF), internal fluid/air exchange, and completion of internal drainage of SRF is utilized. This is followed by endolaser retinopexy unless the break is in the macular or peripapillary region. Scleral buckling is used for traction that cannot be managed by epiretinal membrane dissection. PVR and glial recurrences were previously discussed in Chapters 7 and 8.

INTRAOCULAR HEMORRHAGE

Postoperative intraocular hemorrhage is rare except in the diabetic patient. Diabetic patients develop postoperative hemorrhage approximately 50% of the time. Resected vascular tissue, sclerotomy wounds, iris neovascularization, and incomplete involution of retinal neovascularization are the most frequent causes of postoperative intraocular hemorrhage. As discussed in this chapter, hemorrhage cases should be followed with ultrasound and reoperated only if retinal detachment occurs. If the patient is blind in an only eye or both eyes, reoperation to remove blood should be considered for the better eye.

If indicated, blood removal should be performed in all instances using the full setup and three-incision technique. This permits extrusion, bipolar diathermy, endophotocoagulation, and dissection of any significant ERM to be done. If iris neovascularization is present, blood removal should be performed to accomplish retinal reattachment and/or additional PRP.

CATARACT

Many surgical factors add to the baseline incidence of cataract associated with the ocular diseases requiring vitreous surgery (17). Lens opacities are a frequent but easily manageable postvitrectomy complication. Lens removal should be considered to address the patient's visual needs or if the view of the retina is lost, preventing good management.

The typical endocapsular pars plana lensectomy approach (see Chapter 3) should be used for cases requiring combined vitreoretinal surgery. Phako and posterior chamber intraocular lenses should be used for all other cases. Some cataract surgeons believe that removal of the anterior vitreous cortex at the time of vitrectomy results in posterior displacement of the lens during subsequent cataract surgery.

SUTURE EXTRUSION

On occasion, the 8-0 monofilament nylon sclerotomy sutures will erode through the conjunctiva. Because this is a running suture, it is quite difficult to remove at the slit lamp. It is better to use topical anesthesia and the laser to melt the protruding end. Alternatively, a disposable electrothermal cautery can be used if the lids are retracted securely. If loops of suture erode, they can be severed with a blade or Vannas scissors at the slit lamp in the office. The nylon scleral buckle sutures can be trimmed in the office, but this may result in buckle extrusion. With the use of hard silicone explants, copious antibiotic flushing, and a 1-mm conjunctival flap, infected buckles are extremely rare. If infection occurs, it should be managed by removal of the explant materials and irrigation with saline and antibiotics.

FOLLOW-UP INTERVALS

Typically, vitrectomy patients go home on the day of surgery. The first postoperative visit should be on the day after surgery and the subsequent examination should be in 3 weeks in most instances. It would be unusual to experience any reason to reoperate in the first 3 weeks, and a 3-week follow-up examination discovers the highest incidence of treatable postoperative complications. If this period were extended to 1 month, in the diabetic vitrectomy patient there would be a much higher incidence of NVG. Most PVR recurrences occur in the first 3 weeks. Most rhegmatogenous postvitrectomy retinal detachments will also present by the 3-week mark and can be effectively managed at that time. The first postop day visit is usually sufficient to cover the acute endophthalmitis risk.

If the patient is doing well at the 3-week visit, he or she can be given a 6-week visit unless the patient is a diabetic. The diabetic patient should return in 3 weeks for further examination for iris neovascularization and glial recurrence. In all patients, it is important to emphasize that they check their vision every day and contact the physician immediately if visual loss or pain occurs. It is critical to instruct the office staff about the access these patients must be afforded to postoperative care. The complexity of post-vitrectomy patients simply prohibits the use of a waiting list. As a rule, diabetics should be followed at 6-week to 3-month intervals until they are stable for 1 year. At this point, the interval can be lengthened.

REFERENCES

1. Perry HD, Foulks GN, Thoft RA, et al. Corneal complications after closed vitrectomy through the pars plana. *Arch Ophthalmol* 1978;96:401.
2. Brightvill FS, Myers FL, Bresnick GH. Postvitrectomy keratopathy. *Am J Ophthalmol* 1978;85:651.
3. Aaberg TM, Van Horn DL. Late complications of pars plana vitreous surgery. *Ophthalmology* 1978;85:116.
4. Kenyon KR, Stark WJ, Stone DL. Corneal endothelial degeneration and fibrous proliferation after pars plana vitrectomy. *Am J Ophthalmol* 1976;8:486.
5. Campbell DG, Simmons Rl, Tolentino Fl, et al. Glaucoma occurring after closed vitrectomy. *Am J Ophthalmol* 1977;83:63.
6. Brucker AJ, Michels RG, Green WR. Pars plana vitrectomy in the management of blood-induced glaucoma with vitreous hemorrhage. *Am J Ophthalmol* 1978;10:1427.
7. Herschler J, Agness D. A modified filtering operation for vascular glaucoma. *Arch Ophthalmol* 1979;97:2339.
8. Krupin T, Kaufman P, Mandell A, et al. Filtering valve implant surgery for eyes with neovascular glaucoma. *Am J Ophthalmol* 1980;89:338.
9. Krupin T, Kaufman P, Mandell A, et al. Long-term results of valve implants in filtering surgery for eyes with neovascular glaucoma. *Am J Ophthalmol* 1983;95:775.
10. Moltens ACB, Van Rooyen MMB, Bartholomew RS. Implants for draining neovascular glaucoma. *Br J Ophthalmol* 1977;61:120.
11. Schocket SS, Lakhanpal V, Richards RD. Anterior chamber tube shunt to an encircling band in the treatment of neovascular glaucoma. *Ophthalmology* 1982;89:1188.
12. Schocket SS, Nirankari VS, Lakhanpal V, et al. Anterior chamber tube shunt to an encircling band in the treatment of neovascular glaucoma and other refractory glaucomas: a long-term study. *Ophthalmology* 1985;92:553.
13. Sinclair SH, Aaberg TM, Meredith TA. A pars plana filtering procedure combined with lensectomy and vitrectomy for neovascular glaucoma. *Am J Ophthalmol* 1982;93:185.
14. In press. To come.
15. In press. To come.
16. Sjaarda RN, et al. Distribution of iatrogenic retinal breaks in macular hole surgery. *Ophthalmology* 1995;102:1387–1392.
17. Blankenship G, Cortez R, Machemer R. The lens and pars plana vitrectomy for diabetic retinopathy complications. *Arch Ophthalmol* 1979;97:1263.

21

Surgical Self-Education

Although many excellent courses, articles, and textbooks are available concerning vitreoretinal surgery, improvement in judgment and surgical skills must come about principally through self-education. The complexity of high-technology vitreous surgery on high-risk patients demands a continued assessment of surgical and biologic results. Vitreous surgery requires an excellent training in microsurgery and retinal diseases. Eye bank and porcine eyes can be used for surgical practice (1–6). It is simply poor judgment to begin vitreous surgery or a new technique on the human patient without sufficient practice. After reading the available literature, visiting other surgeons, and attending appropriate courses, progress will be made in the laboratory. When sufficient competency is obtained in the laboratory, the beginning surgeon should assemble the disposables and equipment required for simulated surgery. Regardless of the presence of other vitreous surgeons at the same institution, it is the responsibility of the beginning surgeon to go through this practice surgery approach. It is absolutely the responsibility of each surgeon to make certain that all equipment is available and functioning. Unfortunately, many surgeons fall into the trap of placing this responsibility upon technicians and nurses. Practice surgery in the actual operating room should be repeated on the days preceding vitreous surgery if the case in question has not been approached before or the procedures are done infrequently.

The great complexity of vitreoretinal surgery requires an honest assessment of the surgeon's own capabilities. It is simply inadequate to perform vitrectomy without stereopsis. Many areas of medicine are less demanding in the requirements for stereopsis, and the surgeon should not perform vitreous surgery without stereopsis. Red/green color blindness is a major handicap. It is even important to attempt assessment of one's temperament. Vitreous surgery requires a calm but rapid and efficient approach. A surgeon who becomes very tense and inefficient in times of surgical stress has no place in vitreous surgery. A person so compulsive and rigid that necessary changes in the game plan produce overwhelming stress probably should not be performing vitreous surgery. Although ego and economic factors unfortunately influence some surgeons' decisions, the pleasure is short-lived if the results are poor, resulting in a damaged and unhappy patient and possibly a lawsuit. It therefore becomes important to look realistically at the demands for vitreous surgery in the individual's practice, with an eye toward determining if certain procedures can be done frequently enough to attain sufficient surgical skill.

OUTCOMES ANALYSIS

The collection of preoperative, operative, and postoperative information is essential to the self-assessment of surgical techniques and skills. Although some feel that this is the obligation of so-called academic institutions, it is, in fact, the obligation of each and every surgeon. Some surgeons can achieve a series large enough for publication, but each individual must produce a series for comparison. The importance derives not so much from contributing to the literature as from being apprised of one's own outcomes. Outcomes research begins with careful preoperative evaluation and prospective recording of this information. It is best to have a format on which these data can be recorded, and extensive use of abbreviations and recognized grading systems should be utilized. With the use of a scribe accompanying the examiner, the information can be dictated in abbreviation format and recorded extremely rapidly without the unavoidable errors that occur with trying to recall this later at the time of dictation. Although it is permissible to fill out sheets at this time, if they are secondary to the primary charting method, details tend to be overlooked in a busy practice. It is critical to determine the parameters that one wishes to follow pre- and postoperatively and to record all this information on each patient to permit biostatistical evaluation at a later date.

It is best to compile this information by disease category so that discrete biologic groups may be identified. This compilation can be as simple as single sheets that list patients with a given disease state and entrance criteria, with columns for preoperative, operative, and postoperative findings and especially complications. These sheets should be filled out immediately following each day's examinations so that missing findings can be determined at that point. The surgical part of these forms should be filled out immediately following surgery so that it will not have the inaccuracies inherent in subsequent abstraction from postoperative dictation. Similarly, the postoperative findings should be recorded after each visit, preferably while the patient is still present, so that any missing information can be obtained.

The computers utilized in office practice could make this process more efficient, but useful computerized medical record software is just becoming available, and if one waits until computer skills or capabilities are sufficient, a considerable amount of data and useful information will be lost.

It is essential to determine average success rates from the data forms and to compare complication rates to published outcomes. This should be done at least every 3 months, with a stimulus being provided by a quarterly report, an upcoming paper, or an upcoming lecture. The data then become very helpful in predicting the outcome of surgery for patients and in self-assessment for surgical improvement. Care must be taken to compare similar biologic groups that are selected with given entrance criteria. For example, a vitreous hemorrhage patient should not be compared with a traction detachment patient with respect to visual improvement because simple clearing of the media improves the vision in a different manner from macular reattachment.

SURGICAL DATA

It is important to dictate an extremely complete and honest operative note at the end of each procedure. This should be done describing every aspect of the technique and all surgical findings. While some physicians use surgical forms, they are usually too stereotyped and inflexible for this complex type of surgery. Similarly, while photographs and drawings can complement the description, carefully described surgical findings are very helpful in following the patients in the office. This approach helps not only in outcomes research, but also in understanding complications on an individual basis. In addition to the copies of the operative notes in the hospital and office records, a third copy should be kept in the computer or separate files. These sequential operative notes should then be abstracted with cross-referencing for certain findings or techniques that will benefit from subsequent analysis. For example, all macular hole patients who underwent peeling of the cortex from the optic nerve can be assessed for visual results to determine if optic nerve damage is a complication of this method. Again, a computer-based approach can be quite effective but requires additional work to set up, and its unavailability should not be used as an excuse for not having continuous data monitoring.

It is helpful to have one member of the surgical assistant team monitor these data with the surgeon so as to increase his or her involvement and understanding. If a surgical team member helps by abstracting operative records, it adds impartial credibility and enhances surgical understanding as well. If this same individual is involved in pre- and postoperative clinical photography and other special examination techniques, it increases concern for the patient and understanding of prognostic and management factors.

CORRESPONDENCE

All postoperative follow-up information from referring doctors should be coded immediately into the file sheets as well as on the chart. In this way, a retrospective chart review with all its inherent inadequacies is avoided entirely. The quarterly or pretalk data compilation will uncover many patients who had inadequate follow-up. At this time, the referring doctor should be contacted by phone or postoperative follow-up forms should be mailed to complete all follow-up information. These frequent checkups serve a purpose in stimulating follow-up by the surgeon and referring physicians. Preprinted follow-up forms can be made available to referring physicians, which can act as a stimulus for better data retrieval. Unfortunately, many practitioners do not refract other physician's postoperative patients, making the visual acuity data inadequate. One then must specifically inquire and encourage the use of best-refracted visions.

GROUP EDUCATION

The use of effective outcomes research as described earlier contributes to the quality of presentations to other surgeons and at meetings. It is important to attend meetings frequently with surgeons performing similar work to upgrade medical and surgical knowledge. Unfortunately, the literature is months to years behind in reporting newer methods; more rapid education is possible by attending meetings. If all speakers emphasize this approach to outcomes research with at least a modicum of knowledge concerning biostatistics, better communication is possible. Certainly, everything cannot be studied in a randomized masked study, but accurate compilation of results is nevertheless mandatory.

INTERACTION WITH COMPANIES

The careful analysis of results with different surgical techniques permits better communication with medical equipment manufacturing companies. This should be done not to make the equipment a scapegoat for surgical failure, but to provide constructive advice concerning equipment improvement. It is usually better to go to major equipment manufacturers for prototype equipment than to go to local machine shops. If these devices are made in local shops, they are not accessible to colleagues and are not prototyped with a view to future manufacturing methods. It is very important for the surgeon to have frequent and open communication with companies so as to create a climate of intellectual cooperation that encourages equipment improvement. An extension of this attitude toward the surgical team and colleagues benefits all those involved.

REFERENCES

1. Michels RG. Intraocular fluorescein in experimental vitrectomy. *Ophthalmic Surg* 1977;8:139.
2. Bensen WE. Vitrectomy in rabbit eyes (appendix). In: Machemer R. *Vitrectomy: a pars plana approach.* New York: Grune & Stratton, 1975.
3. O'Malley C. Learning surgery without risk or anxiety. *Ocutome Newsletter* 1977;2.
4. Borirak-chanyavat S, Lindquist TD, Kaplan HJ. A cadaveric eye model for practicing anterior and posterior segment surgeries. *Ophthalmology* 1995;102:1932–1935.
5. Eckardt U, Eckardt C. Keratoprosthesis as an aid to learning surgical techniques on cadaver eyes. *Ophthalmic Surg* 1995;26:358–359.
6. Moorehead LC. Practice vitrectomy. *Arch Ophthalmol* 1980;98:1297–1298.

Appendix A
Abbreviations

ACL   Anterior chamber lens
ALT   Argon laser trabeculoplasty
AVC   Anterior vitreous cortex
BBD   Bipolar bimanual diathermy
BF ERG   Bright flash electroretinography
CME   Cystoid Macular edema
CNV   Choroidal neovascular membrane
CSME   Clinically significant macular edema
ECCE   Extracapsular cataract extraction
EMM   Epimacular membrane
EMTRD   Extramacular traction retinal detachment
ERM   Epiretinal membrane
FP   Frontal plane
ILM   Internal limiting membrane
IOFB   Intraocular foreign body
IOL   Intraocular lens
IOP   Intraocular pressure
MTRD   Macular traction retinal detachment
MVR   Microvitreoretinal
NVD   Neovascularization of disk
NVE   Neovascularization elsewhere
NVG   Neovascular glaucoma
NVI   Iris neovascularization
PAS   Peripheral anterior synechia
PCL   Posterior chamber lens
PDR   Proliferative diabetic retinopathy
PHPV   Persistent hyperplastic primary vitreous
PRP   Panretinal photocoagulation
PVC   Posterior vitreous cortex
PVD   Posterior vitreous detachment
PVR   Proliferative vitreoretinopathy
PFV   Persistent fetal vasculature
RLNV   Retrolenticular neovascularization
ROP   Retinopathy of prematurity
RPE   Retinal pigment epithelium
SRF   Subretinal fluid
SRM   Subretinal membrane

TPPL	Trans–pars plana lensectomy
TPPV	Trans–pars plana vitrectomy
TRD	Traction retinal detachment
UBD	Unimanual bipolar diathermy
VEGF	Vascular endothelial growth factor
VEP	Visual evoked potential

Appendix B
Discoveries and Inventions of Steve Charles

Scientific Discoveries

- 1968: Discovery of the cause of the fixed, dilated pupil of angle-closure glaucoma.
- 1968: Discovery of an afferent pupillary defect during retinal rivalry in amblyopia.
- 1970: Discovery of the presence of the early receptor potential (ERP) in detached retina.
- 1971: Discovery of the role of exposure to ambient illumination in the degeneration of photoreceptors in detached retina.

Surgical Techniques Developed

- Internal fluid/gas exchange, 1973
- Internal drainage of subretinal fluid, 1973
- Bipolar bimanual diathermy, 1974
- Endophotocoagulation, 1974
- Scissors segmentation of epiretinal membranes, 1974
- Anterior loop traction dissection, 1976
- Retinotomy, 1978
- Retinectomy, 1978
- Subretinal surgery, 1978
- Inside-out membrane dissection techniques, 1979
- Scissors delamination of epiretinal membranes, 1979
- Delamination prior to posterior hyaloid face truncation ("en bloc"), 1979
- Needle external drainage of subretinal fluid, 1980

Clinical Concepts

- Glial recurrence in proliferative diabetic retinopathy vitrectomy, 1975
- Retrolenticular neovascularization (anterior hyaloidal fibrovascular proliferation), 1979
- Anterior loop traction, 1975
- Compartmentalization concept (barrier concept), 1979
- PVR enhancing effect of silicone/gas retinal interface, 1979
- PVR enhancing effect of lens/IOL, 1979
- Role of anterior hyaloid face and lens in anterior segment neovascularization, 1979

Equipment Developed

- Internal drain cannula (tapered/bent) for subretinal fluid, 1973
- Spinning illuminated E for controlled low vision testing, 1974
- Coaxial cannula, 1974
- Zeiss endophotocoagulator adapter, 1974
- Subretinal fluid drainer, 1974
- Real-time, gray-scale B-scan ultrasound, 1975
- Real-time color encoding in B-scan ultrasound, 1975
- Real-time central vector in B-scan ultrasound, 1975
- Fenestrated muscle hook, 1975
- 4-mm/20-gauge infusion cannula, 1976
- Filter for fluorescein angioscopy during vitrectomy
- Microretinal retractor, 1976
- Flute needle, 1976
- Irrigating fundus contact lens with integrated handle and fluid connection, 1976
- Bipolar bimanual intraocular diathermy clips, 1976
- Suction only modality of the foot pedal, 1977
- Log III portable xenon endophotocoagulation adapter, 1978
- Modified Sutherland scissors for delamination, 1978
- Infusion sleeve (Charles), 1978
- Subretinal scissors, 1979
- MicroVit proportional scissors, 1979
- Subretinal forceps, 1979
- Illuminated intraocular foreign-body forceps, 1979
- MicroVit (MVS) vitrectomy system, 1979
- Volumetric power gas injector, 1979
- Ocutome air-operated vertical scissors, 1980
- Coherent 900 argon laser endophotocoagulation adapter, 1980
- Microvitreoretinal (MVR) blade, 1980
- Stable head rest for operating table, 1980
- Charles fluid collection drape, 1983
- 9-mm nonslotted tire for scleral buckling, 1983
- Delamination oscillatory cutter system, 1984
- Ocular connection machine, 1986
- Laser imaging workstation, 1986
- Innovit cutter, 1986
- Surgical instrumentation cart, 1986
- Surgeon-controlled positioner, 1993

Patents Awarded to Steve Charles for Work in Robotics and Instrumentation

- USP 3,993,064: One-handed syringe (November 23, 1976)
- USP 4,045,630: Chin-activated switch (August 30, 1977)
- USP 4,395,258: Linear intraocular suction device (July 26, 1983)
- USP 4,493,698: Method of performing ophthalmic surgery utilizing a linear intraocular suction device (January 15, 1985)
- USP D325,086: Ocular unit for eye surgery (March 31, 1992)
- USP 5,176,628: Vitreous cutter (January 5, 1993)

- USP 5,464,025: Self-contained surgical tubing management system (November 7, 1995)
- USP 5,710,870: Decoupled six-degree-of-freedom robot manipulator (January 20, 1998)
- USP 5,784,542: Decoupled six-degree-of-freedom teleoperated robot system (July 12, 1998)
- USP 5,858,345: *In vivo* polymerizable ophthalmic compositions (January 12, 1999)
- USP 5,943,914: Master-slave micromanipulator apparatus (August 31, 1999)
- USP 6,000,297: Master-slave micromanipulator method (December 14, 1999)
- USP 6,016,607: Coordinated X-Y stage apparatus (January 25, 2000)
- USP 6,124,037: Articles coated with *in vivo* polymerizable ophthalmic compositions (September 26, 2000)
- USP 6,180,687: *In vivo* polymerizable ophthalmic compositions and methods of using (January 30, 2001)

Appendix C
Bibliography

Carroll D, ed. *Surgery of the eye.* New York: Churchill Livingstone. (In press.)

Cibis PA. *Vitreoretinal pathology in surgery in retinal detachment.* St. Louis: CV Mosby, 1965.

Fraunfelder FT, Roy FH, eds. *Current ocular therapy, 2nd ed.* Philadelphia: WB Saunders, 1983.

Freeman HM, Hirose T, Schepens CL, eds. *Vitreous surgery and advances in fundus diagnosis and treatment.* New York: Appleton-Century-Crofts, 1977.

Friedman E, L'Esperance F Jr, eds. *Diabetic renal–retinal syndrome 3: therapy.* Orlando, FL: Grune & Stratton, 1986.

Gitter KA, ed. *Current concepts of the vitreous (including vitreous).* St. Louis: CV Mosby, 1976.

Irvine AR, O'Malley C, eds. *Advances in vitreous surgery.* Springfield, IL: Charles C Thomas, 1976.

Jacobiec FA, Sigelman J. *Advanced techniques in ocular surgery.* Philadelphia: WB Saunders, 1984.

Klein RM, Katzin HM. *Microsurgery of the vitreous: comparisons of instrumentation, techniques, and philosophies.* Baltimore: Williams & Wilkins, 1978.

Little H, ed. *Diabetic retinopathy.* New York: Thieme-Stratton, 1983.

Machemer R. *Vitrectomy: a pars plana approach.* New York: Grune & Stratton, 1975.

Machemer R. Aaberg TM. *Vitrectomy, 2nd ed.* New York: Grune & Stratton, 1979.

McPherson A, ed. *Retinopathy of prematurity.* Philadelphia: BC Decker, 1986.

Michels RG. *Vitreous microsurgery.* St. Louis: CV Mosby, 1980.

Peyman GA, Schulman JA. *Intravitreal surgery: principles and practice.* New York: Apple-Century-Crofts, 1986.

Subject Index

Page numbers followed by F indicate figures; page numbers followed by t indicate tables.